LETHAL DECISIONS

LETHAL Decisions

The Unnecessary Deaths of
Women and Children from
HIV/AIDS

ARTHUR J. AMMANN, MD

Vanderbilt University Press
Nashville

This book is printed on acid-free paper.
Manufactured in the United States of America

Library of Congress Cataloging-in-Publication Data on file
LC control number 2016007503
LC classification number RC606.5
Dewey class number 362.19697/92—dc23
LC record available at *lccn.loc.gov/2016007503*

ISBN 978–0-8265–2124–8 (hardcover)
ISBN 978–0-8265–2125–5 (paperback)
ISBN 978–0-8265–2126–2 (ebook)

TO MY WIFE who throughout the thirty-five years of the HIV/AIDS epidemic stood by me, encouraging, listening, and understanding the human toll of a new epidemic that unfolded before us. She partnered with me to establish Global Strategies for HIV Prevention, addressing issues of injustice and inequity among vulnerable women and children in poor countries. She shared in the compassion to help those whose voices could not be heard yet suffered so much. To my children, Kimberly and Scott, who grew up listening to conversations about the HIV/AIDS epidemic and who balanced patience with encouragement for a father who often traveled away from home. To my grandchildren, Sophia, Caleb, Leland, and Avery, who listened to stories about the HIV/AIDS orphaned children and did what they as children could do to help. They were constant reminders of how precious the life of each child must be.

TO THE MOTHERS who always held out hope that the prevention and treatments that were transforming the lives of those in wealthy countries would reach them to save their lives and the lives of their infants. To the thousands who participated in clinical research studies, always giving of themselves and hoping that their participation would help those in their communities and around the world. This book is to honor their disappointments, their lives, their courage, and their sacrifices.

CONTENTS

FOREWORD

In the aftermath of cataclysmic events a witness often comes forth to tell us how it came about and point to pivotal opportunities that would have minimized its impact. Dr. Arthur Ammann, the doctor who identified the first cases of AIDS in children and the transmission of HIV by blood transfusion, is such a witness.

Lethal Decisions is his highly personal account of an ongoing disaster, the global HIV epidemic in children and mothers, and the world's fatally flawed response. Dr. Ammann was uniquely positioned for this role. A medical school professor and expert in the diagnosis of immune deficiencies, he was there at the beginning of AIDS and stayed involved for the life of the epidemic. In my opinion he is the successor to the late Elizabeth Glaser as the conscience of the pediatric HIV epidemic.

Before meeting him in the context of AIDS, I knew of him through his contributions to the medical literature in the area of inherited immunodeficiency diseases. Dr. Ammann and others of his generation were my role models in choosing to become an immunologist. *Lethal Decisions* chronicles his odyssey from doctor and laboratory scientist to the medical and geopolitical frontlines of the HIV epidemic. His medical care of some of the first patients and their mothers led to an intense and enduring commitment. Present at every pivotal moment in the history of pediatric AIDS, his goals were common to those of many doctors in the field: understanding the differences between pediatric and adult AIDS, discovering how to prevent mother-to-child transmission, and learning how to treat children who were already infected. He was instrumental in the establishment of non-profits that addressed these questions, including the Elizabeth Glaser Pediatric AIDS Foundation with its novel Think Tank retreats and the American Foundation for AIDS Research (amfAR).

The 1990s were a time of milestones in HIV treatment and prevention. In the study known as ACTG 076, published in 1994, mother-to-child transmission of HIV was reduced by a dramatic 60 percent, and at the 1996 International AIDS Conference in Vancouver, British Columbia, it became clear that HIV could be suppressed with protease inhibitors as part of an antiviral cocktail. This discovery led to a marked decline in the number of deaths from AIDS in the developed world.

Aware of urgent, unaddressed needs in resource-poor countries and frustrated by the slow pace of intervention by the international community, Dr. Ammann founded Global Strategies in 1998 with the mission of bringing advances in health care to frontiers of the epidemic that were untouched and in fact shunned by other agencies. His goal was to ensure that advances in treatment and prevention reached the most vulnerable children and women living in remote and sometimes war-torn places—poor, stigmatized, and at risk for sexual violence.

In *Lethal Decisions*, Dr. Ammann documents the inexcusable missteps that delayed the translation of advances in care to the resource-poor settings of sub-Saharan Africa where nearly twenty million people had already died by the time Global Strategies was founded. He makes the history of HIV/AIDS in children come alive from its very earliest days to the present, complete with its heroes, heroines, and villains. No one is better qualified to tell this story.

Michael Gottlieb, MD
Los Angeles, California
Dr. Gottlieb identified the Acquired
Immunodeficiency Syndrome (AIDS)
as a new disease in 1981.

ACKNOWLEDGMENTS

It would be a dishonor if I did not first acknowledge the women and children of the epidemic who suffered so greatly from a disease that they too often did not understand. They volunteered for research that often benefited others more than it benefited them. In spite of their suffering, they continued to care for their families while embracing the hope that a means to end the HIV/AIDS epidemic would be found. Prevention and treatment did not come quickly enough for millions of them. I seek to honor them by writing this book, hoping to preserve the memory of their sacrifices that too often included their very lives.

The tenacity of the many dedicated and brilliant scientists from a host of disciplines is acknowledged. They saw the challenge of the HIV/AIDS epidemic, not as something that would bring them personal reward, but as something that they believed science had the capacity to overcome. They described the syndrome of AIDS, discovered the virus that caused AIDS, discovered the treatments that could both prevent HIV transmission and conquer the virus that had already infected millions of individuals. Their endeavors are a tribute to the highest values of science and the ability of scientific discovery to improve the lives of millions worldwide.

I acknowledge the critical role that activists played in being certain that medical discoveries did not languish in the halls of the academy and governments while the HIV/AIDS epidemic continued to take the lives of men, women, and children. They fought against bureaucratic obstacles to bring ARVs to those who were infected. They demonstrated that change is possible and individuals who suffer from a disease can insist on changing the way research is conducted, drugs are developed, and rapid access to life-saving drugs can be accomplished. They did this not only for themselves but also, importantly, for others with additional diseases.

Numerous dedicated community and health-care workers played an essential role in the care of HIV-infected individuals. Many of them earned no income but took on much of the burden of caring for the ill, defending their rights to treatment and nondiscrimination, and educating the public on how to prevent HIV infection. Their task was difficult, and I am grateful for what they set out to do, often without the benefit of the resources that exist in wealthy countries.

The pharmaceutical companies, too often maligned, contributed to discovering miraculous new drugs, overcoming patent issues to provide once-a-day combinations of ARVs that simplified the task of adherence, negotiated World Trade Organization agreements to allow much less expensive generic drugs to be used in poor countries, and contributed ARVs where they were not available to prevent and treat HIV infection when no one else would do it.

During the epidemic, there were leaders in government agencies who recognized the threat of HIV. Those within the CDC helped to define the epidemiology of HIV/AIDS and provided continuing surveillance. Leaders within the NIH defined priorities for critical research targets and funded the most important scientific advances that lead to prevention and treatment. Many of them began at the start of the epidemic and never tired in their role as leaders. They advocated before Congress to provide the funds to continue research for an epidemic that has not yet ended.

I acknowledge the opportunities that were provided to me during my education to engage in research, beginning as an undergraduate at Wheaton College, where I learned the basics of biology, scientific research, and the ethical principles that should guide us all. The professors at New Jersey School of Medicine encouraged me in pediatrics and in research. The University of California San Francisco Medical Center provided me with training through a pediatric residency and later provided opportunities and resources when I was a faculty member. They offered the time, encouragement, and opportunities to present the discoveries of HIV/AIDS to audiences around the world. My immunology fellowship at the University of Minnesota and the University of Wisconsin gave me the tools to diagnose immunodeficiency, which were used to define AIDS in patients in San Francisco and in the first infants and children. I am grateful to my mentors, Drs. E. Richard Stiehm and Richard Hong, who were generous with their time, taught me the science of immunology, and were examples of what could be achieved through respect, dedication, and integrity.

There are those who are infrequently acknowledged but who nevertheless played an essential role in accelerating the discoveries and implementation related to HIV/AIDS. They are the many dedicated and hardworking administrative assistants, laboratory technicians, program managers, and volunteers who knew they were doing something important but whose contributions were not fully recognized.

My work with Global Strategies could not have been successful without the encouragement of numerous collaborators, many of whom were leaders in their own countries ravaged by the HIV epidemic. The financial donations of thousands of individuals, NGOs, and faith-based organizations helped to fund our programs. While each donation was essential, special recognition goes to the exceptional generosity of Google, the Schmidt Family Foundation, the Robert James Frascino Foundation, Bayside Church in Sacramento, First Presbyterian Church in Berkeley, and Christ Presbyterian Church in Edina.

The contributions of many in the media helped to bring public recognition to the HIV/AIDS epidemic and to the discoveries that had the potential to end the epidemic— Lawrence Altman, Laurie Garret, Donald McNeil, and Jon Cohen.

The input and editorial assistance of Sahai Burrowes was essential as we struggled to make sense of the cumbersome and confusing WHO and USPHS HIV guidelines that for years, more often than not, kept more individuals off needed treatment than were put on.

I could not have continued working for the past twenty years without the use of a pacemaker and cardiac stents allowing me to continue our HIV/AIDS treatment and prevention programs in even the most remote regions of the world. I recently had the opportunity to meet the inventor of the portable pacemaker, Earl Bakken, and individuals at Medtronic to personally thank them.

PART 1 The Beginning

In any case the narrator (whose identity will be made known in due course) would have little claim to competence for a task like this, had not chance put him in the way of gathering much information, and had he not been, by the force of things, closely involved in all he proposes to narrate. This is the justification for playing the part of the historian. Naturally a historian, even an amateur, always has data, personal or at secondhand, to guide him. The present narrator has three kinds of data: first, what he saw himself; secondly, the accounts of other eyewitnesses (thanks to the part he played, he was enabled to learn their personal impressions from all those figuring in this chronicle); and lastly, documents that subsequently came into his hands. He proposes to draw on those records whenever this seems desirable and to employ them as he thinks best.

Albert Camus, *The Plague*

Pediatric HIV/AIDS

A MYSTERIOUS NEW DISEASE

It was June of 1981 when the scientific and medical communities first read about a mysterious new immunodeficiency disorder seen in young gay men (Gottlieb et al. 1981). The disease was first reported by Dr. Michael Gottlieb, a physician and immunologist at UCLA, who had identified a number of previously healthy young men who had suddenly developed a variety of opportunistic fungal, viral, and protozoal infections. The infections were of varieties not typically observed in adults, except in cancer patients whose immune systems had been suppressed after receiving large doses of radiation or chemotherapy. The young men whom Gottlieb was treating, however, had no history of cancer or cancer treatments. Gottlieb's initial report created quite a stir, and it soon became apparent that similar cases were on the rise across the country, from Miami to New York City to San Francisco.[1] Due to its prevalence among young gay men, some clinicians initially termed the disease Gay-Related Immunodeficiency, or GRID. In 1982, however, a group of activists and the US Centers for Disease Control and Prevention (CDC) suggested that the name "AIDS" be used instead, and the name stuck.[2]

I knew Michael from the immunology circles that we each traveled in—rather small circles, as there were few immunodeficiency diseases known, except in children, where we were dealing with genetic immunodeficiency disorders on the order of about one in one hundred thousand. Michael's patients were adults, and what he was describing was a severe immunodeficiency in previously healthy individuals. Michael was not prone to exaggeration, so when I read news reports about this new disorder in young gay men, I took it seriously, even though I could not conceive at the time that it had anything to do with children and immunodeficiency disorders.

When the news broke, I was working as a professor of pediatric immunology at Moffitt Hospital at the University of California San Francisco (UCSF) Medical Center, where I had established the first immunology laboratory devoted to the study and diagnosis of genetically acquired immunodeficiencies in both children and adults. There would be an occasional adult with a disease called acquired hypogammaglobulinemia, but this was a genetic disorder that could be easily diagnosed and treated. Much of my laboratory's activity focused on performing immunologic tests, especially measuring patients' levels of T-cells (TDL)—which are derived from the thymus gland

and bone marrow and are known to protect against opportunistic infections—and B-cells, which produce antibodies of different types, collectively known as immunoglobulins, against bacteria, viruses, protozoa, and fungi. My laboratory studied a number of rare immunologic disorders in children, including Ataxia Telangiectasia, Wiskott-Aldrich syndrome, and congenital hypogammaglobulinemia. The most severe disorders were typically characterized by deficiencies in both TDL numbers and function, as well as decreased levels of immunoglobulins. These severe but rare disorders had not been known to occur in formerly healthy adults. However, in 1981, there were increasing numbers of reports added to Gottlieb's groundbreaking discovery, and they were coming from major metropolitan areas in the United States. They had in common severe acquired immunodeficiency, occurring almost exclusively in young gay men who had no apparent cause for the disorder. AIDS appeared to be a new immunodeficiency disorder far removed from any of the forms of immunodeficiency that I had been studying for more than a decade.

During my first ten years on the faculty at UCSF, I had established an immunology laboratory to assist in diagnosing the patients who were referred to me for possible immunodeficiency disorders. In the process I discovered several new immunodeficiency disorders that were unknown, not only to the pediatric community, but also to the general medical community. Thus, in August of 1981, I was not completely surprised when I was invited to a meeting of fellow UCSF faculty members to discuss the strange new immunodeficiency disease that seemed to be spreading among young gay men nationwide.

The discussion group was called together by Dr. Marcus Conant, a dermatologist who was seeing an increased number of patients with Kaposi's sarcoma (KS), a rare cancer that classically occurred in middle-aged men of Mediterranean descent but was now being observed with increasing frequency in the newly described AIDS disease (CDC 1981a).[3] The group, which met regularly for lunch at the UCSF Faculty Club, was made up of an eclectic mix of individuals from various departments. Considering the significance of what was happening, and how this entirely new disease would move from a handful of patients to a major worldwide epidemic, the beginnings of the discussion group now seem inauspicious.

On November 6, 1981, Dr. Conant sent the ad hoc group a memo outlining the immunologic studies of the disease, which would be performed in my laboratory. I truly believed at that time that the number of patients who required studies would be limited, but I also felt it was important to document the degree of immunodeficiency and agreed to include a repository of blood samples from all patients suspected of having the acquired immunodeficiency. Thus began an organized approach to the evaluation of suspected AIDS patients, laying the groundwork for a repository of blood samples that, following the discovery of the human immunodeficiency virus (HIV) in 1983 as the cause of AIDS, would be tested to prove that the 1981 patients, many of whom had died by 1983, were indeed infected with HIV (Barre-Sinoussi et al. 1983; Broder and Gallo 1984; Chermann et al. 1983; Gallo et al. 1983).

From the very beginning of the Faculty Club meetings and throughout the early years of the AIDS epidemic, the original members of the ad hoc group worked collaboratively to define the epidemiologic, clinical, and laboratory features of AIDS, and from that point forward all members of the group would dedicate their professional careers to the AIDS epidemic. It was an extraordinary time of collaborating between individuals from different medical disciplines, gradual piecing together of different presentations about AIDS, and unraveling of a mystery that would eventually be attributed to a single cause.[4]

KEY PLAYERS

I particularly remember Paul Volberding, an energetic young research fellow in hematology and oncology, who was looking forward to an exciting career at UCSF. His AIDS patients began coming to him in increasing numbers with a variety of hematologic problems as well as KS. Paul had the essential combination of interest in pursuing the cause of disease coupled with compassion for the patients he saw, almost all of whom were deteriorating before his eyes due to immunodeficiency complications. It was not surprising that Paul was not only a key player in documenting the efficacy of one of the first drugs to treat HIV but also the individual who formed one of the first compassionate and comprehensive AIDS clinics in the United States to address the emerging epidemic (Fischl, Richman, Grieco, et al. 1987; Groopman and Volberding 1984).

Marcus Conant was a dermatologist with a large and thriving dermatology practice in San Francisco and at UCSF. As I got to know Marcus, I was impressed with his tenacity and determination to go beyond just the dermatologic manifestations of his patients to try to get at the cause. Marcus also seemed well connected politically, and I learned that he would use his political influence to be certain that AIDS was not ignored, either by the medical community or politicians. Marcus had started to observe a marked increase in the number of patients suffering from KS who were not of classical origin, middle-aged men of Mediterranean extraction.[5] Instead, these were young men who were referred to him to evaluate lesions that were appearing on the skin, mouth, and esophagus and which could have metastasized to other areas of the body.

William Wara, a radiation oncologist, joined the group because he, too, was observing an increasing number of patients with malignancies, ranging from KS to unusual lymphomas. His medical experience broadened the spectrum of the subspecialties in which patients with AIDS were being seen and highlighted the association of immunodeficiency and malignancy.

John Greenspan was an oral biologist who was observing a dramatic rise in the number of young gay men coming to his clinic with oral lesions called oral hairy leukoplakia, a relatively rare disease causing lesions on the mouth and tongue. John brought flair to the group with his distinct English accent but, more importantly, he broadened the spectrum of AIDS as he and his collaborators persisted in defining the various manifestations of the disease, eventually discovering the association of Epstein-Barr virus (EBV) with hairy leukoplakia (D. Greenspan 1985; J. S. Greenspan et al. 1985).

We continued to meet almost weekly, each of us consciously realizing that as more and more individuals were reported with AIDS, we were participants in the evolution of a new disease. On occasion, and with some trepidation, we would speculate as to whether the epidemic might expand to other populations and other countries. In this way the meetings became almost prophetic as questions of "What if this were to happen?" were soon answered with ever-increasing reports of new populations manifesting the clinical and laboratory features of AIDS. But in those beginning days of the

AIDS epidemic I felt somewhat removed, thinking that this new disease was confined to young adult males and could not occur in infants and children. My role remained to document the immunologic profile of this new disease and to process how such a disease could occur and whether it would remain confined to a specific population of individuals in the adult community.[6]

The challenges that lay before our group seemed urgent, and it was perhaps for this reason that we never paused to establish an official name. As we continued to discuss the evolution of this mysterious disease that was fast becoming a major epidemic, the effort to find a common etiology among all of the patients increased. The growing number of individuals who required immunologic evaluation was beginning to put pressure on my laboratory. Nevertheless, I agreed to offer the immunologic tests to assist in identifying and following patients who were being diagnosed with AIDS.

During the months that followed, concern about the increasing numbers of young gay men with AIDS came from many different individuals in the medical field. On March 22, 1982, a meeting was called at San Francisco General Hospital, where many of the AIDS patients were being evaluated. The University of California was not receptive to having these patients at their main hospital on "The Hill," as we often referred to the medical center. They feared that if referring physicians knew that individuals with AIDS were being admitted to the University hospital, they might not refer other patients. The meeting at San Francisco General was with Drs. Volberding, Wara, Drew, Sande, Gerberding, and me, all of whom were drawn into the AIDS epidemic either because we were seeing patients or because we were seeing the complications of AIDS. This particular meeting was the beginning of the attempt to precisely define the extent of the problem. Did it involve, for example, only the gay community? And how did the other risk factors that were being observed, such as KS, fit into the picture of the acquired immunodeficiency syndrome? At this early stage of the AIDS epidemic, it was clear that patients were presenting with very advanced immunodeficiency and primary clinical manifestations of opportunistic infections. Were there earlier manifestations of the syndrome?

FUNDING EMERGES FOR HIV/AIDS RESEARCH BUT NOT WITHOUT CONTROVERSY

Early in the epidemic there was a paucity of funds to conduct research into the cause and treatment of HIV/AIDS. I was a professor of pediatrics and immunology at the UCSF Medical Center in charge of the Pediatric Clinical Research Center, which gave me a limited amount of flexible funding to investigate immunodeficiency disorders in children. I had established a laboratory that had the capacity to measure all aspects of immune function. It was this laboratory that was called upon to do the first immunologic studies in both adults and children who presented with AIDS in 1981 (Ammann, Abrams, et al. 1983; Ammann 1983; Weintrub et al. 1983).

I was not the only one struggling with obtaining funds to conduct research into this new syndrome primarily affecting gay men in San Francisco. Depending on which clinical presentation of AIDS caused patients to seek medical help, they were referred to specialists in infectious disease, hematology, oncology, oral biology, or dermatology— each of the doctors in these subspecialties needed funds for research. The problem was that there were no funding agencies that foresaw the impact of the AIDS epidemic, and they were reluctant to invest funds in a new disease.

Dr. Marcus Conant was seeing a dramatic increase in patients with AIDS and KS in his dermatology office at UCSF, and he wanted to know if there was a relationship between KS and HIV/AIDS. Conant had direct access to Willie Brown, Jr., who at that time was the head of the California state legislature. Brown was sympathetic to funding AIDS research, and he decided to gather together the clinicians who were seeing patients with AIDS, including myself, as I was now seeing children with the same disorder. A masterful politician, Brown felt he could get state funding for research on AIDS—but he needed a detailed research plan from those immersed in the California epidemic.

In May 1983, Willie Brown called for a meeting in his office in Los Angeles and invited investigators from the University of California, San Francisco, Los Angeles, and Irvine to put together a comprehensive research proposal with the anticipation that state funding would be available. Those from UCSF included Drs. Conant, Volberding, Greenspan, Levy, and I. We left San Francisco on a 5:30 a.m. flight to Los Angeles. When we arrived, we worked intensely, with Conant as the leader. Sometime during the middle of the meeting, Willie Brown entered the room and in his eloquent way outlined the importance of what we were doing and what else needed to be done. We could only sit in amazement at his political prowess. Apparently, he had already announced to the press that he was going to give money for AIDS research, even though it had not officially been approved by the state legislature. It was a great political move. Even if the money was never made available, he would still get the credit for making the move to provide the first state funding for AIDS research.

It wasn't long before others in the university system found out about the availability of special funding through Willie Brown. They were extraordinarily upset that a small group of upstart investigators would have the audacity to go straight to the legislature to obtain funds for AIDS research. Accordingly, they decided that the money would not go directly to the investigators but would instead go through what they called "The Cancer Coordinating Committee," a group with no experience in AIDS research and composed of individuals who seemed more intent on slowing the funding process than in making research money quickly available.

In the end, Willie Brown put together a $2.9 million package of state funding to compensate for the lack of federal funding for AIDS in California. The legislature approved the total amount, and California Governor George Deukmejian signed the bill in October. But the University of California hierarchy, including Dr. Rudi Schimd, Dean of the UCSF Medical Center, allowed the funds to languish in the coffers of the Cancer Coordinating Committee. When the committee was criticized by the AIDS community, they responded by fabricating reasons that they hoped would satisfy the public. Cornelius Hopper, who was the assistant to the University of California president, said that the delays came about because the researchers did not submit detailed enough proposals . . . academic politics had nothing to do with the decision, and they planned to disperse the money by November 30th, a whole six months after the meeting in Willie Brown's office in Los Angeles. Speaker Brown was furious with the university and asked for an investigation of the delay. He stated, "California has a public health emergency and these funds are critical if existing AIDS research is to continue . . . the university's bureaucrats must stop treating these funds as gravy to be ladled out to ambitious faculty members who suddenly see a professorship or Nobel Prize lurking somewhere in the tragedy of AIDS."[7]

In his 1987 book *And the Band Played On*, Randy Shilts, a *San Francisco Chronicle* writer at that time, recalls the event: "the tale of the University of California's withholding funds appeared in the *San Francisco Chronicle*. Dr. Art Ammann, an eminent pediatric immunologist, was one of the handful of doctors with the courage to go public, saying AIDS research is being punished for committing a 'bureaucratic offense' against the University hierarchy" (Shilts 1987).

Although clinical researchers and the activist community expected that the release of funding at a state level would be immediately followed by dramatic increases in funding at the national level, especially from the National Institutes of Health (NIH), it did not happen quickly—there were those at the NIH who did not believe that AIDS would become a major public health problem and, in all likelihood, felt they needed to protect their own funding for other diseases. Fortunately, there was a cadre of researchers at the NIH who were investigating specific clinical manifestations of AIDS and would move the NIH agenda forward into investigating this new disease. They, too, encountered roadblocks, many of which had to do with "turf" battles and how the NIH had been organized to address new diseases.

STRIKING IMMUNOLOGIC ABNORMALITIES IN YOUNG MEN

It was on September 8, 1981, that I witnessed what I had never seen before. There, prominently posted on the whiteboard as I entered my laboratory, were five individuals' immunologic lab results. The tests showed that all five patients had low TDL levels and function but elevated levels of immunoglobulins—a striking pattern of immunodeficiency that did not fit with any existing genetic immunodeficiency disorder. I remember asking, "Who are these new patients?" I did not recognize their names and had never in my career seen such severe immunodeficiency in five patients evaluated at the same time. They were, in fact, blood samples from the clinics of Marcus Conant and Paul Volberding and belonged to young gay men who were suspected of having AIDS. It so happened that the results were posted along with those of three children who had also been referred to me for evaluation of immunologic function. I did not conceive at that time that there was a common etiology among them.

As I considered the three children's immunologic results, my thoughts went to another immunodeficiency disease. I was aware of only one similar disorder, which occurred solely in children with a genetic enzyme deficiency: purine nucleoside phosphorylase deficiency, which I had discovered in 1976 (A. Cohen et al. 1976). It was characterized by similar low levels and function of TDL and elevated immunoglobulins. But this disorder was so rare that it was only seen in one out of 100,000 to 200,000 births, and it only occurred in infants and children, not in adults. The rarity of purine nucleoside phosphorylase deficiency made it highly unlikely that all three of the children could have the same disorder. This mysterious new immunologic pattern in young adult males suggested to me that there must be some new, non-genetic cause of AIDS. Along with much of the medical and scientific community, the ad hoc group of physicians at UCSF puzzled over whether there was a single cause of this new disease and, if so, what it was. Aside from the fact that many of the patients were gay, the group continued to come up empty-handed with a potential cause of AIDS. Ultimately, it would be the addition of unique and tragic cases involving infants and children that finally led the investigators to one of the most important pieces in the epidemic puzzle. This piece had been there very early in the epidemic—there had to be an undiscovered infectious agent being transmitted sexually or by blood, or both.

RACHAEL

Early in 1982, I was asked to evaluate an extremely sick girl named Rachael Bellow, who had been born at UCSF Medical Center in 1979.[8] Rachael was kept in the intensive care nursery (ICN) for several months due to severe breathing problems. She was eventually discharged, but three years later she was brought back to the hospital for evaluation, as she had only reached the size and physical development of a one year old.

After years of seeing the problems that premature infants were left with after prolonged stays in the ICN, I knew that deciphering what was happening was not going to be easy. Premature infants frequently suffered from chronic lung disease, neurologic disorders, and what was generally called failure to thrive—a nonspecific designation that simply described slowed growth and development.

My very first glance at Rachael's tiny, wasted body told me that she was suffering from not just one specific problem, but the chronic effects of multiple illnesses. Rachael's abdomen protruded unnaturally due to an enlarged liver and spleen, which was visible from across the room without even performing a physical examination. She also had swollen parotid glands along with enlarged lymph nodes in her neck, underarms, and groin. It struck me as unusual to see such a young child with swollen parotid glands, and since they were coupled with the obviously swollen lymph nodes, I began to think that Rachael had either a malignant disease or an infectious disease. The outline of her bones was visible through her pale skin, and she displayed the telltale redness of diaper rash, most likely due to a chronic fungal infection.

I began to gather whatever information I could get from a physical examination and the medical records. An X-ray demonstrated multiple pulmonary infiltrates that apparently were making it difficult for her to breathe. Rachael was gasping for air by taking short, rasping breaths. She looked up at me with pleading eyes, as if begging for something to be done, but also with the air of suspicion common among children who have experienced the constant prodding and testing characteristic of prolonged hospital stays.

I learned that Rachael had been born to Susan Bellow, a prostitute and intravenous drug user (IDU) in San Francisco. Rachael was born prematurely at twenty-six weeks of gestation and weighed only 860 gm. She had acquired cytomegalovirus (CMV) infection and had also been infected with Staphylococcus epidermis. By order of a court, Rachael was now living in the protective custody of a foster mother. There was no evidence that Rachael had suffered neglect or abuse at the hands of her birth mother; rather, Susan had simply not been able to properly care for Rachael's needs due to her profession and lifestyle. It was evident that Susan sincerely cared for Rachael, visiting her frequently in the foster home to check on her well-being.

Rachael's foster mother stated that Rachael had been chronically ill almost since the first day she was placed in her care. The infant's symptoms were exhaustive: Rachael suffered from difficulty breathing, a chronic cough, frequent diarrhea, recurrent fungal infection in her diaper area, frequent ear infections, and fungal infections of the mouth that were difficult to clear. All these conditions prevented her from sleeping or feeding well and, as a result, she had barely gained any weight over the past three years. Based on Rachael's vast collection of symptoms and clinical features suggesting lack of resistance to infection, it seemed logical that I was asked to determine whether she might have been born with a form of genetic immunodeficiency.

My initial evaluation included laboratory tests of Rachael's immune system. These tests uncovered a peculiar immunologic pattern that was strikingly similar to the one being observed in adult AIDS patients, but it was not characteristic of any patients with genetic immunodeficiency disease, other than the extremely rare purine nucleoside phosphorylase deficiency. Rachael's TDL levels were markedly suppressed, and TDL function was severely deficient, while her antibody levels were unexpectedly high. After testing Rachael for purine nucleoside phosphorylase deficiency and confirming that she did not have a genetic immunodeficiency, I was puzzled and wondered whether perhaps she had yet another form of genetic immunodeficiency that had not yet been described.

I was also puzzled about the CMV infection. Could it cause the chronic lymph node swelling and enlargement of the liver and spleen as well as swelling of the parotid glands? CMV occurred as an acute infection, but I had not seen a chronic form of CMV infection that was associated with all of Rachael's additional abnormalities, especially the immunodeficiency. For a fleeting moment I wondered whether Rachael might have the immunodeficiency disorder similar to what I had been studying in adult patients with AIDS. But how could I reconcile an acquired immunodeficiency in an infant with a similar acquired immunodeficiency in young gay men?

Seeking any clues as to what might have caused Rachael's illness, I took a closer look at her medical and family history. Rachael's birth mother revealed that she had two other daughters, a two-year-old and a one-year-old, both of whom were also living in foster care. I thought if Rachael was indeed afflicted with a new inherited immunodeficiency disease, the other two girls, Esther and Sally, might display the same clinical features and immunologic pattern. However, when I located the children and consulted with their pediatricians, I found that only Esther displayed some of the unique clinical symptoms of AIDS. She suffered from swollen lymph nodes and parotid glands, and a chest X-ray revealed a distinct infiltrate throughout her lungs.

These symptoms were difficult to explain, as Esther's medical history showed no evidence of anything that might have brought on these symptoms. Her doctors theorized that Esther might have an EBV infection, which can cause infectious mononucleosis and other acute symptoms in older children. Laboratory tests confirmed that Esther did have EBV, but there were no reported cases of EBV infection that resulted in persistently swollen lymph nodes, parotid enlargement, infiltrates in the lungs, and immunodeficiency. Could Esther's illness also be due to chronic CMV infection? There were no known cases of chronic CMV infection causing severe immunodeficiency, so that diagnosis seemed unlikely. Esther's doctors simply could not come up with a theory that sufficiently explained her symptoms. However, upon comparing blood samples taken from Susan's three children, I found that while only Rachael and Esther displayed clinical symptoms, all three girls had the same immunologic pattern of elevated immunoglobulins and deficient TDL that I was observing in adult patients with AIDS, but at greatly varying degrees of severity.

I began to wonder if there was some way that an inherited immunodeficiency disease could be transmitted to all three of the girls. I spoke to my good friend Charlie Epstein, a pediatric geneticist at UCSF, to help me think through possible inherited mechanisms to explain a disease that affected only females. Several theories were proposed, but none sufficiently explained what I was witnessing, and it soon became clear that the missing piece to this puzzle might lie in the medical history of the girls' father. I asked Susan if the father of each of the girls was the same. Susan was adamant—there was only one father. Nevertheless, I obtained permission from Susan to run further tests on the three girls, which clearly disproved Susan's claims that all three girls had the same father. In fact, genetic testing showed that each girl had a different father. As such, immunologic tests on Susan seemed in order. These tests ultimately revealed that the girls' mother had the same immunodeficiency pattern found in the gay men with AIDS whom I had been studying.

Here was the first possible link: the mother was an intravenous drug abuser and a prostitute. Could she have acquired the infectious agent sexually or as a consequence of intravenous drug use and transmitted it to all three of her infants during pregnancy? It was not out of the question. Almost two decades before the AIDS epidemic began, I had studied infants born to mothers who had acquired rubella during pregnancy (Stiehm, Ammann, and Cherry 1966). In congenital rubella syndrome, the virus was passed from the mother to the infant, causing congenital abnormalities and marked elevation of antibodies in the infant's blood. CMV was also known to be transmitted from an infected mother to her infant (Kibrick and Loria 1974). But neither of these two factors caused severe chronic immunodeficiency. It was becoming ever clearer that Rachael's birth mother must have harbored some infectious agent—perhaps acquired through intravenous drug use or transmitted sexually from her multiple sexual partners—that resulted in her immunodeficiency and in turn caused immunodeficiency in her daughters. If that were true, then the infectious agents in Susan and her daughters might be the same as an infectious agent in male homosexuals with AIDS.

As her doctors continued to puzzle over Rachael's case, her condition worsened progressively during the year. She died in her foster home at the age of forty-eight months, suffering from acute infections and malnutrition. Upon hearing this news, I knew it was essential to establish the cause of death and obtain additional blood and organ samples. This would allow for future studies which could be used to isolate an infectious agent and determine if treatment would be available for the other children. But Rachael's body had already been sent for autopsy to a pathologist who was likely unaware of the importance of blood and tissue samples in discovering a possible link between AIDS in adults and AIDS in children, so late at night, I drove thirty-five miles from San Francisco to the Sonoma County pathologist's office to get tissue autopsy samples. I carried an insulated container of dry ice to freeze the tissue samples. Walking into the autopsy room after that solemn journey would be one of my strangest and most uncomfortable experiences throughout the epidemic, but the importance of my mission overwhelmed my feelings of unease. I drove back to UCSF that night and safely stored the tissue samples in the freezer on the fourteenth floor of the research building. Several weeks later the pathologist informed me that autopsy results revealed that Rachael had died of Pneumocystis carinii (PCP) (now renamed Pneumocystis jiroveci), commonly seen in patients with severe immunodeficiency, including AIDS (Gottlieb et al. 1983).

CHARLES

The same year that I wrestled with the cause for an immunodeficiency disorder in three children born to an intravenous drug-using and prostitute mother, I was asked to evaluate an infant named Charles Minot. Charles was born on March 6, 1981, at UCSF. He had severe anemia as a consequence of Rh hemolytic disease and was placed in the ICN. While in the nursery, Charles received more than twenty blood transfusions from nineteen different donors. Charles eventually left the hospital seemingly well, but when I was called to see him when he was fourteen months old, he was critically ill.

Charles was admitted to the hospital at UCSF. He had ongoing recurrent respiratory infections, a fungal infection of the mouth that did not respond to treatment, recurrent ear infections, hemolytic anemia, neutropenia, and a persistently enlarged liver and spleen. I was asked to provide an immunologic evaluation to determine whether Charles had an immunodeficiency disorder underlying his poor health. After performing a physical examination and reviewing Charles's medical history, I requested that tests of his immune function be obtained and a bone marrow sample taken for culture of infectious organisms. After years of caring for immunodeficient children, I had learned that routine tests for infection-causing organisms such as bacteria and fungi sometimes failed to detect an infectious agent and could only be found by culturing bone marrow.

When the immune function tests were returned, they showed that Charles had a low TDL count and, importantly, elevated levels of immunoglobulins, a pattern that was becoming all too familiar from studies of adult patients with AIDS. Based on these results, Charles's doctors requested functional tests of his immune system. These tests showed that Charles was severely deficient in both function and number of TDL, and he was therefore unable to respond to infections. It explained his multiple clinical abnormalities and recurrent infections, but there was no family history of a genetic immunodeficiency disorder. So, at the time, the cause of the immunodeficiency was not clear to me or his physicians. Charles was discharged from UCSF to be followed by his local pediatrician and to return for further evaluation.

One month later, the laboratory reported that from Charles's bone marrow they had cultured an unusual organism known as Mycobacterium avium intracellulare (MAI), which was being reported in AIDS patients (Zakowski et al. 1982). Although MAI was considered to be an opportunistic infection, I had never seen it cultured from any of the children with severe genetic immunodeficiency whom I had seen over the past several decades.

As improbable as it seemed, it was no longer impossible to ignore the similarities among the Bellows children, Charles Minot, and the adult patients with AIDS I had been studying. There had to be some sort of infectious agent acquired sexually and transmitted both sexually and by blood, either from intravenous drug abuse, from an infected mother to her infant, or, as in Charles's case, from a blood transfusion.

AIDS and Blood

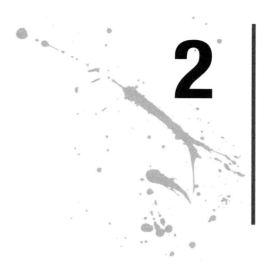

2

THE TRANSFUSION CONNECTION

In 1982, CDC investigations provided additional support for the hypothesis that AIDS was transmitted through blood products. The CDC reported that hemophiliac patients who had received commercial plasma concentrated from multiple donors were developing AIDS (1982d). This caused some suspicion, but as commercial plasma was being administered in multiple doses to thousands of hemophiliacs each year, it was difficult to understand why only a few had developed AIDS if blood products were indeed the cause of the disorder. Nevertheless, taken together, the evidence for transmission of AIDS through blood transfusion was suggestive enough to convince me and some of my colleagues to investigate whether Charles had contracted AIDS from one or more of his twenty blood transfusions obtained from nineteen separate donors.

Charles's donor blood had come from Irwin Memorial Blood Bank, which was the official provider of blood to UCSF and other hospitals in San Francisco. Herb Perkins, the director of the blood bank, was always concerned about the safety of blood transfusions, and it would take his cooperation to examine the list of those who had donated blood for Charles when he was in the ICN. But to make a link between receiving a blood transfusion and AIDS would require detailed analysis of all individuals who had donated blood to Charles and determining whether one or more had features of AIDS during donation or had developed AIDS following donation. Fortunately, in San Francisco there were many who were concerned about the rapid expansion of the AIDS epidemic. One of those individuals was Dr. Selma Dritz, the head of the San Francisco Public Health Department. Without the cooperation of Perkins and Dritz, and subsequently Harold Jaffe from the CDC, the link between AIDS and blood transfusion could never have been made so quickly ("AIDS: A Lethal Mystery Story," *Newsweek*, December 27, 1982, 63–64).

I was given permission to view the full list of Charles's blood donors and then cross-check the medical records of all nineteen of them with Dritz.[1] It was a difficult and painstaking search, but it was not in vain; one of the blood transfusions that Charles received had come from a donor who was well at the time of blood donation but had become very sick with the symptoms of AIDS over the following year. The donor ultimately died of AIDS the same month that the immunological investigations were being performed on Charles. It was a crucial and alarming discovery, as it implied that individuals who were unaware that they had AIDS could donate blood and unknowingly transmit the disease to others.

Despite the fact that we still had no clue as to what caused AIDS, I felt compelled to report Charles's case to both the medical community and the public. But I needed the CDC's help to confirm our suspicion. Help came from Harold Jaffe, an investigator at the CDC who would go on to become one of the important figures in defining the epidemiology of the AIDS epidemic. By 1982 there were already more than sixteen hundred reports of AIDS throughout the United States (CDC 1982c). Upon hearing of my investigation, Jaffe agreed to immediately fly from Atlanta to San Francisco to help review the data. We convened at my UCSF office, a space so small that we were forced to spread the records across the floor, covering every inch of available space. The data had to match up perfectly to credibly demonstrate a connection between blood transfusions and AIDS, and Jaffe and I worked into the late hours of the night to meticulously compare the names of those who had donated blood to Charles with names recorded in the AIDS registry of the San Francisco Public Health Department. By early morning of the next day, we were certain of our preliminary conclusion—young Charles Minot had indeed acquired AIDS from a blood transfusion.

NEW QUESTIONS AND A DIFFICULT DECISION

A host of new questions was generated. Was there sufficient evidence to report the link between a blood transfusion and AIDS? Should we report our discovery? If so, to whom? With millions of blood transfusions given each year, would alerting the public cause unnecessary alarm? What were the blood banks supposed to do with this information? Would there be panic among blood-donor recipients? After all, Jaffe and I still did not fully understand what AIDS was, let alone what caused it, and we could only diagnose patients through the association of clinical signs and symptoms and immunologic tests. Nonetheless, we both felt that it was our scientific and ethical obligation to report our findings. This would allow a thorough investigation of whether there were similar instances of AIDS transmitted by blood transfusions elsewhere in the United States.

After deciding to alert the public health community, Jaffe urged that the association between blood transfusion and AIDS be published in the CDC's *Morbidity and Mortality Weekly Report* (*MMWR*). However, the *MMWR* was not commonly read by the average physician or clinician, particularly not by doctors in surgical sub-specialties who frequently administered blood transfusions, and it was certainly not read by the general public. Therefore, given the ramifications of the association of AIDS and blood transfusions and our deep concern about preventing additional patients from acquiring AIDS through blood transfusions, Perkins, Dritz, and I decided to hold a press conference that would coincide with the release of the *MMWR* report on December 10, 1982 (CDC 1982a). We then hoped to publish our findings in a medical journal with high visibility and broad readership.

I first reached out to the *New England Journal of Medicine* (*NEJM*), the most widely read medical journal in the United States, which prided itself in publishing breaking medical research that was important to public health. With the now well-documented rapid increase in the number of patients reported with AIDS, I felt that they would certainly want to publish the details of the case calling for further investigations into the association between AIDS and blood transfusions. To my disappointment, in spite of the international public health implications of our findings, the *NEJM* rejected the article under the "Ingelfinger Rule" (Culliton 1972). Ingelfinger was the lead editor of the journal, and his policy was that previously published medical information could not be subsequently published in the *NEJM*, a somewhat arrogant position for a journal that represented itself as a leader in reporting medical advances. Ingelfinger considered the *MMWR* as a previous medical publication and refused to yield in spite of objections from Jaffe and me and from Jim Curran at the CDC. The decision was unfortunate and resulted in months of delay before the general medical community was informed about the risks of AIDS from blood transfusion.

Discouraged but undaunted, I next submitted the report to *Lancet*, a British weekly medical publication with the same level of readership as the *NEJM* but with a greater international focus. *Lancet* initially rejected the report, claiming that AIDS was a problem confined to the United States and not of concern elsewhere. It caused me to pause. Perhaps, I thought, I had come to the wrong conclusion. The suggestion that such disparate populations of individuals—young homosexual men, intravenous drug users (IDUs), pregnant women, and now some individuals who had received blood transfusions—could develop AIDS from the same cause seemed aggressive, but I felt there was too much at stake to not be persistent.

At the time of *Lancet*'s refusal, it was not yet known that AIDS would become a global epidemic. But this time I refused to take the medical editor's no for an answer, countering that if this disease could indeed be transmitted through blood products, it was only a matter of time before it would have serious worldwide implications. *Lancet* eventually relented and published the article on April 30, 1983 (Ammann, Cowan, et al. 1983).

As I anticipated, the article received incredible attention, not least of which came in the form of criticism regarding the many questions that remained open-ended, the most important of which was whether there really was an infectious agent that could destroy the immune system and result in AIDS. And even if there were, what could be done about it? Investigating this question was, of course, of critical importance. Indeed, one of the purposes of the publication was to stimulate intense research on the issue. Although blood transfusion-associated AIDS would become the focus of heated debate and intense research competition during the next few years, no test for HIV would be approved for use in blood banks until 1985 (Schochetman and George 1994). Until then, the focus was placed on how to screen blood donors to reduce the risk of AIDS patients donating blood and transmitting the disease.

In the absence of a specific test to diagnose HIV, various screening methods were proposed and tested. Some blood banks, including Irwin Memorial, decided to be more aggressive in their screening of potential donors' medical histories and refused donations from high-risk individuals, such as those having multiple sex partners. There was some precedence for this solution, as intravenous drug users had already been prohibited from donating blood due to the threat of transmitting hepatitis. Nonetheless, these actions also presented political problems, as questions were raised about whether aggressive screening was in fact a form of discrimination, particularly as AIDS was most commonly found in gay men with multiple sexual partners. Some members of the gay community recognized that the danger of spreading AIDS far outweighed any concerns of discrimination and encouraged their constituents to refrain from donating blood. However, throughout most of the United States there was an immediate outcry against aggressive screening from members of the gay community who feared that they would be stigmatized as the transmitters of the disease and as practitioners of a promiscuous lifestyle. This opposition was unfortunate and was one of the first examples of what was subsequently called HIV/AIDS denialism, referring to exemption of certain aspects of the AIDS epidemic from established public health guidelines (Casarett and Lantos 1998). Although concerns about discrimination against homosexuals were realistic, the public health concern of transmitting a potentially fatal disease via blood transfusion was more than legitimate and certainly seemed to outweigh other concerns. Many blood banks also opted to refuse donations from Haitians, a population linked to an increased risk of AIDS, but as the Haitian population was not well-organized politically, there were fewer protests from that demographic, so being of Haitian origin remained listed as a screening risk factor for blood donors (Curran and Jaffe 2011; Pitchenik et al. 1983; Schochetman and George 1994).

A different solution was pioneered by Edgar Engleman, who was at the time the director of the Stanford University Blood Bank. Knowing that most AIDS patients had very low CD4 counts, the subset of TDL that are most affected in AIDS, Engleman tested the CD4 levels of all donors after they gave blood. If donors displayed a low CD4 count, he would subsequently destroy their donations. Engleman did not disclose his actions to donors or patients, but any ethical questions raised by his methodology were clearly outweighed by the fact that his actions likely prevented hundreds of individuals from acquiring AIDS (Lifson et al. 1985; Richter 2013).

Yet another solution was that of directed donations, a quite controversial practice by which individuals undergoing elective surgery could preselect specific blood donors, such as members of their family (Schochetman and George 1994). Opponents of this practice questioned whether it was actually safer than normal donation procedures, with the strongest resistance coming from individual physicians, especially surgeons, who routinely transfused high volumes of blood and feared that a system of directed donations would not meet their needs. Some physicians would outright refuse to cooperate if a patient requested a directed donation. One such physician was an orthopedic surgeon at UCSF who publicly claimed that directed donations were no safer than randomized donations. A few months after he made that claim, I happened to be seated next to him on a flight en route to a meeting. He was wearing a cast. We started chatting about the recent procedure on his broken leg following a skiing accident. I was not surprised to hear him confess that he had preselected blood donors in advance of his surgery in order to ensure his own safety if blood transfusions became necessary.

In the end, all of the methods for screening blood donors who were likely to have AIDS were nothing more than stopgaps. The only true solution would be to identify the cause of AIDS and develop a blood test to detect the presumed infectious agent. As time went on, more and more laboratories and researchers entered the race to identify the deadly infectious agent, giving rise to an intriguing story of competition, frustration, backstabbing, and eventual victory when HIV was discovered as the cause of AIDS in 1983 (Barre-Sinoussi et al. 1983; Chermann et al. 1983; Gallo et al. 1983). Until then, another dramatic story unfolded, as the interests of the blood banks and the health concerns of the public came to a sensational clash (Feldman 1999).

The Blood Banking Industry in Denial

3

TRUST US, OUR BLOOD IS SAFE

Even before I published the groundbreaking report in *Lancet*, linking blood transfusions and AIDS and hinting that transfusion of blood products was potentially unsafe, resistance from the blood banking industry was emerging. Within a year of the 1982 report, the CDC had received hundreds of reports of conditions resembling AIDS in patients who had undergone blood transfusions for elective surgeries, as well as in hemophiliac patients who had been treated with transfusions of factor VIII blood concentrates (CDC 1982c, 1982d; Curran and Jaffe 2011). This evidence strongly suggested that there were safety issues with blood products, but as investigators had not yet been able to identify a consistent infectious agent that was the cause of AIDS, it was difficult to determine appropriate next steps.

In 1982, Bruce Evatt, a hemophilia specialist at the CDC, called a meeting in which he presented the results of the CDC's investigations into what he considered to be unusual cases of AIDS (Evatt 2006). These cases did not fall into either of the majority high-risk groups of young gay men or intravenous drug users, and the only commonality among the cases was the fact that the patients had received blood products and transfusions from high-risk individuals. Top-ranking members of the blood banking industry were in attendance and were undeniably made aware of the possibility of transmitting AIDS through blood products. However, the blood banking industry would prove itself irresponsible in their delays that followed.

The blood banking industry is made up of a large number of blood banks throughout the United States and is responsible for the procurement and distribution of blood products. These entities include small independent blood banks such as Irwin Memorial in San Francisco, blood banks owned by universities like Stanford or hospitals like Cedars-Sinai, and the largest blood banking association in the entire country, the American Red Cross. In conjunction with the CDC and the Food and Drug Administration (FDA), these blood banks are responsible for protecting the public with safety measures that include blood typing and testing of blood for transmissible infectious agents (Schochetman and George 1994).

While the blood banking industry is regulated by the FDA, it is also very much a private industry, and while most blood banks are technically nonprofit organizations, they are certainly profitable. By 1982, the blood banking industry was responsible for more than 3.5 million blood transfusions annually, making it a multi-billion-dollar industry (this number pales in comparison to the industry's profits today) (Starr 1998). At that time, it cost approximately fifty dollars to procure a unit of blood, which covered the costs of recruiting donors, storing and testing blood products, and separating blood donations into sub-products. As more attention was given to proper safety procedures, the price of procurement skyrocketed. In 1982, by the time a hospital had charged a patient for the administration of blood, the price had seen a hefty markup from $400 to $600 per unit (Forbes et al. 1991; Starr 1998).

It was discouraging but not surprising that the blood banking industry's concern for public safety was ultimately outweighed by economic motivations. Oddly, most states exempted blood banks of any legal liability for negative repercussions resulting from blood transfusions. Thus, many blood banks were primarily worried about the potential loss of income that would result from lower sales of blood products and not about lawsuits for negligence or the safety of blood products. They also feared that if they acknowledged AIDS could be transmitted through blood products, the public would misinterpret the message to mean that the act of donating blood was in itself dangerous. In the end, these economic considerations prompted the blood banks to resist taking any significant action following the meeting in 1982. Tragically, over the next few years, the CDC continued to identify cases of AIDS that were transmitted via blood transfusions. These AIDS cases likely could have been prevented if the blood banks had taken immediate action (Leveton, Sox, and Stoto 1995).

THERE IS NO DANGER BECAUSE WE SAY SO

What began as passive resistance to implementing better screening procedures soon transitioned into active and outright denial that AIDS could be transmitted in blood products, as the blood banking industry sought to prevent a public panic. The FDA's Blood Products Advisory Committee, the American Red Cross, the American Association of Blood Banks, and the Council for Community Blood Centers all started to insist at public forums that there was no documented evidence that sufficiently linked blood transfusion with AIDS, issuing a joint communiqué against directed donations.[1] Three organizations emphasized that there was no scientific basis for the assumption that blood from donors selected by patients is safer than that available from volunteers at community blood banks. They inferred that such a practice might be hazardous because it could pressure selected donors to be untruthful about their eligibility to meet donor requirements.

Their statement was clearly targeting the use of directed donors. The communiqué went on to state, "It appears at this time that the risk of possible transfusion-associated AIDS is on the order of one case per million patients transfused." This estimate was completely false and failed to consider the long incubation period between acquiring HIV and developing symptoms of AIDS, which made it virtually impossible to accurately estimate the number of individuals who had acquired AIDS from blood transfusions. Further communications throughout 1983 stated that, even if all suspected cases of blood transfusion-associated AIDS were accepted as correct, the total number of cases was still extremely low. In a strange twist of events, some of the larger blood bank associations released communications to their constituent blood banks stating that if the blood banks took certain precautionary measures, they could significantly reduce the number of cases of blood transfusion-associated AIDS. The discrepancy in their communications was obvious—denying a risk of transfusion-associated AIDS while maximizing precautionary steps to prevent it.

The vague and weak safety recommendations offered by associations like the American Red Cross were clearly motivated by issues of politics, economics, and confidentiality. Confidentiality would remain a great concern throughout the entire epidemic, as questions were raised about the ethics of publicly identifying donors who had AIDS or individuals who had contracted AIDS from blood transfusions. These questions made it very difficult to obtain medical records detailing patients' histories of blood transfusions and their HIV status. In an attempt to absolve themselves from the responsibility of informing blood transfusion recipients that they had been given a blood product from a donor with AIDS, the blood bank associations issued a joint statement in 1984 recommending that "the decision to tell patients or family members that they have been transfused with products donated by individuals who later developed AIDS should be made by the patients' physician." This recommendation represented a critical step backward from the accepted procedures of informing individuals who had been exposed to sexually transmitted infections (STIs), environmental hazards, dangerous products, and the like and all but assured that individuals who received a blood transfusion from a donor found to have AIDS would never be notified. The overly complicated involvement of multiple entities, including cumbersome and slow-moving government organizations such as the FDA and the Department of Health and Human Services (HHS), was certainly not to the benefit of the public, and as a result transmission of AIDS by blood transfusions continued.[2]

I was shocked by the blood banking industry's stance of resistance. While working with Herb Perkins at Irwin Memorial Blood Bank, I had come to expect that most blood banks would be responsive to the threat posed by this devastating disease. Although my experience with Perkins was encouraging, it became ever more obvious that the primary concern driving most people in the blood banking community was their economic preservation and liability. In contrast to the medical research community, which rushed to put all its energy into identifying the infectious agent that caused AIDS, the American Red Cross and other blood banks chose to funnel their efforts, and their vast financial resources, into convincing the public that blood transfusions were completely safe. With no effective screening procedures in place, blood banks continued to accept donations from individuals who had AIDS or who were asymptomatic but potentially infected with early-stage HIV (Leveton, Sox, and Stoto 1995; Schochetman and George 1994; Feldman 1999).

GOVERNMENT DECEPTION

I soon found that the blood banking industry was not the only entity that attempted to deceive the public about AIDS. On June 14, 1983, Margaret Heckler, secretary of HHS, stated at the US Conference of Mayors, held in Denver, Colorado, that "the disease is spread almost entirely through sexual contact, through the sharing of needles by drug abusers, and less commonly by blood or blood products, including transmission in utero." Specifically regarding blood transfusion-associated AIDS, Heckler recommended somewhat indifferently, almost as an afterthought, that "members of groups at increased risk for AIDS should refrain from donating plasma or blood products." She made no recommendations that blood banks actively take more aggressive approaches to donor screening to prevent the spread of AIDS. As if one ineffectual and ill-informed bureaucracy supported another, Heckler's quotes as secretary of HHS were widely circulated in the American Red Cross recommendations on AIDS and blood donations. I should not have been surprised that the FDA was not more helpful. On March 24, 1983, FDA Director of Biologics John Petricciani circulated a memorandum to all national blood collecting agencies recommending that they institute educational programs to inform people at high risk for AIDS that they should refrain from blood donation. This was yet another inadequate approach, falling far short of instituting any specific requirements. Petricciani also sent a letter to all national plasma collecting agencies, making the bizarre recommendation that if plasma were collected from a high-risk donor, it should merely be labeled as restricted "for use in manufacturing non-injectable blood products only," rather than being destroyed altogether.[3]

While it was certainly an uphill battle, I found that there were some crucial allies in the fight against the government's and the blood banking industry's resistance. One was Donald Francis, an epidemiologist at the CDC who argued early in 1983 that if emerging evidence suggested that AIDS was spread in a manner similar to the hepatitis B virus, it indirectly suggested that AIDS had a viral cause as well (Feorino et al. 1985). Another was the media, in this case *Time Magazine*, stating in a March 28, 1983, article titled "Battling a Deadly New Epidemic": "Pediatric immunologist Arthur Ammann of the University of California at San Francisco has presented the most compelling evidence of parental transmission of AIDS: a 30-year-old drug-addicted prostitute whose four daughters all developed symptoms of the immune disorder. The fact that each baby had a different father and that the mother has no sign of a hereditary disease suggests that the cause was not genetic. Our only option is an infectious cause." In contrast, Dr. Joseph Bove from Yale University declared on national television that same year that there was zero evidence of transmission of AIDS through blood transfusions. Fortunately, Francis continued his campaign and, at a meeting between the CDC and the blood banks, pounded on the table and angrily declared, "How many deaths do you need before you do something about this problem?" (Shilts 1987).

Another group greatly concerned with blood transfusion-associated AIDS was the National Hemophilia Foundation (NHF) (Johnson et al. 1985; MSAC 1983). I personally had not taken care of any children with hemophilia, other than in my residency training. But I was well aware of the number of transfusions that they required and the need for constant administration of factor VIII, an essential blood-clotting protein, to control the bleeding. Hemophiliac patients received regular administrations of concentrated factor VIII obtained from blood plasma pooled from multiple donors, and a number of them—both children and adults—had developed AIDS. It set off alarm bells among the hemophilia community as well as in the NHF. In 1983, Alan Brownstein, executive director of NHF, stated that "hemophiliacs serve as an early warning system for the safety of the blood supply. The message we were trying to communicate . . . was that we were blinking a yellow warning about a blood supply and we didn't want the industry to wait for a red light to take action." That same year, the NHF distributed its own rec-ommendations for preventing AIDS that were specifically geared toward hemophiliac patients. These recommendations greatly disturbed the blood banking industry, as the NHF openly acknowledged that AIDS could be transmitted in blood products. The NHF also recommended direct questioning and screening of individuals in high-risk groups such as gay men, intravenous drug users, and Haitians and made recommenda-tions based on the not-yet-confirmed assumption that AIDS was transmitted via virus (Johnson et al. 1985).

Bruce Evatt from the CDC continued working on the increasing reports of patients with hemophilia who appeared to have AIDS as a result of receiving factor VIII–containing blood products to prevent bleeding. His first case was referred to him in 1982. Evatt was working closely with the NHF to convince blood banks and govern-ment authorities to do something to screen blood products donated from individuals who were in risk categories for AIDS. Evatt and the NHF were having trouble con-vincing the same groups and individuals that I had worked with and who were denying that blood transfusion was associated with AIDS. This included those who attended the meetings Evatt organized—the American Red Cross, the FDA, the NIH, the American Association of Blood Banks, the National Gay Task Force, the Pharmaceutical Manufacturers Association, the Council of Community Blood Centers, and the State and Territorial Epidemiologists. In spite of his zeal and pleas that additional restric-tions should be added to blood donations, Evatt would be disappointed. In the end, a political decision was made not to add additional restrictions to blood donations. This decision was influenced by the blood banking industry, which feared loss of revenue, and the gay community, which felt that restrictions would lead to further stigmatization of homosexuals. Tragically, during the period of debate from 1981 to 1984, more than 50 percent of the patients with hemophilia in the United States became infected with HIV, and during the decades that followed, many of them died (Evatt 2006).

Evatt knew that there was tension between the CDC and the FDA regarding who should make recommendations on the safety of blood products. In 1983, he and his associates at the CDC decided to disregard protocol and publish their own recommen-dations for donating blood. They felt that in addition to the mounting cases of AIDS in patients with hemophilia, my report of transfusion-associated AIDS published in the *MMWR* was a clear warning for all individuals receiving transfusions and warranted urgent action. Writing about the history of AIDS in hemophilia, Evatt stated that the December 1982 transfusion case provided evidence that could no longer be ignored: "In our opinion, urgent changes in blood policy are needed to reduce the risk" (Evatt 2006).

Nonetheless, the blood banks and various government agencies maintained their hard stance of denial through 1984; no amount of science and data seemed to convince them to overcome their political concerns (Deresinski et al. 1984; Schochetman and George 1994). For an additional three years, they continued to waver. Not even the 1983 joint discovery of HIV as the cause of AIDS by Luc Montagnier from the Pasteur Institute and Robert Gallo from NIH resulted in a clear and urgent call for developing an antibody test to screen blood donors. In 1984, research antibody tests were made available that could diagnose individuals with HIV, even if they had not yet started to manifest the symptoms of AIDS. My hopes that the HIV antibody test could be quickly implemented for screening blood donors were dashed when the use of the antibody test for commercial purposes was delayed until March 1, 1985 (FDA 2014). This meant that I could use the antibody test to diagnose HIV infection in individuals with AIDS for research purposes, but blood banks could not use it to screen blood donors for HIV to protect blood transfusion recipients from becoming infected with a lethal virus such as HIV. Regardless, the blood banks could easily have contracted with laboratories to do screening tests on blood donors rather than choosing to wait a full year, resulting in even more HIV infection in blood-donor recipients, until the FDA finally mandated that blood banks use HIV testing on blood donors. At times I felt hopeless, thinking about the number of individuals who would unnecessarily contract AIDS from blood transfusions as a consequence of the unnecessary delays.

Additional allies were needed to change the bureaucracy mindset. I saw what the gay community activists were accomplishing by insisting that this was an epidemic that could not be ignored. I knew it would take individuals who were directly affected—either those who had personally contracted AIDS or those whose loved ones had—to call attention to the issue of blood-product safety through their own tragic stories. One such heartbreaking testimony was found in the case of three-year-old Sam Kushnick.

A Personal Tragedy

4

A LATE NIGHT CALL FROM LOS ANGELES

Late on the night of October 12, 1983, I received a desperate phone call from a couple named Helen and Jerry Kushnick. The Kushnicks had been referred to me by their cousin, who had been my professor at the New Jersey College of Medicine. The Kushnicks emotionally explained that their three-year-old son Sam was critically ill in the Intensive Care Unit at Cedars-Sinai Hospital in Los Angeles. Believing that their son might have blood transfusion–associated AIDS, they begged me to fly down to Los Angeles that very night. I was battling a fairly severe flu virus at the time, and the last thing I wanted to do that night was catch a redeye to LA. The Kushnicks were very persuasive, and I would later witness their persistence on behalf of HIV prevention time and time again. Somewhere around midnight I boarded a commuter flight to LA.

Jerry Kushnick met me at the airport and drove me to Cedars-Sinai Hospital. As we walked toward the Intensive Care Unit, I passed through hallways emptied of people and lined with original artwork from wealthy donors, not quite the hospital that I had been accustomed to working in. I first examined Sam and then his twin sister Sara, who was not hospitalized. Sara appeared to be perfectly healthy, but since birth, Sam had grown at a significantly slower rate than his sister and had suffered from multiple respiratory and ear infections. After I reviewed Sam's medical records, I was struck by the similarities between Sam and Charles Minot. Like Charles, Sam had received numerous blood transfusions as an infant in the ICN and now had low TDL counts. He had also been diagnosed with PCP, the opportunistic infection commonly seen in advanced AIDS patients (CDC 1981a, c). I pored over Sam's hospital records until after 4:00 a.m. There was no question in my mind that Sam had AIDS. Before I left the hospital, I glanced once more at Sam, and a helpless feeling returned as I realized that Sam would soon die from the complications of AIDS, and there was nothing I could do about it.

There was much to learn about Sam's family.[1] I learned that Helen and Jerry had only recently been married, and Sam and Sara were their first children. Helen became pregnant with the twins in 1980, and the entire course of the pregnancy and delivery was marked by a series of medical errors. Throughout the pregnancy, Helen gained excessive weight very rapidly, but her obstetrician failed to diagnose her twin pregnancy. At the eight-month mark, Helen's membranes ruptured prematurely, and she had to be rushed to Cedars-Sinai Hospital. There was no wheelchair available upon arrival, so she had to walk to the maternity ward. When she was placed in a hospital bed, the bed broke, and she nearly fell to the floor. She was administered several drugs to slow her labor, but this caused her blood pressure to drop significantly, to the point where a Cesarean section became necessary.

When the twins emerged from Helen's womb, Sam and Sara each weighed only three pounds. Both infants were placed in the ICN, where they developed multiple complications, but only Sam required blood transfusions. Ironically, some of the transfusions were only necessary to replace the blood that was being taken for countless blood tests. Sam ended up receiving more than twenty blood transfusions from at least thirteen different donors. After Sam and Sara were released from Cedars-Sinai, Sam began to suffer from multiple infections, and by the time he was three years old, he was critically ill—a story that I now recognized as intimately linked with AIDS. In my mind, there was no question of the diagnosis.

The Kushnicks were anxious and aggressive, which had led the Cedars-Sinai physicians to label them as "hyper-concerned parents." Moreover, they were powerful figures in the entertainment industry, and the medical staff was reluctant to deliver bad news to such wealthy and influential individuals. It was just one of the many tragedies in their story. Much could have been done to prevent Sam from developing such an advanced stage of AIDS if the Kushnicks had only been told the truth earlier.

After speaking with the attending physician, I found that he also suspected AIDS but was reluctant to say anything to the Kushnicks. I called Helen and Jerry into a small, poorly-lit room strewn with crumpled pieces of paper, half-empty coffee cups, and partially eaten snacks. I broke the news and watched their faces turn pale. Sadly, there was not much encouragement to offer, as there was no treatment for AIDS available at the time, or even a way to test for AIDS, leaving the Kushnicks concerned that Sara might be infected as well. However, Sara had never received any blood transfusions or experienced any of the same symptoms as Sam, so I was able to give them some reassurance that she probably did not have AIDS, as it was not known to be contagious between siblings without direct exposure to blood.[2]

The Kushnicks offered to drive me to the airport, stopping along the way for a somber meal at one of the few restaurants open in the early morning hours. Upon arriving home at 10:00 a.m., I collapsed into bed and fell asleep. Within a few hours, I awoke to the phone ringing. It was Jerry Kushnick calling to tell me that Sam had passed away. For the moment, all I could say was that I was sorry.

This unfathomable tragedy spurred the Kushnicks to become two of the most influential public figures in the story of blood transfusion–associated AIDS, as well as strong advocates for the pediatric AIDS research movement. Paradoxically, while their personal lives were crumbling following the shock of Sam's death, their professional and financial lives were skyrocketing. The couple owned a theatrical management company, and in 1975 they identified a promising but unknown young comedian named Jay Leno. After sponsoring many small storefront shows in the early days of Leno's career, the Kushnicks came to be his primary representatives. They eventually pushed for Leno to take over hosting *The Tonight Show* from Johnny Carson in 1992, which shot them to the top tiers of the Los Angeles entertainment industry's power structure.

The Kushnicks' influence and power in the entertainment industry proved to be instrumental in making the public aware of blood transfusion-associated AIDS, thereby pushing the blood-safety agenda forward. I found that they could get access to influential people and politicians who were otherwise almost impossible for me to see. I accompanied Helen to appearances on *20/20*, *The Donahue Show*, and *Good Morning America*, where she discussed the blood banking industry's slow response to the threat of AIDS. My role was to document the threat of AIDS-related blood transfusions, as well as the rapidly increasing epidemic among other populations of individuals at risk. Helen was interviewed for articles in the *Wall Street Journal* and *People Magazine*, and she was also able to obtain meetings with members of Congress, the CDC, and heads of major blood banks, including the American Red Cross. She wrote a letter to Nancy Reagan asking her to take up the cause of pediatric AIDS, and she called upon Congressman Henry Waxman, Chair of the Subcommittee on Health and Environment, to increase funding for research on blood transfusion-associated AIDS.

In 1984, Helen arranged for us to meet with Richard Schubert, then president of the American Red Cross, in Washington, DC. As Helen and I expressed our concern that safety procedures were not being put in place to protect the public, the inevitable question arose: would Schubert consider the current blood supply safe enough to transfuse to himself or a family member? Without a moment's hesitation, he stated that his belief was that current procedures would assure complete safety of blood products. In contrast to the meeting with Schubert, Helen did have some success in convincing two CDC officials and physicians—Assistant Secretary for Public Health Edward Brandt and James Mason from the CDC—to locate the records of Sam's donors to investigate how Sam may have been infected. Helen's aggressiveness persisted throughout her ongoing battle against blood transfusion-associated AIDS and her fight for increased recognition of pediatric AIDS. In honor of the contributions that Helen made to pediatric AIDS awareness, C. Everett Koop, the US surgeon general under President Ronald Reagan from 1982 to 1989 who was acknowledged for his own outstanding contribution to the cause, dedicated his Report on the Surgeon General's Workshop on Children With HIV Infection and Their Families, held in Philadelphia in 1987, to the memory of Samuel Jared Kushnick, stating "how much his life has counted and how well his voice is heard."

On a more personal level, I saw Helen's tenacity and refusal to accept discrimination exhibited immediately following Sam's death, when there was the threat of backlash against Sam's twin, Sara. In 1983, the early stage of the AIDS epidemic, there was much confusion and a lot of guessing about how AIDS was transmitted from person to person. Sara attended a private school in Beverly Hills, and a number of parents started telling the head rabbi that they wanted Sara taken out of school for fear that she would somehow transmit AIDS to their children. By the time these complaints were brought to Helen's attention in 1984, a diagnostic test for HIV had been developed, and Sara had been tested and found to be HIV-free. With this knowledge in hand, Helen asked the rabbi to give her the name of every parent who had complained. She then called them one by one to discuss their concerns.

First, she informed them that Sara had been tested and found negative for HIV. She asked if their children had been tested, and of course the answer in every case was no.

Next, she asked women if their husbands had been tested, as it was certainly possible that they might have had a sexual relationship outside of the marriage. This was enough to cause most of the parents to sheepishly withdraw their concerns, and Sara was allowed to attend school.

In the years after Sam's death from AIDS, I saw additional tragedies unfold in the Kushnick family. Jerry died of colon cancer and Helen of breast cancer. Only Sara survived. In the end, the Kushnicks' is a story of a family that experienced a tragedy completely out of their control but turned it into a battle to protect others against similar devastation. Aided by their high-level connections, influence, and wealth, the Kushnicks did much good work to accelerate public awareness and concern regarding the safety of transfused blood products. It is hard to say whether more could have been done had they survived. However, looking back, I see the events of thirty years ago as an example of how difficult it can be, in spite of scientific evidence and personal tragedy, to move large and cumbersome institutions and the individuals working within them into action to protect the public from dangers. Sadly, we repeatedly witness the tragic consequences of such institutional gridlock, as in the recent case of lead-contaminated water in Flint, Michigan.

BABY STEPS TOWARD RECOGNIZING THE RISKS OF TRANSFUSIONS

In January of 1985, a positive step in the pediatric AIDS agenda was finally taken when the American Red Cross officially recognized that newborn infants were particularly susceptible to complications of blood transfusions, including the transmission of AIDS and other infectious agents. I attended the ad hoc committee meeting on pediatric transfusion practices at the American Red Cross headquarters in Washington, DC, which was also attended by high-ranking individuals representing local blood banks and national blood bank associations.[3]

The meeting began with a summary of the previous two years, with the blood bank representatives striving to explain the work they had done to minimize the risk of blood transfusion-associated AIDS and, more generally, the risk of transmission of all infectious diseases in infants. The claims were not convincing and were met with criticisms that both the blood banks and the federal regulatory agencies had failed to provide timely and adequate protection to susceptible individuals. This failure was brought on by their refusal to accept early scientific evidence that AIDS could be transmitted through blood transfusions and also by their misuse of grossly inaccurate statistics, often based on partial epidemiological studies, in an effort to falsely reassure the public. Furthermore, much of the delay in introducing more aggressive donor-screening procedures was a result of including advisors from special interest groups that did not want the issue of blood-transfused AIDS to be associated with a gay lifestyle, while simultaneously excluding consumer groups from policy-making meetings. Several speakers, including myself, pointed out that when it came to pediatric patients, especially newborn infants, even the transfusion of blood products that were considered safe for adults carried potential hazards due to newborns' underdeveloped immune systems. I was proud to point out that the Irwin Memorial Blood Bank in San Francisco, under the leadership of Herb

Perkins, had been screening blood donors for CMV and excluding CMV antibody-positive blood from being used in newborns, and this same blood bank had been the first to acknowledge the risk of blood in the transmission of AIDS (Drew et al. 1982). The representatives of the blood bank industry were vigorously urged to relinquish their defensive posture regarding the safety of blood products and were asked to finally commit their efforts to investigating the association of blood transfusions and AIDS and protect the public from blood-borne diseases.

The meeting concluded with a number of crucial outcomes. First, the committee determined that the right to privacy versus the right to individual protection had been dangerously confused and misinterpreted, as the inability to question individuals about their sexual orientation allowed high-risk blood donations to be accepted with greater ease. Second, the committee created clearer recommendations to prevent the transfusion of blood containing CMV antibodies, a possible indicator of AIDS, to infants. Although the FDA had not yet officially approved an antibody test for HIV, I recommended its rapid approval and that blood products be screened for antibodies to HIV by utilizing research-based studies rather than waiting for a formal FDA-approved test.

BREAKDOWNS IN MAKING BLOOD TRANSFUSION SAFE

The blood-transfusion AIDS epidemic was allowed to rage as long as it did as a result of breakdowns in political, ethical, and legal safeguards meant to protect the public. The political breakdown stemmed from a refusal to accept early evidence of the connection between blood transfusions and AIDS in hemophilia patients, as well as in patients who had received blood transfusions from donors who were subsequently identified as having AIDS. The legal breakdown stemmed from the blood banks' lack of liability for any harm suffered by recipients of blood products who had been assured that receiving a blood transfusion was safe. Even though HIV had not yet been identified, there was ample scientific evidence that screening donors through their medical history or surrogate laboratory tests could greatly decrease the inadvertent donation of infected blood. Finally, the ethical breakdown stemmed from the multimillion-dollar blood banking industry's concern for its own economic preservation outweighing its concern for public safety and from the AIDS activists insisting that confidentiality superseded the safety of the blood supply. Altogether, these factors led to an unacceptable delay in implementing practices that could have prevented thousands of deaths.

Today, blood donations are tested for seven infectious agents, and in many developing countries, an additional three. The laboratory tests to detect these infectious agents are much more sensitive and sophisticated than when blood was originally tested prior to the AIDS epidemic. But the lessons learned from the false assurances of the 1980s should be a reminder to remain vigilant (Gallman 2015). The recent political move that loosened the restrictions on who can donate blood raises concerns that once again politics will supersede the safety priority of blood transfusion. The exclusion of certain risk groups from donating blood is meant as a safeguard to protect those who require blood transfusions from perhaps additional, yet unknown infectious diseases and should therefore not be compromised. The recent Ebola virus epidemic is a reminder that we can never be complacent about the hazards of transmission of infectious diseases. I consider donating blood a privilege and not a right, meant to protect individuals such as the ones I cared for from an infection with either known or unknown agents. In the balance of rights, those who have no choice but to receive a blood transfusion for their health must be given precedence over those who volunteer to donate blood. A warning from the World Health Organization (WHO) should be taken seriously: "It should be recognized, however, that all blood screening programs have limitations and that absolute safety, in terms of freedom from infection risk, cannot be guaranteed" (WHO 2009, 2).

Finding the Cause of AIDS

5

IF IT'S A VIRUS, WHAT KIND IS IT?

The most crucial piece in the puzzle of the AIDS epidemic was identifying the cause of AIDS, which would allow scientists to make an accurate diagnosis of the disease, understand how the disease was spread, and develop methods for prevention and treatment. The symptoms and physical findings that the scientific and medical community had observed strongly suggested that AIDS was caused by a virus that attacked the patient's immune system, but a number of other potential leads were pursued in earnest, each with its own group of staunch supporters.

One lead that was considered frequently throughout the early stages of the epidemic was CMV infection (Bachman et al. 1982; Drew et al. 1982; Drew et al. 1985). Antibodies to the virus were found in a high percentage of adults with AIDS, as well as in some children with AIDS (Ammann 1983). It was known that CMV could be transmitted by blood transfusions and from mothers to infants, and many children who were born with CMV had elevated immunoglobulins. My personal view, as I entered the debate, was that chronic CMV infection in both children and adults was not associated with immunodeficiency. Speaking with Perkins at the Irwin Memorial Blood Bank while testing blood donors for CMV, I learned that almost 50 percent of San Francisco blood donors had antibodies to CMV by the time they reached age forty. If CMV were the cause of AIDS, it should have been observed decades earlier and should have occurred in the vast majority of individuals infected with CMV. Ultimately, we determined that as the antibody was not present in all patients with AIDS, CMV infection could not therefore be the cause of AIDS.

But one prominent immunologist could not let go of a possible link between CMV and AIDS in infants and children. In a 1983 meeting at the New York Academy of Sciences, which was heralded as the world's first major conference on AIDS, I was asked to present our first cases of AIDS in children and describe their laboratory abnormalities and clinical symptoms (Ammann, Wara, and Cowan 1984). Dr. Robert Good, an internationally recognized immunologist with whom I had taken a one-year research fellowship at the University of Minnesota in Minneapolis, stood up after my presentation and vehemently objected, stating that he had observed countless numbers of children with features of AIDS—deficient TDL function and elevated immunoglobulins—and all had CMV infection. He insisted that I was simply re-describing CMV infection in an attempt to jump on the AIDS bandwagon. Good was known for having a strong ego and wanting to be first in the field of immunology. I was not certain if his comments were based on valid scientific observations or simply on being upset about not having first described AIDS in children. Regardless of his reasoning, I countered that patients with only CMV infection had normal TDL immunity and lacked opportunistic infections, whereas AIDS patients had TDL deficiency, multiple opportunistic infections, and many lacked antibodies to CMV. I then challenged Dr. Good to present his data on the infants whom he claimed had CMV, opportunistic infections, and abnormally low levels of TDL. The proceedings of the meeting were published in 1984, after HIV had been discovered and antibody tests were available to confirm HIV infection. As I read through the published proceedings, I noticed that Good had removed his 1983 comments from the published comments, clearly having been unable to meet my challenge (Ammann, Wara, and Cowan 1984).

Another contender for the cause of AIDS was a drug called amyl nitrate, which was commonly used in the gay community to enhance sexual experiences. However, the use of amyl nitrate could not explain all AIDS cases. Although mothers who gave birth to babies with AIDS might have used the drug, their babies hadn't, and it wasn't conceivable that an effect of a drug such as amyl nitrate could be transmitted in utero. There were also many hemophiliac patients who had blood transfusion-associated AIDS who had no history of drug use. Amyl nitrate was ultimately dismissed as a potential cause of AIDS.

A final lead that I pursued was the Haitian connection to AIDS (Altema and Bright 1983; Pape et al. 1983). Why Haiti? Was there something unique in the Haitian culture that linked other known associations with AIDS? It was a long shot, but by now nothing was to be discounted as a potential clue to the cause of AIDS. I lived close to the Haight-Ashbury neighborhood in San Francisco and often walked through the area on my way to UCSF. In the mid-1960s, drug use was increasing and the "summer of love" and "flower children" had arrived. Sexual freedom was increasing, as were STIs. While the various movements characteristic of the 1960s were not as visible in the early 1980s, lifestyle changes persisted in Haight-Ashbury. Bearing first-hand witness to the behaviors of drug users, I wondered if there was something in common in the use of drugs, multiple sexual partners, or perhaps a virus that could be transferred from one drug user or sexual partner to another. But what could that virus be, and what was the connection among all the various populations known to be affected by AIDS, including children, drug users, hemophiliacs, gay men, prostitutes, and Haitians?

I knew of a bookstore on Haight Street that specialized in offbeat books. In an effort to understand the Haitian connection, I searched through the stacks of books, looking for descriptions of Haitian voodoo and black magic practices. I was successful in finding several books about voodoo magic in Haiti and discovered that blood sacrifices from animals such as chickens and roosters were a frequent practice. At that time, researchers did not yet know that HIV had originated from monkeys and then crossed over into humans (Sharp and Hahn 2010). Regardless, my research didn't reveal evidence of monkey or human blood sacrifices, especially considering there were no monkeys in Haiti that could have been used for these rituals. In the end, my investigation, though an intriguing cultural diversion, yielded no additional clues to help explain the reason the Haitian population was at a higher risk of contracting the disease.

THE RACE TO DISCOVERY

In the 1970s, immunology and infectious disease research were expanding rapidly as separate subspecialties, with exciting advances being made in both fields. Many investigators focused their energies on linking the association of viruses and cancer. It had been well known for many years that certain viruses could cause cancer in animals, so many researchers were attempting to find similar viruses that occurred in humans and could potentially be cancer-causing as well. One such researcher was Dr. Harold Varmus, a well-known virologist at UCSF. Varmus began his postdoctoral studies in 1970 in Michael Bishop's laboratories at UCSF. It was there that Varmus and Bishop performed their breakthrough oncogene research that, in 1989, would win them both a Nobel Prize (Raju 2000). Varmus and Bishop were talented scientists and good thinkers but were not directly involved in the early AIDS epidemic.

I was intent on utilizing the stored blood samples and frozen organs I had obtained from deceased AIDS patients to isolate what I and many others felt had to be a virus associated with AIDS. But I had no expertise in the field of virology, let alone the laboratory skills to identify an unknown virus. The blood samples and tissues had been frozen for several years, but antibodies and traces of virus remain stable over very long periods of time, so they still had the potential to provide a wealth of scientific information. In addition, with the increase in the number of patients with AIDS, weekly samples of fresh blood could be obtained. I was determined to enlist the help of anyone who had the capability to identify a new infectious agent in the multiple tissue and blood samples that I had stored, and I was willing to provide these samples to any credible researcher who might use them to determine the existence of a unique AIDS virus. I was convinced Varmus could do it, so I arranged a meeting.

Varmus and I had never met in spite of working at the same medical center, but our first meeting in 1983 confirmed Varmus's reputation as being smart, energetic, and completely intent on being the first to discover the association of viruses and cancer. I briefly detailed the story of AIDS and, convinced that AIDS was caused by a virus, explained what I hoped he could provide once given the frozen blood and tissue samples, as well as the fresh blood samples. Varmus hesitated briefly, then told me that while the problem was a very interesting one and certainly important, there was simply "no money in it," meaning, of course, that there were no funds for research. The discovery of HIV would thus be left to three other researchers working with retroviruses—Luc Montagnier in Paris at the Pasteur Institute, who would be credited with first discovering HIV; Robert Gallo at the NIH in Washington, DC; and later by Jay Levy at UCSF (Barre-Sinoussi et al. 1983; Gallo et al. 1983).

Years later I ran into Varmus, who by then had become director of the NIH after receiving the Nobel Prize for his discovery of the association between cancer and retroviruses (Bishop et al. 1973; Varmus et al. 1975; Marshall 1993). I congratulated him on his accomplishments and briefly recounted the story of our first meeting at UCSF, finding his earlier statement amusing, considering that hundreds of millions of dollars from NIH were now being directed by Varmus into AIDS research. Apparently, Varmus did not find it so amusing, and he simply countered that he did not recall any such conversation. However, the individuals who were working feverishly toward discovering the association of retroviruses to AIDS were in fact engaged in a ferocious competition and had the Nobel Prize in their sights. Discovering the cause of such a devastating international epidemic was practically a guaranteed ticket to taking center stage at the Nobel Prize award ceremony.

I soon realized how naïve I was about the intensity of the competition. On September 14, 1983, a major conference on identifying a potential virus that might be the cause of AIDS began at Long Island's Cold Spring Harbor Laboratory. I was asked to present my pediatric data to the group at an afternoon session. Pediatric AIDS was a topic that intrigued many in the scientific community due to the strong support it lent to the theory that AIDS must be transmitted by some sort of virus. During the first evening of presentations, a French scientist named Luc Montagnier from the Pasteur Institute took center stage for a mere twenty minutes. He was a somewhat quiet and seemingly insecure individual, presenting his data in a low voice and, considering its future importance, a somewhat subdued fashion. During the presentation, Montagnier appeared as a silhouette against a large projected photograph depicting a cell containing particles of what he called lymphadenopathy-associated virus (LAV) isolated from an AIDS patient. Montagnier stated that his group had found antibodies to LAV in nearly 75 percent of patients with pre-AIDS and in 20 percent with AIDS. I remember being very impressed with Montagnier's data and wondering whether he would actually be the first researcher to have discovered the virus that caused AIDS.

Following Montagnier's presentation, I left the conference room still thinking about the significance of what I had heard. I entered the hallway, passing two individuals whom I did not recognize who were engaged in an extremely heated discussion. The two scientists were Sam Broder, a researcher at the National Cancer Institute (NCI), who was playing a critical role in the development of the early treatment for AIDS, and Robert Gallo, who was on his way to—or according to some, had already succeeded in—discovering the association of AIDS and what he was calling the human T-cell lymphotropic virus 3 (HTLV-3). Interestingly, a few months earlier Gallo had called me to ask for blood samples from pediatric patients with AIDS. Gallo's laboratory had discovered the early association of human retroviruses with cancer (human T-cell leukemia virus, HTLV-1 and -2), and he believed HTLV might be the cause of AIDS. But I had decided that the symptoms of HTLV-1 and HTLV-2 were not similar enough to AIDS to warrant parting with the precious blood samples. Now, seeing Gallo in person for the first time as he and Broder were engaged in an intense discussion, I couldn't help but stop to listen to the conversation, mostly because Gallo was so agitated and speaking in such a loud voice. Gallo was shouting to Broder, "*I'm* going to be the first one who discovers the virus that causes AIDS, not someone else. It's going to be *me*." I would later learn that there was an intense competition between Montagnier and Gallo that would continue for years and would ultimately result in an incompletely resolved debate over who truly discovered HIV. Most scientists, and apparently the Nobel Prize committee, agreed it was most likely Luc Montagnier, and in 2008, Montagnier and his coworker Françoise Barre-Sinoussi were awarded the Nobel Prize for their discovery of the virus that causes AIDS.

The dispute regarding the discovery of HIV was also carried over to a dispute of who should own the potentially highly profitable patent for detecting antibodies to HIV. Both Gallo and Montagnier filed for a patent on an antibody test, and the Pasteur Institute brought suit against the United States government in 1985. It took two years of fighting to resolve the issue. In 1987, the United States and France agreed to share royalties, and President Ronald Reagan and Prime Minister Jacques Chirac announced at a joint press conference that Gallo and Montagnier had independently identified HIV as the cause of AIDS. Some felt that the patent dispute resulted in the Nobel Prize committee denying Gallo a prize for codiscovering the AIDS virus (Harden 2012).

In 1985, Simon Wain-Hobson from the Pasteur Institute and Lee Ratner, a research fellow with Gallo at the NCI, analyzed the nucleotide sequences of Gallo's HTLV-3, Montagnier's LAV, and Levy's later-described ARV, proving that the three viruses were not just strikingly similar, but in fact belonged to the same retroviral family (Ratner, Gallo, and Wong-Staal 1985; Wain-Hobson, Alizon, and Montagnier 1985). In 1986, the International Committee on Viral Taxonomy renamed all three viruses the Human Immunodeficiency Virus (HIV) (Coffin et al. 1986). In retrospect, it is remarkable that amid the intense competition and all the egos involved, two major laboratories—one at the Pasteur Institute in Paris, France, one at the NCI in Washington, DC—discovered HIV within a remarkably short period of time.

The discovery of HIV was crucial, as it allowed for the development of an antibody test that could be used to diagnose and describe the worldwide epidemiology of HIV/AIDS. It also allowed epidemiologists and clinicians to identify the routes of HIV transmission, confirming what my colleagues and I had observed at the very beginning of the epidemic in 1981 and early 1982, when I studied blood samples from twelve patients with AIDS at my UCSF immunology laboratory: sexual transmission, transmission from mother to infant, and transmission via blood. Transmission from breast milk would not be discovered until later, when breast milk was obtained from mothers in low-income countries who had no other option than to breastfeed their infants (Mok 1993).

In June 1984, my colleagues and I began collaborating with Levy at UCSF to use his HIV antibody test on blood samples of children with various immunodeficiency disorders. I wondered whether AIDS in infants and children might have been present years earlier and, if so, whether other pediatric immunologists and I had missed the diagnosis. Levy agreed to study our stored blood samples from infants and children who had various genetic immunodeficiency disorders and chronic infections. The blood samples dated back to 1968 and had been obtained when I was an immunology fellow at the University of Minnesota and the University of Wisconsin with Drs. Good and Hong, respectively. I continued to store blood samples following my move to UCSF in 1971. Upon studying these samples, including the most recent ones from children with AIDS, and comparing them to blood samples from adult patients with AIDS, Levy discovered that the AIDS samples tested positive for HIV, while the samples from patients with other genetic immunodeficiency disorders were negative. These results strongly suggested that HIV was the true cause of AIDS in these pediatric patients (Ammann 1983, 1985; Ammann et al. 1985).

Saving Lives

Preventing HIV Infection of Infants

6

COULD HIV TRANSMISSION BE PREVENTED?

Within weeks of my 1982 report of the first child who had acquired AIDS via blood transfusion, the CDC's *MMWR* reported four cases of children with immunologic features and clinical histories consistent with the acquired immune deficiency syndrome (1982a, b). Included was one of the four female siblings I had studied in 1982. The transmission in these four children was not linked to the transfusion of blood, but rather to their mothers, who were prostitutes and intravenous drug users. The children were reported to the CDC by myself and two separate well-known pediatric immunologists—Jim Oleske in Newark, New Jersey, and Arye Rubinstein in the Bronx, New York (Oleske et al. 1983; Rubinstein et al. 1983). Both were recognized for their outstanding accomplishments in research and teaching in pediatric immunology. Oleske was at the New Jersey College of Medicine, the school from which both he and I had graduated, although at different times. The AIDS epidemic in children, which they were now discovering on opposite coasts of the United States, was bringing us together to solve the mystery of how these children had developed AIDS. Arye Rubinstein, an immunologist and allergist with experience in pediatric and adult immunodeficiencies, was at Albert Einstein College of Medicine in the Bronx. The *MMWR* report ended with identifying an additional twelve infants suspected of having acquired AIDS from their mothers. All of the children we reported had at least one thing in common: they were all the children of mothers who abused intravenous drugs. The comments in the *MMWR* ended with, "Transmission of an 'AIDS agent' from mother to child, either in utero or shortly after birth, could account for the early onset of immunodeficiency in these infants." Here were three pediatric immunologists, located in different regions of the United States, who were witnessing the expansion of the AIDS epidemic into children. Even at this early date, we questioned whether it might be possible, assuming an infectious agent was causing AIDS, that infection of infants might be preventable with treatment. But it was not until five years later that an initial research study in mice would provide the first solid hint that this would be possible.

FIRST STEPS TO PREVENTING HIV TRANSMISSION FROM MOTHERS TO INFANTS

The first real step toward what is today known as Prevention of Mother-to-Child Transmission of HIV (PMTCT) was reported in 1987 by Ruth Ruprecht (Ruprecht et al. 1990; Sharpe, Jaenisch, and Ruprecht 1987). Ruprecht demonstrated in a mouse model that the drug zidovudine (ZDV), when administered to pregnant mice, could markedly retard the onset and course of a retrovirus-induced central nervous system disease in fetuses. The results provided the first evidence that antiretroviral therapy (ART) during gestation and in the perinatal period might prevent the transmission of a human retrovirus such as HIV from infected mothers to their infants.

In much of the scientific community, there was widespread concern that drugs like ZDV, which inhibited RNA viruses such as HIV, would prove to be too toxic to be clinically useful. Following HIV infection of a cell, the HIV RNA is converted to DNA by an enzyme called reverse transcriptase (RT). HIV then "hijacks" the cell's own machinery to reproduce itself. ZDV works by blocking the RT enzymatic function and prevents HIV from multiplying. Many scientists feared that ZDV would also produce severe toxicity to normal cells and RNA molecules, which are some of the most fundamental molecules in living cells. This was a long-standing issue in the field of cancer research, as many of the anti-cancer drugs that were proved to be potent in a laboratory setting were simply too toxic to be tested on humans (Toltzits et al. 1991).

At the time, few pharmaceutical companies were engaged in developing anti-HIV drugs, primarily due to profit concerns. The market for anti-HIV drugs was perceived to be relatively small, with disproportionately high financial risks. Pharmaceutical companies feared that if they did discover a successful drug, the strong and vocal community of HIV activists might exert political pressure to provide the drug at a low cost or even for free, thus jeopardizing their profits. Thankfully, pharmaceutical companies such as Burroughs Wellcome moved ahead with antiretroviral (ARV) drug development and gained FDA approval of ZDV in 1987. Burroughs Wellcome went on to provide the drug for infected children, which was critically important in determining if ZDV could prevent mother-to-child HIV transmission. In 1987, Margaret Fischl, Paul Volberding, and their colleagues reported in the *NEJM* the first successful treatment of patients with HIV using ZDV (Fischl, Richman, Grieco, et al. 1987). ZDV became the first ARV to be approved by the FDA for the treatment of HIV infection, raising hope that there would be hundreds of thousands of HIV-infected individuals who could be treated before their HIV progressed to AIDS.

Administering ZDV to women during pregnancy to determine whether the drug might prevent HIV transmission from infected pregnant women to their infants was a different story, however, in spite of Ruprecht's observations in her mouse model. Several obstacles stood in the way of a study in HIV-infected pregnant women. First, the appropriate dose of ZDV for pregnant women and infants was not known. Also, there were no liquid formulations of ZDV, which would be necessary for the treatment of very young infants. At the time, most pharmaceutical companies only tested drugs on adult patients. Again, this was primarily due to economic concerns, as the pediatric market was viewed as too small to generate the profits necessary to offset the costs of additional testing. As a stopgap measure, pharmaceutical companies suggested that dosing for infants should be determined simply by calculating the infant drug dose relative to an adult dose. Pediatricians had unfortunately been forced to do this for decades with other medicines, not knowing if the calculated dose would be effective, ineffective, or even toxic.

Second, there was the question of whether it would be ethical to treat a pregnant woman and her fetus with a drug that could potentially produce toxicity to the cells of both the mother and the developing fetus. Some scientists feared that ZDV could produce fetal abnormalities or even cancer in unborn infants (Gogu, Beckman, and Agrawal 1989; Toltzis et al. 1991). Third, there was no evidence from other clinical studies in humans that ZDV could prevent transmission of HIV from one infected individual to another. Fourth, there was skepticism that even if the drug were effective in controlling HIV in adults, it would not be sufficient for the treatment of HIV-infected pregnant women and the prevention of HIV transmission to a fetus.

Finally, the presumption that the administration of ZDV to a pregnant woman could prevent the transmission of HIV to her unborn infant came with its own seemingly contradictory observations. Based on epidemiologic studies, only 30 percent of infants who were born to HIV-infected mothers were born with HIV, with 70 percent of infants escaping infection entirely ("Report of a Consensus Workshop" 1992). Therefore, some questioned whether it made sense to treat all HIV-infected pregnant women with a drug that was in fact only necessary for 30 percent of infants. Nonetheless, the number of HIV-infected pregnant women was increasing at alarming rates worldwide, and many of these mothers were transmitting the virus to their infants. As these numbers grew, it became ever clearer that the risks of treating HIV-infected pregnant women with ZDV were far outweighed by the importance of preventing an escalating epidemic of HIV-infected infants and children.

On April 6–7, 1987, the Surgeon General's Workshop on Children with HIV Infection and Their Families was held at Philadelphia Children's Hospital to discuss the pros and cons of moving ahead with a clinical trial to evaluate the potential of ZDV for prevention of mother-to-child HIV transmission. The meeting was chaired by Surgeon General C. Everett Koop, who was a staunch defender of aggressive HIV research but also demanded that research adhere to fundamental ethical principles. At the meeting, strong arguments were made in favor of designing a clinical trial of ZDV in pregnant women to prevent HIV transmission, overriding counterarguments regarding ZDV's potential toxicity. I had reservations about the ability of a drug such as ZDV to inhibit the transmission of HIV from infected mothers to infants. The drug was not an extremely potent one in inhibiting the growth of HIV, and while patients in the Fischl study had not progressed to developing opportunistic infection when treated with ZDV, the virus was not eradicated. This time, I must admit, I was the skeptic who rather pointedly asked whether the unknown potential toxicities of ZDV warranted moving ahead with a clinical trial of mothers and their infants at this time. Cathy Wilfert, an infectious disease pediatrician from Duke University and a strong and compassionate advocate for children, countered with a cogent argument in favor of moving ahead. She reminded everyone that the HIV infection rate of infants was increasing worldwide and, if unimpeded, HIV could become a major cause of early infant mortality. Ultimately, Cathy would turn out to be correct, and ZDV would be successful.

There was little preliminary knowledge on how to design a clinical study of prevention of mother-to-child HIV transmission. It had never been done before, and many questions were still unanswered when the study design was finalized. For example, during pregnancy, when is a fetus first infected with HIV? Should ZDV be administered during the entire pregnancy or only after the first trimester when the fetus is more developed and at the least risk for developing congenital abnormalities? How long should ZDV be administered after delivery once it is started during pregnancy? Was it necessary to administer ZDV to the mother alone, or should it also be administered to the infant, and if so, for how long?

Using the best knowledge they had, and recognizing that there were many pieces of missing information, the scientists devised a treatment plan and decided that the first administration of ZDV should start at fourteen weeks into gestation, which was believed to be beyond the most vulnerable period for potential fetal toxicity. From that time on the mother would receive oral ZDV, and during labor and delivery intravenous ZDV would be used to ensure that a high level of the medicine would cross through the placenta to the infant. Assuming that a single exposure to ZDV via the mother would not be sufficient to prevent infants from becoming infected, the study called for the administration of oral ZDV to the infant for six weeks after birth. Finally, the mothers would forgo breastfeeding, an additional source of HIV transmission to the infant, and feed their infants formula instead.

LINGERING CONCERNS

There were a number of lingering concerns with the study, not least of which was the fear that these infants would suffer negative health consequences farther down the road. One repeatedly raised example of long-term consequences of the administration of a drug to pregnant women was the use of the drug diethylstilbestrol (DES) (McFarlane, Feinstein, and Horwitz 1986). DES was a synthetic form of the hormone estrogen that was given to some pregnant women between 1940 and 1971 to prevent miscarriage, premature labor, and related complications of pregnancy. While the drug did not cause immediate toxicity, the female children of women who took DES during pregnancy had an approximately forty times greater risk of developing a cancer of the lower genital tract two to three decades after exposure. The lesson learned from the DES experience was seriously considered, and the strategy for the study included evaluation of both short- and long-term toxicities of ZDV in mothers and infants. Plans for the study moved ahead with the acknowledgement that the infants would have to be carefully evaluated and monitored after birth to ensure that they had suffered no fetal abnormalities or congenital deformities.

A final area of debate surrounded the use of a placebo in pregnant women and their infants (Angell 1997; Lurie and Wolfe 1997). The study was designed so that HIV-infected pregnant women would be randomly assigned to either ZDV or a placebo. The use of a placebo is an accepted scientific means of studying new therapies. This method reduces the number of research subjects required to obtain a result so that, if effective, the drug is available to patients more quickly. The use of placebos in children and pregnant women had historically been highly controversial, and given the international visibility of HIV, the debate surrounding the use of a placebo in the ZDV study was even more contentious than usual (Varmus and Satcher 1997). However, the rationale for the use of a placebo seemed sound—if ZDV were effective, the number of mothers and infants required to prove it would be smaller, and the study could be completed more quickly. This would allow ZDV to be available sooner for hundreds of thousands of HIV-infected pregnant women and their infants. In addition, if ZDV were ineffective but toxic, fewer mothers and infants would be exposed to the drug.

THE DISCOVERY THAT SHOULD HAVE ENDED
THE PEDIATRIC HIV/AIDS EPIDEMIC

In 1991, pediatric clinical researchers funded by the NIH took a courageous step forward and sponsored a clinical trial called the AIDS Clinical Trial Group 076 (ACTG 076) (Connor et al. 1994). The study began to enroll HIV-infected pregnant women and their infants and initiated treatment with ZDV, as outlined in the 1987 Philadelphia meeting. Treatment was started at fourteen weeks gestation and continued until labor and delivery, at which time the mother was switched to intravenous ZDV. The infants received a six-week course of ZDV following birth.[1]

The ACTG 076 study was conducted under the scrutiny of an independent board of clinicians and scientists known as the Data and Safety Monitoring Board (DSMB). The DSMB had the responsibility of monitoring the study and deciding at any point whether it should be stopped early, either because of toxicity to the mothers and infants or because sufficient preliminary data would prove the efficacy of ZDV in preventing HIV transmission from mothers to infants. By 1994, the ACTG 076 trial had enrolled sufficient numbers of HIV-infected pregnant women and their infants that the DSMB could begin to examine the study results to ensure that there were no safety issues and to determine if there might be early evidence of efficacy. Following an analysis of the preliminary results, the DSMB called for a halt to the study, not because there were any safety issues, but because the reduction in HIV transmission had been so dramatic. When compared to the placebo group, the mothers and infants who had received ZDV showed a 60 percent reduction in the transmission of HIV. This was a remarkable result. For the first time in the history of the HIV/AIDS epidemic, a drug was shown to prevent the transmission of HIV from one infected individual to another. The optimism that at last the pediatric AIDS epidemic could be brought under control was now in full swing. On February 21, 1994, the *New York Times* ran an article by Lawrence Altman titled "In a Major Finding Drug Curbs HIV Infection in Newborns."

Although this was the first study to show that a drug could stop the transmission of HIV from one individual to another, the story did not generate the level of enthusiasm anticipated. In fact, like so many headline news stories about children, it seemed to gradually disappear over time. The lack of a public response was surprising, as the study had important implications for the potential worldwide prevention of HIV transmission between sexual partners, in health-care workers following needle accidents, and in girls and women following rape and sexual abuse. But what disturbed me the most was the notable absence of voices from the adult HIV activist community calling for the immediate availability of ZDV for all HIV-infected pregnant women. It was as if they had forgotten their own pleas for immediate provision of treatment for HIV infection. Not willing to accept this puzzling silence, in July 1994 I flew to Washington, DC, to meet with Phil Lee, the director of HHS at the US Public Health Service (USPHS), who knew me from his days as chancellor at UCSF Medical Center. In the past, the USPHS had publicly announced nearly every important advance in HIV treatment in adults. I begged Lee to do the same with the ACTG 076 results, which had important implications for preventing new HIV infection in infants and children and potentially ending the epidemic of HIV infection in infants (Conner et al. 1994; Montaner et al. 2014).

Not surprisingly, as with many discoveries throughout the history of the AIDS epidemic, the ACTG 076 study result was not universally embraced, and certain individuals apparently did not share in the enthusiasm. The first of those was Sydney Wolf's Public Citizens Group, a public advocacy group in Washington, DC, that took on various health-related legal and ethical issues (Lurie and Wolfe 1997). They claimed that the use of a placebo in pregnant women and children was unethical. Marcia Angell, editor of the *NEJM*, also stated in an editorial that it was unethical to use placebos in studies that included infants, in spite of the fact that the *NEJM* had published the results of the study (Angell 1997). In response, Joseph Saba (from UNAIDS) and I crafted an op-ed piece to be published in the *New York Times*, in which we justified the use of a placebo in this particular study as urgently necessary, considering how rapidly the HIV/AIDS epidemic was expanding ("A Cultural Divide on AIDS Research," September 20, 1997). We noted that when the study was performed, there was no evidence that ZDV could prevent HIV transmission and that without a placebo the study would have required the enrollment of hundreds, if not thousands, more women and children, thus delaying the study results and the availability of an effective drug to hundreds of thousands of HIV-infected pregnant women and their infants. Cathy Wilfert also defended the use of placebo and resigned from the editorial board of the *NEJM* in protest against Marcia Angell's editorial. Oddly, the use of placebo in HIV-infected pregnant women and their infants soon ended. Once it was shown that an ARV could prevent HIV transmission from mother to infant, my fellow scientists and I felt that it would no longer be necessary or ethical to use placebos in future studies involving HIV-infected women and children. (A more detailed discussion of the ethics of placebo use in research studies can be found in Chapter 26.)

Lurking in the background of this debate, however, were influential naysayers waiting for an opportunity to speak out against placebo use in any study of drugs in HIV-infected women and children. A movement referred to as "the denialists" by the HIV/AIDS research and clinical community was beginning to take hold. As with many other issues in the AIDS epidemic, I found myself pulled into defending what we felt had been unequivocally proven by science.

The Denialist Movement 7

UNDERSTANDING HIV/AIDS DENIALISM

Denialism took many forms, from scientists denying that HIV was the cause of AIDS, to governments denying that their countries had an HIV/AIDS epidemic, to individuals denying how they contracted HIV. The denialist movement was important to the pediatric AIDS epidemic, primarily because it had a profoundly disproportionate negative impact on HIV-infected pregnant women and their infants worldwide. Fortunately the influence of those who denied that HIV caused AIDS did not persist. While adults, even those who were HIV infected, could make their own decisions regarding the cause of AIDS, HIV-infected women and infants, who were primarily in low-income countries and vulnerable to the control of indifferent or nefarious individuals, lacked the power to overcome the negative forces of denialism. Once the movement took hold in the United States, it spread to the rest of the world as it was taken up by a few influential political and media figures. Believing in the denialist theories meant not only denying that you were infected with HIV but also turning your back on the potent ARVs that could halt progression of the virus to AIDS and eventual death. When I first heard about the denialist theories, I thought their impact would be limited to just a few individuals and did not believe they would lead to some HIV-infected infants being denied treatment with ARVs.

The denialist theories played into the growing culture of conspiracy theories in the United States (Russel et al. 2011; Salmon et al. 2015). The HIV/AIDS epidemic had seemingly appeared out of nowhere, and HIV infection rates were skyrocketing overnight, ultimately affecting tens of millions of people worldwide. The epidemic had spawned an enormous research industry and, in the process of developing dozens of drugs to treat HIV infection, many individuals and pharmaceutical companies had become wealthy. Even the research community and academic institutions, which often suffered funding deficiencies, began to see a dramatic increase in funds for HIV research, covering all aspects of science, from epidemiology to behavioral. In the 1990s, funds devoted to HIV-related research reached annual sums of more than $1 billion. On the surface, it is not difficult to see why some would choose to subscribe to a theory claiming that the epidemic was a conspiracy fostered by the usual suspects—the government, pharmaceutical companies, the FDA, and the AMA.

The denialist movement was initiated by Peter Duesberg, a tenured professor of molecular and cellular biology at the University of California, Berkeley. Duesberg had initially gained recognition for his research linking retroviruses to cancer, but he would ultimately be identified as the pivotal person who put an academic and intellectual stamp of approval on the denialist hypothesis that HIV was not the cause of AIDS (Duesberg 1990, 1996).

Duesberg began to promote his theories in 1987, first simply claiming that retroviruses were harmless and not the cause of AIDS. He had never done any true research on HIV/AIDS or on any of the anti-HIV drugs such as ZDV but rather relied on an armchair analysis to make his claims (Duesberg 1996). However, Duesberg was able to capitalize upon his early career achievements in his work on cancer and retroviruses: he was elected to the prestigious National Academy of Sciences and received both a Fogarty Scholarship and an Outstanding Investigator Grant from the NIH. In 1996, Duesberg published a book titled *Inventing the AIDS Virus*, in which he boldly claimed that there was insufficient evidence to prove that HIV existed or, even if it did exist, that it was the cause of AIDS. This claim was at odds with all of the epidemiological evidence at that time, as numerous studies around the world had proved the association between HIV, individual infection, and transmission to others.

In order to support his theories, Duesberg devised an alternative theory. He proposed that AIDS was caused by (non-intravenous) drug use and malnutrition, a hypothesis he created simply from linking observations that patients with AIDS were often drug users who hailed from backgrounds of poverty. However, none of the patients in those studies had ever displayed anything close to the severe degree of immunodeficiency or the complications of opportunistic infections and malignancies that were seen in AIDS patients.

I realized that Duesberg's theories disregarded scientific data, including studies that were able to isolate HIV and define its molecular structure. He chose to ignore the evidence that millions of HIV-positive individuals around the world went on to develop AIDS and that HIV could be transmitted from infected mothers to their infants, and he failed to recognize the thousands of patients who had acquired HIV through blood transfusions but displayed none of the supposed risk factors of drug use, poverty, or malnutrition that he had proposed as the cause of AIDS.

Duesberg took his theories even further, going so far as to claim that ZDV might in fact be the cause of AIDS, even though AIDS was discovered six years before ZDV was used. His claims that ZDV could act as a carcinogen failed to point out that almost lethal doses of ZDV had to be given to mice to produce this effect. Duesberg further claimed that ZDV was the cause of the immunosuppression seen in AIDS patients. The more I read about his theories, the more concerned I became that infants and children would be the most susceptible to treatment denial. When he attacked ZDV, he attacked the only known means of preventing HIV transmission from infected pregnant women to their infants.

Duesberg's primary means for spreading his theories to the public was the Internet, but a few of his publications were accepted in obscure scientific journals. In 1991, Duesberg published an article in the *Proceedings of the National Academy of Sciences* espousing his theory that HIV was not the cause of AIDS. This prompted an outcry from a number of scientists who felt that scientific journals should not facilitate the spread of unsubstantiated theories. As Duesberg gained access to other scientific journals, the damage resulting from his theories broadened. He began to hone his attack on AIDS by inventing terminology such as "passenger virus" to explain why HIV was found in patients with AIDS (Duesberg and Rasnick 1998). In July of 2009, the journal *Medical Hypotheses*, which was under pressure from credible scientists who were shaming it for granting Duesberg access to the medical literature, published a retraction of his previous publication (Duesberg et al. 2009). As the years went on, Duesberg continued to publicly declare that HIV was not the cause of AIDS, even as it became ever clearer that he was contradicting the entire worldwide scientific community. Ultimately, Duesberg's theories were widely discredited.

DENIALISM SPREADS INTERNATIONALLY

One of the most influential and internationally visible individuals to happen on the denialist literature that was sweeping the Internet was Thabo Mbeki, who served from 1999 to 2008 as the second post-apartheid president of South Africa, a country that had one of the largest and fastest-growing HIV/AIDS epidemics in the world. Mbeki was a highly educated individual. Both of his parents were teachers and activists, his father a staunch supporter of the African National Congress and the South African Communist Party. Mbeki had received a bachelor's degree in economics and a master's degree in African studies from the University of Sussex in England. Mbeki also loved the Internet. He frequently surfed the Web in search of diverse and obscure resources to enhance his reputation as an interesting and charismatic speaker, often sprinkling his speeches with quotes from the *New York Times*. In what would prove to be a tragic find, his online research eventually led him to the denialist movement.

Most everyone in the AIDS community was shocked when they heard that Mbeki, president of one of the richest countries in Africa, yet one with the largest number of HIV-infected individuals in the world, was becoming involved in the denialist movement. Initially, it appeared that Mbeki would take an active stance in the fight against HIV/AIDS. At the 1995 International Conference for People Living with HIV/AIDS, held in South Africa, Mbeki acknowledged that an estimated 850,000 South Africans were infected with HIV. However, his position changed drastically during the next five years, and at a similar conference in 2000, Mbeki avoided the issue of HIV altogether, instead stressing poverty as the cause of AIDS. It seems unlikely that Mbeki embraced denialist theories due to a lack of knowledge, and it has been suggested that the drastic shift in his position was motivated by political and economic concerns. Denialism, by associating AIDS with poverty and malnutrition, provided Mbeki with grounds to argue that South Africa required funds from international organizations to stop the epidemic. By embracing the idea that HIV was not the cause of AIDS, Mbeki could also avoid paying for the production and distribution of ARVs in South Africa (Schneider and Fassin 2002).

Some insight into Mbeki's adoption of denialism can also be gained by examining his writings and speeches regarding HIV, the cause of the epidemic, the influence of the international community, and the involvement of Western countries in South Africa's affairs (Schneider and Fassin 2002). Mbeki accused Western countries of characterizing Africa as a continent of hopelessness, promiscuity, and ongoing disease. He played on the suspicions held by many in South Africa that black Africans had been deliberately infected with HIV so that Western pharmaceutical companies could profit from the sales of expensive ARVs. In some of his writings, he went so far as to portray HIV/AIDS scientists as latter-day Nazi concentration-camp doctors and claimed that the thesis that HIV caused AIDS was comparable to "centuries-old white racist beliefs and concepts about Africans." Mbeki's rhetoric resulted in unnecessary HIV infection and the deaths of thousands, estimated by some to be over 300,000, and more than 35,000 newly infected infants as he continued to blame outside influences for the AIDS epidemic in the country for which he had assumed political leadership (Sarah Boseley, "Mbeki AIDS Policy 'Led to 330,000 Deaths,'" *Guardian*, November 26, 2008).

Mbeki carried out his attack on HIV with the assistance of cabinet members such as Manto Tshabalala-Msimang, who served as Mbeki's minister of health from 1999 to 2008. She received her medical training at the First Leningrad Medical Institute in the Soviet Union from 1962 to 1969 and trained in obstetrics and gynecology in Tanzania before returning to South Africa. If it were not for the tragic consequences of her continued support of denialism, her treatment plans for HIV could be viewed as laughable: she refused to develop a public plan for treating HIV-infected individuals with ARVs, which she claimed to be toxic, and instead promoted holistic treatments consisting of beetroot, garlic, lemons, beer, and African potatoes (Ploch 2011).

Mbeki also relied on denialists from the United States and Germany to further his crusade against HIV treatment. Many denialists, including American David Rasnick and German Matthias Rath, were invited to testify about the cause of AIDS at conferences in South Africa ("South African Treatment Action Campaign" 2009). In 2008, Rasnick and Rath declared the risks and potential toxicity of ART, urging AIDS patients to forgo treatment and adopt instead a regimen of vitamins and nutritional supplements that they, of course, were marketing in South Africa. They were eventually ordered by the government to cease and desist, but only after the Treatment Action Campaign (TAC), a South African activist organization representing HIV-infected individuals, initiated a lawsuit against the Rath Foundation on the grounds that they were conducting unapproved clinical trials ("South African Treatment Action Campaign" 2009). It turned out that Rath and Rasnick were recruiting poor, black, HIV-positive South Africans to take vitamins and supplements instead of ARVs. It is believed that these trials resulted in as many as twelve deaths.

The impact of Mbeki's denialist theories and policies would soon be revealed. By the year 2000, it was estimated that of the thirty-four million people worldwide living with HIV/AIDS, twenty-four million lived in Sub-Saharan Africa. In South Africa alone, it was believed that eleven thousand individuals became infected with HIV each day, and from 1990 to 1998, the rate of HIV infection in pregnant women increased from less than 1 percent to as high as 35 percent. Other African countries had undertaken successful HIV prevention and treatment campaigns, such as Ugandan President Museveni's ABC (Abstinence, Be Faithful, Condoms) campaign, which was credited with decreasing the HIV seroprevalence in Uganda from about 15 percent in the early 1990s to about 5 percent in 2001 (Murphy et al. 2006). The calamity of South Africa was that it was perfectly positioned to become the world's leader in the fight against HIV. South Africa boasted one of the highest GDPs on the entire African continent and had many highly educated health-care workers and doctors, the best education structure in all of Africa, and the best health-care infrastructure in sub-Saharan Africa. Mbeki's fatal denialism slowed the implementation of HIV prevention and treatment (Bateman 2007; Gisselquist 2008; Bond 2004). Instead of helping, his denialism resulted in the deaths of hundreds of thousands of individuals, including infants, from AIDS (Boseley, "Mbeki AIDS Policy"). In 1999, in one of the most glaring examples of denial and abuse of political power, Mbeki claimed that there were insufficient funds to provide ARVs for HIV-infected pregnant women, yet he purchased two diesel-electric submarines for military defense at the cost of $30 million—enough money at that time to treat fifteen million HIV-infected pregnant women or infants to prevent HIV infection (Van Der Westhuizen 2005).

DENIALISM IN THE MEDIA

Although Duesberg can be viewed as the founder of the denialist movement, he was not an isolated aberration in the scientific community. He was joined by a number of peers, as well as activists and media personalities. One was Neville Hodgkinson, a British health journalist working for London's *Sunday Times*. During the 1990s, Hodgkinson published numerous inaccurate and inflammatory statements, later repeated in *Mothering Magazine*, espousing denialism and attacking both HIV as the cause of AIDS and the use of ZDV for prevention of perinatal HIV transmission. I was furious when I read Hodgkinson's vitriolic attacks that seemed to target the global population of defenseless HIV-infected pregnant women and infants. Hodgkinson was adept at making circular arguments—if HIV did not cause AIDS, but ZDV was being used to treat HIV, then infants were being exposed to a toxic drug unnecessarily. Many of Hodgkinson's publications were based on outright exaggerations and partial truths designed to appeal to conspiracy theorists. Some of his more outrageous statements included the claim that the harm done by ZDV had been extensively documented and that "a minority of infants born to HIV-positive mothers show elevated levels of HIV antibodies." He also emphasized that many infants lose their HIV-antibody positive status when they are eighteen months old, failing to note that by eighteen months all infants lose antibodies transferred from their mothers, including antibodies to polio, measles, and other infectious agents. In other words, it was a normal biologic process (Hodgkinson 2001).

In 2001, Hodgkinson published an article titled "Poisoning Our Babies: The Lethal Dangers of Zidovudine" in *Mothering Magazine*. By this time, a full seven years had passed since it was first reported that ZDV could reduce mother-to-child HIV transmission by 60 percent, and ZDV had gone on to save thousands of infant lives worldwide. Hodgkinson, however, failed to reference one single instance of an infant who avoided HIV infection as a result of receiving ZDV in utero and after delivery.[1]

One of the most well-known denialists, who had both money and easy access to the media industry, was Christine Maggiore, a successful businesswoman who had developed a multimillion-dollar import-export business. A routine medical exam in 1992 revealed that she was HIV-positive. Maggiore initially became involved with organizations supporting HIV/AIDS activism, but in 1994 she met Peter Duesberg and quickly adopted denialism. Maggiore soon founded Alive and Well, an organization that questioned the science behind the discovery of HIV and the tests used to identify HIV-infected individuals. She refused to take any retroviral drugs and encouraged others, including HIV-infected pregnant women and mothers, to do the same.

Maggiore was a prominent and well-known figure throughout the United States, particularly in Los Angeles, and she was easily able to promote her denialist message. Various media channels were eager to publish controversial stories, especially the kind that got public attention and promoted sales yet did not require them to consider the disastrous implications of publishing false information. They promoted the articles with provocative titles such as "Molecular Miscarriage: Is the HIV Theory a Tragic Mistake?" and "Zidovudine in Babies: Terrible Risk, Zero Benefit." Once again I was frustrated with the media's callousness in contributing to denialism, believing, perhaps naïvely, that they had an ethical responsibility to fact check their stories when so many lives were at stake. But there was no limit to how far the media would go. When Maggiore became pregnant in 2001, she still refused to take ARVs, flaunting her decision by posing on the cover of *Mothering Magazine* with "ZDV" in a circle with a slash through it drawn on her pregnant abdomen, under the title "HIV+ Moms Say NO to AIDS Drugs" (Gorski 2009).

When Maggiore's daughter, Eliza Jane, was born, Maggiore refused to have her tested for HIV and insisted upon breastfeeding ("Court Upholds Mother's Right" 1998). Several years later, when asked about Eliza Jane's health, Maggiore stated that Eliza had "never had respiratory problems, flu, intractable colds, ear infections, nothing. So our choices, however radical they seem, are extremely well-founded" (Ornstein and Costello 2005). Only seven weeks later, on May 16, 2005, Eliza Jane died. An initial autopsy, which was released to the public, showed that she had died of PCP and HIV encephalitis, clear indicators that she had HIV. Maggiore and her husband, Robin Scoville, responded first by suing the county of Los Angeles for violating their daughter's privacy and civil rights by releasing the autopsy report and next by hiring their own independent review of the autopsy report. The independent review came to the conclusion that Eliza Jane had died of an allergic reaction to an antibiotic that had been used to treat her infections. In 2006, the California State Medical Board opened proceedings against Paul Fleiss, Eliza Jane's pediatrician, accusing him of gross negligence in his care of several patients, including the daughter of the AIDS dissident. Because he failed to administer ZDV to Eliza Jane and allowed Maggiore to breastfeed, Fleiss was charged with failing to provide standard medical practices for the care of HIV-infected infants. The medical review board initially revoked Fleiss's medical license, an appropriate response. However, the board subsequently chose to stay the action in favor of a five-month probation, during which time Fliess was merely subject to regular monitoring of his practice and was required to take continuing medical education classes. Fliess was alive, but Eliza Jane was dead ("Did HIV-Positive Mom's Beliefs Put Her Children at Risk?" 2005; Gorski 2009). On December 27, 2008, Maggiore died of pneumonia at the age of fifty-two. To the bitter end, she denied that HIV was the cause of her symptoms and refused to take ARVs. As she was under the care of a physician at the time of her death, no autopsy was performed, but she was added to the growing list of HIV-infected denialists who were dying of AIDS having refused any treatment. Their deaths were quietly swept aside, contributing to the subterfuge of the denialist movement and further confusing the public about the fatal consequences of HIV as well as the success of ART to extend the lives of the majority of HIV-infected individuals indefinitely (Ornstein and Costello 2005; Wilson 2009).

DENIALISM IN THE COURTS

The theories of denialists like Duesberg and Hodgkinson spread and had a significant impact on the welfare of infants and children, which led to a number of important court cases in the 1990s. One of the most important was the case of Kathleen Tyson. One day in April 1999, I received a phone call from the district attorney in Eugene, Oregon, who said that he had been referred to me by a local pediatrician who had trained with me at UCSF. He explained that he hoped I could testify as an HIV expert in an upcoming court case. He was unable to offer any reimbursement, but upon hearing the details of the case, I immediately agreed to pay my own expenses and provide *pro bono* testimony.

The case involved Kathleen Tyson, her husband David, and their newborn son, Felix. While pregnant with Felix, Kathleen was told that a routine blood test indicated she was infected with HIV. It was unclear how she acquired the virus, as she had no history of blood transfusion and denied injecting drugs or having any sex partners outside of her marriage. Kathleen's physician instructed her to take a combination of ARVs to protect her unborn infant from acquiring HIV, to which Kathleen initially agreed. However, early into treatment she experienced negative side effects from the drugs and soon stopped taking them. Instead, she turned to the Internet for further information, where she stumbled upon denialist theories. When Felix was born, he was tested for HIV and thankfully found to be negative. In order to ensure his continued safety, Kathleen's doctors recommended that Felix receive ZDV treatment and that Kathleen abstain from breastfeeding, a known source of HIV transmission to infants. However, Kathleen refused both suggestions. Her physicians reported her to Child Protective Services, and she was charged with intent to harm her infant son.[2]

The trial, which was held in Eugene and heard by Judge Maurice Merten, attracted an enormous amount of media attention, making it an ideal case for both denialists and breastfeeding advocates to acquire publicity. The Tysons hired attorney Hilary Billings, who was known for an earlier case in which she had represented a young Maine woman named Valerie Emerson, whose right to withhold ZDV from her four-year-old son was upheld in court. Sadly, Valerie's son would die just a few years later ("Court Upholds Mother's Right" 1998).

With backing from the International Coalition for Medical Justice, Billings marched out as many pro-denialism witnesses as possible, including a scientist with a dubious reputation named David Rasnick, who had received his PhD from Georgia Tech University and claimed to be an expert on HIV due to his twenty years of work on proteases and protease inhibitors (PIs), enzymes related to HIV only because drug-induced inhibition of these enzymes prevented the HIV virus from growing. Although he, like most denialists, had never conducted any research on HIV and had most likely never even seen a patient suffering from AIDS, he was extremely articulate in expressing his theories. By means of clever deception remarkably similar to flim-flam artists, Rasnick was often sought out to testify in highly visible court cases on behalf of the denialist cause (Scudellari 2010).

In preparation for the trial, I spent a great amount of time poring over the denialist literature. As I did so, I became more and more astounded by how overwhelmingly confusing their theories were. How could anyone believe them? Moreover, the theories were completely unsubstantiated, and most denialists themselves did not have any credible expertise either through research on HIV/AIDS or through caring for patients dying of the complications of the disease. During my own testimony, I detailed the dangers of an HIV-infected mother breastfeeding and the high probability that Felix would become infected if the mother persisted. I concluded with the point that the denialists were essentially asking an innocent and defenseless infant to take the risk of acquiring HIV and thereby sacrificing his life in order to prove their theory.

However, I soon realized just how clever and deceptive the denialists could be. Throughout the case, the media listened to all the evidence and testimony that was presented by both sides. After the first day of testimony, one journalist approached me and said, "You know, what they're saying sounds right." I was gaining a first-hand view of how easy it was for the denialists to distort facts and take advantage of the public's naïveté and propensity for conspiracy theories. Rasnick, for example, was masterful in his deceptive testimony. Standing at the front of the courtroom holding a vial of blood, he paused for a moment and then bluntly stated that nobody could see any virus in this blood and asked the court if they could. Surely, I thought to myself, no one would believe what he was saying because it was so obviously ridiculous—no one could see electricity, either. But in fact, he went on to say, nobody had ever seen the virus that was called HIV. He claimed that the virus that the public had seen, in glossy high-powered microscopic photographs provided by scientists, was merely a virus cultured in laboratories, not isolated from any blood. This was a gross distortion of the facts, as HIV had certainly been taken from blood and was only cultured in the laboratory in order to increase the number of viruses for microscopic examination. Rasnick also detailed the requirements for performing an HIV antibody test, pointing out that blood had to be diluted in order for the test to work properly: "What kind of virus is there where you have to dilute the blood to show that the virus is present? Does that make any sense to you?" he asked the court. Of course, this statement failed to recognize that *all* antibody tests are performed on blood dilutions, whether the test is for polio, hepatitis, measles, or HIV.

As more and more witnesses approached the bench to testify on behalf of the denialists, I became more and more alarmed. The arguments in favor of breastfeeding under any circumstance were quite extraordinary. One doctor provided a list of at least one hundred diseases that would not occur if breastfeeding were provided. Another individual testified that individuals who were not breastfed had lower IQs than those who were breastfed. At that point, I looked carefully at Judge Merten, wondering whether he had been breastfed and what was going through his head. Within a few seconds, Merten announced that he had heard enough about the benefits of breast milk and that he presumed the next witness would tell him that breast milk was the miracle cure to all diseases.

After two days of testimony, it became clear that the denialists had gone too far when, mid-testimony, Judge Merten announced that he had heard sufficient evidence from both sides. He would allow the testimony from the denialists to continue and be recorded, but he would retire to his room adjacent to the court. He asked the court clerk to simply knock on his door and tell him when the last testimony was completed. At this point, I breathed an inward sigh of relief, confident that Merten would not rule in favor of the denialists. When Judge Merten returned, he ruled that Felix could continue to live with Kathleen and David under protective custody, but that they would be closely monitored and that Kathleen could not breastfeed Felix ("Judge Refuses" 1999; McCarthy 1999). The judge also ordered that Felix receive a brief course of ZDV. I took a deep breath of relief. Felix's life would be spared from a fatal HIV infection. But lingering in my mind was the concern about how many more additional victims would succumb to HIV infection at the hands of the denialists.

The decision to allow Felix to live with his parents was a risky one. The ease with which the Tyson parents had been deluded by information that they found on the Internet, and the degree to which they supported the denialists who testified in their favor, raised questions as to whether they would truly adhere to the court order. All of the information that was coming from Africa, where HIV-infected women had to breastfeed their infants because they lacked formula and clean water, indicated that breastfeeding accounted for about 30 percent of the infant HIV infections in developing countries (Mok 1993). Even a single episode of breastfeeding carried a high risk of transmitting the virus. HIV-infected mothers in the United States could choose to safeguard the lives of their infants by providing formula instead of breast milk.

In the end, the Tyson trial was deemed a loss for the denialists. However, other court cases with very different and tragic outcomes occurred, often involving innocent infants and children. As I witnessed some of these tragic cases evolve, my thoughts often turned to the international HIV/AIDS epidemic that was affecting hundreds of thousands of infants. I wondered what chance the children in low-income countries would have if even in the United States—a country of abundance—not all children could be protected.

COUNTERING DENIALISM INTERNATIONALLY: THE DURBAN DECLARATION

In 2000, the thirteenth annual meeting of the International AIDS Society (IAS) was scheduled to be held in Durban, South Africa. It would be a large gathering of thousands of AIDS activists, advocates, scientists, and politically influential individuals from around the world. Before the conference, I had been speaking with AIDS advocate Peter Hale and a number of colleagues about whether this was the appropriate forum to attempt putting an end to denialism in Mbeki's home country and worldwide. We began to compile a list of thousands of individuals in the international medical community who would publicly stand up against denialism and place their signature on what would come to be known as the Durban Declaration, a document clearly stating that HIV was the unambiguous cause of AIDS.[3] With a tight timeline and an ambitious goal, Peter and I worked day and night to compose the document in time for the conference. With the help of prominent scientists such as Simon Wain-Hobson from the Pasteur Institute and Robin Weiss from the University College of London, the Durban Declaration was finalized. The document explained how both AIDS and HIV were discovered and detailed the wealth of scientific evidence associating the two. The Durban Declaration concluded on a note of encouragement and optimism. The final sentence read, "Science will one day triumph over AIDS, just as it did over smallpox. Curbing the spread of HIV will be the first step. Until then, reason, solidarity, political will, and courage must be our partners" ("The Durban Declaration" 2000). Ultimately, the Durban Declaration was signed by more than five thousand individuals from eighty-four countries, including health-care workers, clinicians, researchers, scientists, and Nobel Prize winners. It was published in *Nature*, a prominent scientific journal, and distributed by journalists around the world to their governments and ministries of health. It has remained the seminal document defining the origin of HIV, the cause of AIDS, and in defeating HIV denialism ("The Durban Declaration" 2000; "Durban Declaration on HIV and AIDS" 2000).

In the United States and around the world, the denialist movement had a disproportionately negative impact on the AIDS epidemic, considering how few people actually adhered to its false theories. Globally, it led to hundreds of thousands of unnecessary deaths. Denialism proved to be most dangerous when it was taken up by figures with broad political influence and media access, such as Christine Maggiore, Thabo Mbeki, and individuals with university appointments, such as Peter Duesberg. The impact upon women and infants was particularly onerous. Fabricated arguments about the toxicity of ZDV resulted in funding delays and loss of precious time, as researchers and clinicians were forced to devote some of their valuable resources to defending the use of ARVs to prevent infant deaths, rather than focusing on additional research.

I would have expected the medical community to take all possible measures to protect helpless infants from HIV, regardless of their parents' beliefs, but a disappointing number of so-called scientists, physicians, and alleged legal experts agreed to testify on behalf of denialists, even when the life of an infant hung in the balance. It remains unclear whether each of these doctors actually subscribed to the denialist mythology, which is hard to believe given the wealth of opposing evidence, or whether they merely succumbed to the lure of money, politics, and media attention.

Support from some misguided members of the scientific community allowed denialism to gain inroads into the non-scientific community by giving denialism an air of credibility where conspiracy theories already had a certain appeal. Denialism played upon some members of the population's suspicion of their government, and in the case of AIDS, the belief that governments and scientists conspire to use the population for financial gain or unnecessary research. A frequent claim heard during the AIDS epidemic was that scientists and pharmaceutical companies were manufacturing false scientific claims in order to obtain money and prestige from their research. Another claim was that the government was conspiring to stigmatize and persecute the denialists. It is not hard to see how suspicion of government and science helped spread denialism, but it is still difficult to understand why the movement was not stopped by the overwhelming body of opposing evidence.

The lessons I learned from the denialist movement reinforced my belief that vigilance against denialism in all forms should be taken seriously. While the voices and impact of the radical denialists eventually faded, new forms of denialism—more subtle, less obvious, and sometimes perpetrated by more powerful and politically influential individuals—were born. In the years of the HIV/AIDS epidemic that followed the Durban Declaration, treatment continued to be withheld from many HIV-infected women and their infants based on a denial of the science, which had proven that all HIV-infected individuals required early initial treatment. Millions of HIV-infected pregnant women around the world would progress to AIDS, and millions of infants would become infected unnecessarily, sacrificed to economic and unvetted ethical interpretations of research in poor countries. Tragically, the new denialists of scientific evidence did not come only from the fringes of science but also from prominent and powerful individuals representing academic and government institutions who had once declared that treatment and prevention were urgently needed to slow the HIV/AIDS epidemic in women and children. Power and money, as will be seen, corrupted the potential for momentous clinical research discoveries to bring a quick end to the global pediatric AIDS epidemic.

PART 2 Pediatric AIDS Becomes a Reality

Michelle's death marked, one might say, the end of the first period. That of bewildering portents, and the beginning of another, relatively more trying, in which the perplexity of the early days gradually gave place to panic.

From now on, it can be said that the plague was the concern of all of us.

Albert Camus, *The Plague*

Born of Necessity

8

The Pediatric AIDS Foundation

A DINNER CONVERSATION: THE DISCOVERER
OF AIDS AND AN ANONYMOUS WOMAN

On September 21, 1988, I received an unexpected and urgent phone call from Dr. Michael Gottlieb, the physician who had originally discovered AIDS in 1981 (Gottlieb et al. 1981). I knew Gottlieb from his position on the Scientific Review Board of the American Foundation for AIDS Research (amfAR), where I was responsible for reviewing pediatric research grants. Gottlieb also knew that I was the director of the Pediatric AIDS Research Program at the UCSF Medical Center and had been at the forefront of the discovery of AIDS in children.

During the phone conversation, Gottlieb explained that an anonymous individual in Santa Monica was interested in starting a pediatric AIDS foundation. Gottlieb described her as "very influential and very serious," as well as dedicated to the cause of adding pediatric AIDS to the overall AIDS research agenda. He asked if I could fly from San Francisco to Los Angeles to meet the secretive person for dinner. Within hours, I was on United Airlines flight 23 to Los Angeles. I met Gottlieb and the mystery woman at the Globe, a fashionable restaurant owned by Dudley Moore and named for the Golden Globe Award Moore had received. When I first spotted Gottlieb and the anonymous donor, I was struck by the woman's diminutive stature and seemingly shy and apprehensive demeanor. In later years, I would learn many times over that this initial impression was not at all indicative of her true character. Over the course of the meal, the donor's interest in pediatric AIDS evolved.

Her story, like so many that I had heard in the realm of pediatric AIDS, was a tragic one, and one that was intimately related to blood transfusion–associated AIDS at Cedars-Sinai Medical Center. This was the same hospital where I had met Sam Kushnick's parents in 1983, just hours before Sam's death. Sam had likely become infected with AIDS after a 1980 blood transfusion. I learned later that, in a strange coincidence, a blood transfusion from the same hospital at the same time had infected three other individuals: the mysterious person who sat before me at dinner and her young daughter and son. I would also find out later that the woman was Elizabeth Glaser, a young schoolteacher and the wife of Paul Glaser, who had gained fame playing Starsky in the 1970s cop thriller television series *Starsky and Hutch*.

In August 1981, Elizabeth gave birth to her first child, Ariel. Complications during the birth required Elizabeth to receive an emergency transfusion of seven units of blood. This occurred a full year after Sam Kushnick and others had also received HIV-contaminated blood transfusions at Cedars-Sinai. After recovering in the hospital and returning home, Elizabeth happened to read about a new deadly disease known as AIDS and the possibility of transmission via blood transfusions. Alarmed, Elizabeth called her physician, who incorrectly assured her that she did not need to be concerned. Elizabeth focused on caring for her newborn and, unfortunately, decided to breastfeed her young daughter. Three years later, Elizabeth gave birth to her second child, a son named Jake. By the time Jake was born, Ariel had started to show symptoms of increasing and unexplained illnesses. An astute UCLA pediatrician, E. Richard Stiehm, who was caring for Ariel, was aware of the increasing number of children with AIDS and the association of blood transfusion and AIDS. In fact, Stiehm had been my mentor in immunology at UCSF in 1966. Together we published my first manuscript in a medical journal, which happened to be on the subject of intrauterine infection with a virus, but on that occasion it was the rubella virus (Stiehm, Ammann, and Cherry 1966). Stiehm was suspicious that HIV may be the cause of Ariel's illness but was unable to prove it until an antibody test was available to diagnosis HIV infection in 1985. The Glasers then had Ariel tested and were horrified to find that she was infected with HIV. The entire Glaser family was tested, and Elizabeth learned that she, Ariel, and Jake were all infected with HIV—Elizabeth via blood transfusion, Ariel via breastfeeding, and Jake through in utero transmission.

Ariel's health was deteriorating rapidly, and Elizabeth was alarmed to learn that there was no treatment available for her daughter. Equally disturbing was that there was very little treatment research being done on pediatric AIDS, and there was no foreseeable funding for this research. ZDV was not approved by the FDA until 1987, but even then it was only approved for adults; testing had not been done to determine a precise dosage for infants, nor was there a formulation of the drug that could be taken by infants (FDA 2014). Desperate, Elizabeth battled with the FDA but was never able to get ZDV for Ariel—she died in the summer of 1988 at the age of seven (Glaser 1993).

This heartbreaking experience, coupled with the knowledge that both she and her son Jake were also infected with HIV, prompted Elizabeth to start asking questions about pediatric AIDS research. The answers she received were disheartening, as she found that there was no meaningful research or progress being made in this area. She was initially frustrated by the US government's slow response to pediatric AIDS, but frustration turned to terror when she realized what this slow response could mean for her HIV-infected son. Moreover, Elizabeth herself faced imminent death unless AIDS research started to move forward much more quickly. Armed with a $500,000 donation from Paul's aunt Vera List, Elizabeth took matters into her own hands and channeled all her energy into establishing a pediatric AIDS research foundation. She turned to Gottlieb for advice, and he recommended that she meet and talk to me as the physician/scientist most knowledgeable about pediatric AIDS (Ammann, Wara, and Cowan 1984).

Seated around the table at the Globe restaurant, oblivious to everything around us, Elizabeth, Michael, and I discussed how we could most quickly establish a foundation dedicated to the prevention and treatment of pediatric AIDS. We contemplated two approaches: first, establishing a brand new foundation, and second, utilizing the structure of an existing foundation. Both approaches had pros and cons. The most expedient course would be to raise money through a new pediatric AIDS foundation but administer that money and grant support through an already established foundation. Michael's and my existing connections made amfAR the most logical choice.

At 10:30 PM, I excused myself from dinner and left to catch a United Airlines midnight flight back to San Francisco, still wondering who the anonymous woman I had just had dinner with might be. Within days of our meeting, on September 8, 1988, Michael Gottlieb, as the chair of the Science Policy Committee of amfAR, wrote the following to members of the board of directors:

> I have met several times with a donor who wishes to remain anonymous and is interested in furthering pediatric AIDS research through amfAR. This person wishes to make an initial donation of $250,000 and may soon be in a position to contribute up to $2 million. The donor is also exploring additional funding sources, which could raise the sum considerably . . . I believe that this could be an important direction for amfAR scientific programs, mainly targeting funding to a specific granting program (e.g., HIV/AIDS in children). This particular program has the potential to stimulate much-needed activity in pediatric AIDS research and to improve the quality of research being done.

AmfAR's cofounder, Dr. Mathilde Krim, and its board of directors graciously agreed to review and administer the funds raised by the foundation without taking any percentage of the money donated. Little did Michael and I realize the impact that our decision at that brief dinner would have for women and children in the worldwide HIV/AIDS epidemic.

THE PEDIATRIC AIDS FOUNDATION IS FORMED

The Pediatric AIDS Foundation was officially established in 1988 (Glaser 1993; EGPAF 2016b). During those early days, Elizabeth enlisted the help of two of her closest friends, Susie Zeegen and Susan DeLaurentis, to get the foundation up and running. The three women would hold planning meetings around Elizabeth's kitchen table, so they nicknamed themselves the "Kitchen Cabinet." This casual work environment would in later years spark a sense of curiosity and admiration in Washington, DC, political circles. Throughout the foundation's first year, Elizabeth chose to remain anonymous due to the significant stigma associated with HIV at that time. She feared that a backlash in the entertainment industry could negatively affect Paul's career, and she also feared for Jake, who was currently attending elementary school. Therefore, on the foundation's first formal letterhead, Elizabeth's name was conspicuously absent. In the upper right-hand corner, however, there was a colorful drawing of flowers and hearts, labeled "Hope for Children with AIDS." The logo had been drawn by Ariel before her premature death, and it has been kept as the foundation's logo to this day.

The number of people formally associated with the initial structure of the foundation was relatively small. The board of directors consisted of Elizabeth Glaser as the chairperson, Elizabeth's close friends and cofounders Susie Zeegen and Susan DeLaurentis, attorney Peter Benzien, and accountant Lloyd Zeiderman. Thanks to Elizabeth's connections in the entertainment industry, an executive advisory board was formed to increase the visibility and funding of the newly formed foundation. The advisory board consisted of luminaries such as Steven Spielberg, William Brock, Bob Burkett, Kitty Dukakis, Michael Eisner, and Susie Field. Later, the foundation would add additional notable individuals, perhaps some in name only, but many who were active in the future of the foundation, such as Elton John, Michael Ovitz, Jonathan Tisch, and Pete Wilson.

EXPERTS ARE ENLISTED FOR THE CAUSE

To develop and drive the research agenda for pediatric AIDS, the foundation needed expert help. As well connected as the founder and co-founders were to individuals in the entertainment industry and potential funding sources, they needed a scientific agenda with clear-cut goals that would directly address the paucity of research in pediatric AIDS. Following Gottlieb's introduction, Elizabeth and the cofounders asked if I would take on the task—I agreed. It was an extraordinary opportunity to do things differently, to short-circuit the long and arduous task of asking individuals to apply for research money, reviewing their research proposals, and then, often more than a year later, finally providing the funds. Now, with a source of funding that could bypass time-consuming tangles and be immediately awarded, coupled with the ability to define the critical research targets, progress in pediatric AIDS was truly possible.

I agreed to chair the Health Advisory Board, which was formed to interact with amfAR to ensure that pediatric AIDS research remained a priority. At that point in the AIDS epidemic, I knew the scientific achievements of many of the most outstanding researchers in the United States and Europe who were working on both the adult and pediatric epidemic. I contacted those with whom I had collaborated, both nationally and internationally, and who were actively working on the emerging pediatric AIDS epidemic. Initial members of the Health Advisory Board were Mary Boland, a nurse at the New Jersey College of Medicine, who provided a broad clinical perspective on the needs of mothers and infants with HIV; Yvonne Bryson, a pediatric infectious disease specialist and an AIDS researcher at UCLA, who was one of the first researchers to become deeply involved in determining immunologic factors that might prevent transmission of HIV from mothers to infants; Phil Pizzo, a pediatric cancer specialist at the NCI, who oversaw pediatric oncology and pediatric AIDS research and had both influence and insight into the workings of the NIH; Gwen Scott, a pediatric infectious disease specialist at the University of Miami, who had been introduced to the pediatric AIDS epidemic by caring for many HIV-infected women and children of Haitian descent; E. Richard Stiehm, a pediatric immunologist at UCLA and also Jake Glaser's pediatrician (a fact that I initially did not know), a highly esteemed immunologist, and the individual who had trained and influenced me to sub-specialize in pediatric immunology; Arye Rubinstein, the pediatric immunologist who discovered AIDS in children of intravenous drug users in the Bronx, New York, while at Albert Einstein School of Medicine and who further defined the clinical and immunological features of children with AIDS; Michael Gottlieb, who discovered AIDS and focused on adult medicine but had a broad perspective on the HIV/AIDS epidemic and a compassionate view of what needed to be accomplished to move the pediatric agenda forward; and Jim Oleske, a pediatric immunologist who discovered AIDS in the children of intravenous drug users in Newark, New Jersey, while at the New Jersey College of Medicine and who continued to contribute to the diagnosis and care of children with AIDS.

Thanks to Elizabeth's tireless determination, the foundation was quickly up and running, soon raising hundreds of thousands of dollars in grants. I began promoting initial priorities for pediatric research and organized a meeting held on December 15, 1988, at the NIH. Scientists from different specialties were selected to attend and contribute to defining pediatric AIDS research priorities: Mitchell Golbus represented obstetrics; Steven Wolinsky was an expert in HIV diagnostics; Phil Pizzo represented pediatric malignancies and AIDS; Norval King was known for his work in animal models; Tom Waldman was an internationally recognized immunologist; and Richard Sweet was an expert in obstetrical research. The group identified perinatal HIV diagnosis, improved diagnostic methods, treatment approaches for HIV-infected children, maternal factors associated with HIV transmission, and animal models as research priorities.

Everyone felt that this was the beginning of the much-needed prioritization of pediatric AIDS research. I eagerly summarized the recommendations from the meeting, wrote up the requests for applications (RFAs) for research studies to be conducted and approved, and submitted them to amfAR to distribute for funding. This was the first time that grant requests specific to pediatric AIDS had been sent to the research community. The process was rapid, efficient, and effective. And, of course, extraordinarily exciting. The pediatric grants were reviewed simultaneously with adult research grants in order to ensure cross-fertilization of intellectual knowledge throughout all aspects of the research. Once grants were approved, the Scientific Advisory Committee (SAC) of amfAR, of which I was chair, directed the funds to fill in critical gaps in pediatric AIDS research. Funding was initially focused on understanding why only 30 percent of children born to HIV-positive women acquired the virus, as well as evaluating drugs that could be administered during pregnancy to prevent HIV transmission.

INCREASING THE VISIBILITY OF PEDIATRIC HIV/AIDS

Elizabeth and the Pediatric AIDS Foundation were well aware that if research were to continue and to accelerate addressing new priorities in pediatric AIDS, significant amounts of funding would be needed. One of the foundation's first large fundraising events was the "A Night to Unite" gala at the National Building Museum in Washington, DC, in July 1989. The gala was one of many that I attended throughout the early years of the HIV/AIDS epidemic, and the scale of the event was indicative of Elizabeth's and the Health Advisory Board's connections in the entertainment industry and national politics. In what was probably the first bipartisan fundraising event for AIDS, each attendee received a joint invitation from both Democratic Senator Howard Metzenbaum as well as his Republican colleague Orrin Hatch, both of whom gave keynote speeches at the gala. Cher provided the entertainment, spurring on friendly political discourse by joking that she would first sing a song for the Republican crowd and then a song for the Democrats. Such cross-party collaboration was a major step that many in the AIDS community had longed to see for years, especially as the more conservative political faction had initially been hesitant to take on the issue of HIV/AIDS.[1]

The gala was co-chaired by Kitty Dukakis and Sandy Brock (the wife of Bill Brock, Ronald Reagan's secretary of labor) and attracted a great mix of highly visible, monetarily endowed individuals including Ted and Susie Fields, Alan Alda, Mohammed Ali, Marlee Matlin, Meredith Baxter Birney, Dana Delaney, and Julianne Phillips (the former wife of Bruce Springsteen). The event garnered much media coverage, although I found it odd that the media gave disproportionate attention to the societal rank and fashion choices of the attendees rather than focusing on the issue at the heart of the event, HIV infection of children and the lack of treatment, research, and resources to address it. But the event did raise a significant amount of money, so to that end, it was a great success. Tickets were sold for $1,500 each, and the gala ultimately raised more than $1 million specifically for pediatric AIDS research.

During most of the event, I stood at the back of the auditorium with Elizabeth, who squealed and jumped up and down like a young girl, unable to contain her excitement at the sight of well-known political figures and entertainers bringing her dream to life. I wondered how long Elizabeth could remain anonymous and, indeed, whether she needed to. The attendance of such highly visible individuals made it impossible to deny the issue of pediatric AIDS, and it seemed that it would be difficult at this point for anyone to discriminate against Elizabeth or her family.

Throughout the epidemic, Elizabeth's personality was essential to pushing the Pediatric AIDS Foundation's agenda forward. Driven and aggressive, Elizabeth knew how to cut through any bureaucracy to get to the key issues, no matter to whom she was speaking. Her life was at stake, as were the lives of an increasing number of infants born with HIV. Her tenacity was largely due to her own personal tragedy; Elizabeth was all too aware that ZDV had been available for a full three years before Ariel's doctors were allowed to give her the drug under a special FDA compassionate-use protocol. These were three long years during which Ariel's life could have been extended. Ariel received only two months of ZDV treatment before she died from complications of HIV infection (Stiehm and Vink 1991). Elizabeth herself was operating on a fundamentally different timeline. At this point, there were still no drugs available to reverse the progression of AIDS, only to slow it down. Elizabeth knew that she was going to die of AIDS, and as a result, she did not mince words. At the end of every meeting, she demanded to know a date when she could expect to see the results of whatever had been discussed. Many times I heard her follow up with the chilling statement, "I don't have time to wait for an answer." When Elizabeth requested funding or assistance, there were only two possible responses: yes or no. Fortunately, Elizabeth heard yes more frequently.

Elizabeth was well liked, and her stern and direct demeanor toward politicians and regulators was tempered by softness in her personal relationships. She frequently sent handwritten notes to her colleagues to express her love and appreciation for their work. She was forgiving of individuals who volunteered their time but who lacked the experience to move the pediatric AIDS agenda forward quickly, and she frequently said, "They're doing the best that they can."

As the Pediatric AIDS Foundation gained visibility, Elizabeth also gained increased access to members of Congress and other politicians. My contribution was my credibility in the scientific and advocacy community, as well as my broad interaction in multiple fields of medical research, and I could therefore provide the much-needed access to the scientific components necessary to move the research agenda forward and insure credibility. Working together, rapid progress could be made.

In March 1989, Representative Barbara Boxer invited Elizabeth and me to attend a congressional hearing on the changing face of AIDS. Other representatives, including Nancy Pelosi, Henry Waxman, and Ted Weiss, were also present. Numerous individuals from the pediatric and adult AIDS research communities testified at the hearing, including Tom Coates from UCSF, whose specialty was behavioral sciences; Don Francis from the CDC, who had been vocal at a meeting of activists at the CDC, demanding that something be done about the safety of blood products; Margaret Haggerty, director of pediatrics at Harlem Hospital, where she represented some of the most marginalized women and children in the epidemic; Jean Maguire, executive director of the AIDS Action Council; and David Werdegar, director of public health in San Francisco. Those who testified made the unified case that the epidemic was increasing in all populations and that more government attention was needed across the board. These expert voices were heard loudly and clearly, and many of the congressional members became strong supporters of AIDS research, maintaining their engagement for many years thereafter.

However, not all meetings were so successful. One meeting stood out as particularly odd. In 1992, Elizabeth and I met with then director of the FDA, Dr. David Kessler. We hoped Kessler would demand that pharmaceutical companies perform safety and efficacy studies of ARVs in infants and children, which thus far they had failed to do. Pharmaceutical companies feared that the studies would take too long or that adverse reactions might occur in children that were not seen in adults, and approval of drugs would therefore be delayed, costing the companies hundreds of millions of dollars. This failure had proved to be a crucial roadblock to FDA drug approval for treating infants and children. I was perplexed that the FDA did not force pharmaceutical companies to study drugs in children. FDA requirements stated that a drug could not be approved to treat a specific disease unless it had been evaluated and tested in the entire population who had the disease, including children. Nevertheless, the FDA had never enforced the rule, so 80 to 90 percent of drugs had never been studied in children (Gendell 1997; Thaul 2012). Instead, dosing for children was determined by comparing the recommended adult dose to the weight of the infant or child. If no liquid formulation was available for children, it was often recommended that a drug be administered with food, syrup, or honey. These methods completely ignored the possibility that drugs were often metabolized or absorbed differently in children and that using this approach could under- or overdose an infant. This was a critical issue, and Elizabeth and I were determined to have Kessler use his bully pulpit position, if not his full authority as head of the FDA, to require pharmaceutical companies to test drugs in children at the same time as adults.

The meeting with Kessler started with the usual pleasantries, and after just a few minutes of conversation, Kessler ushered us over to a more informal conversation area. To our amazement, Kessler took off his shoes, stretched out on a crumpled couch, and began calmly listening to our pleas. After hearing Elizabeth's tale of her own personal losses and her plea for the FDA to push for simultaneous studies of ARVs in adults and children, Kessler replied that although he was sympathetic to the issue as he himself was a pediatrician by training, he was fully engaged with other issues such as tobacco control and breast-cancer treatment. Kessler did not outright refuse to take on our cause, but neither Elizabeth nor I walked out of his office feeling that our concerns would become a priority for him. In an ironic twist, years after Elizabeth's death, Kessler became president of the Pediatric AIDS Foundation.

It was not until 1990 that Elizabeth finally broke her silence and revealed her identity in an appearance before the House Budget Committee, during which she asked for increased funding for pediatric AIDS research. This was a crucial turning point that allowed Elizabeth to become a national spokesperson for pediatric AIDS, expanding on her efforts within the entertainment and political worlds. As far as I could tell, her revelation had no negative repercussions, either for Paul's career or for Jake's school life, but the positive impact was very apparent. Sadly, however, Elizabeth was also beginning to learn in an often unbearably hard way that it was all too easy for individuals to ignore the AIDS epidemic unless and until it affected them on a personal level. Fortunately, successes countered some of the discouragement. As a result of ongoing fundraising events, speaking engagements, and media coverage—including a fourteen-page cover story in *People Magazine*—the public came to know Elizabeth's story and thereby to understand and sympathize with the pain and suffering of HIV-positive mothers and children (Glaser 1993; Ellis 1994).

Elizabeth's audience continued to broaden, and her impassioned pleas were heard by thousands. Few could forget her speech at the Democratic National Convention in New York City on July 14, 1992, when she passionately declared, "I am in a race with the clock. This is not about being a Republican or an Independent or a Democrat. It's about the future—for each and every one of us." She also made clear that she continued to be motivated by her daughter Ariel, despite her own illness. Before all at the convention and millions of TV viewers, she said, "She taught me to love when all I wanted to do was hate. She taught me to help others when all I wanted to do was help myself."

Over the next few years, Elizabeth continued to advocate and battle for pediatric AIDS research, but it was clear that she was slowly being overcome by her own battle against HIV. Elizabeth was under treatment with ZDV, the only treatment available at the time. I frequently accompanied Elizabeth on her travels to and from Washington to explain what was urgently needed for the pediatric AIDS epidemic. On some of those trips, Elizabeth felt unwell due to the side effects of ZDV, which made her nauseous. Often when we were driving between meetings, Elizabeth's nausea would become so overwhelming that I would have to pull over to the side of the road until she felt better. If we were anywhere near one of the hundreds of Dunkin' Donuts lining the highways of the East Coast, I would run inside to get one of Elizabeth's favorite donuts, which for some odd reason would always settle her stomach. As a physician, I was also able to help administer Elizabeth's injectable medications. Over the years, I became increasingly impressed with Elizabeth's stamina and motivation and what one person could accomplish in spite of illness.

Unfortunately, Elizabeth's doctors realized she was developing resistance to her HIV medication. As Elizabeth's health deteriorated, I began visiting her every month in her Santa Monica home. With each visit, it seemed like Elizabeth had suffered a new loss in her physical and mental functions. Despite Elizabeth's attempts to avoid discussing the subject, those close to her were forced to face the inevitable—Elizabeth would soon die, just like many of the other HIV-infected patients who had developed AIDS. There was simply no effective treatment at the time that could halt the relentless onslaught of the virus.

As Elizabeth's condition worsened, I knew that it was time to raise the subject of her legacy. I felt strongly that one of the most important of Elizabeth's potential legacies should be the development and support of a cadre of young, smart, and aggressive scientists who could focus on research relevant to pediatric AIDS. I had discussed the issue of creating an Elizabeth Glaser Scientist Award, but Elizabeth was embarrassed at the suggestion. However, those who knew and loved her thought it was important that Elizabeth be remembered, not by investing in expensive buildings or programs that with time might be forgotten, but rather in sponsoring a generation of bright young researchers who could carry on Elizabeth's mission with passion and ingenuity.

I continued to visit Elizabeth regularly through the final days of her life. Just one year earlier, I had survived a sudden cardiac arrest; this confrontation with my own mortality gave me strength as I watched Elizabeth come to terms with her own impending death. One evening in November 1994, I sat alone with Elizabeth in her living room. On the table before us sat a bottle of saquinavir, the newest and most powerful ARV, a PI that was known to be more potent than ZDV and able to control the onslaught of HIV by preventing the complications of immunodeficiency, thus potentially preventing death. I watched Elizabeth's hands tremble as she nervously took the first tablet with an almost religious aura. I felt as if I could read the thoughts racing through her mind: "Could this be the miracle drug that will control this infection and allow me to survive and continue to advocate for HIV-infected children?" However, in a tragic repeat of young Ariel's death, the new medication came too late, and Elizabeth's condition continued to worsen.

THE LOSS OF AN ESSENTIAL ADVOCATE

The last week of November 1994, I received a phone call from Susan Zeegen, one of the cofounders of the Pediatric AIDS Foundation. She asked if I could go to Boston to accept the Harvard AIDS Institute Leadership Award on Elizabeth's behalf. Elizabeth was too ill to accept, and neither of the cofounders of the Pediatric AIDS Foundation could go in her place. I agreed and arrived in Boston on a cold winter day. The leadership award ceremony was held on December 1—World AIDS Day—at the Harvard Faculty Club. Max Essex, chairman of the Harvard AIDS Institute and a well-known AIDS researcher, provided the welcoming comments, and Harvey Feinberg, dean of the Harvard School of Public Health, provided the closing remarks. I was somewhat intimidated, not only by the responsibility of speaking on Elizabeth's behalf, but also by the Harvard Faculty Club's appearance, an old Boston academic atmosphere likely going back two hundred years, with white-gloved, tuxedoed waiters at the dinner tables and paintings of famous faculty members scattered over the walls. It was a far distance both in miles and character from the cafeteria-like faculty club in San Francisco where in 1981 I and four other UCSF faculty members had first met to address the emerging AIDS epidemic, and even further from the kitchen in Santa Monica where Elizabeth and her friends had established the Pediatric AIDS Foundation.

I started my acceptance speech on behalf of Elizabeth by stating, "Elizabeth could not be here to speak tonight. That responsibility has been given to me. It is something that I agreed to do knowing that I cannot fully speak for her, because I have not experienced the pain of AIDS in the personal manner that she has." I spoke of Elizabeth's many accomplishments and the impact that the foundation had achieved through her, and I closed with words from the musical *Les Misérables*: "Will you join in our crusade? Who will be strong and stand with me? Somewhere beyond the barricade, is there a world you long to see? Do you hear the people sing? Say, do you hear the distant drums? It is the future that they bring when tomorrow comes" (Ammann 1995).

I would see Elizabeth alive for the last time just a few days later when I quietly sat alone with her in her large bedroom, the fireplace flickering. Elizabeth could no longer speak, so I simply held her hand and thanked her on behalf of all the children who now had hope that they might live long and healthy lives. Elizabeth died on December 3, 1994.[2] Her memorial service was held at Pepperdine University on a bluff overlooking the Pacific Ocean. I had written a speech, but it was difficult to truly prepare for the emotional service. Elizabeth was a person who had spoken of hope throughout her entire lifetime, yet her own life came to a close without her hope being fulfilled—only the knowledge of certain death. Paul, the Pediatric AIDS Foundation cofounders, myself, and many others who knew Elizabeth gave speeches, each presenting his or her own unique view, together painting a cohesive portrait of a human being with both strengths and flaws. Jake, her HIV-infected son, played the piano and sang Elizabeth's favorite song. At the end of the service, each person released a balloon into the air. As I watched the balloons rise and slowly float away, I thought about how tightly we hold on to so many things in life to reassure ourselves of security, but some things we must release. In the face of the AIDS epidemic, I felt that it was essential to hold on to the memories of individuals like Elizabeth Glaser in tandem with the thousands of mothers who suffered from AIDS and the individual children with AIDS whose faces I could still see. Too quickly, the HIV/AIDS epidemic became one of anonymous numbers and devoid of faces, contributing to the desensitization of individual suffering and, eventually, unjustifiable delays that failed to control the HIV epidemic among children. Elizabeth died because potent antiviral drugs were not available. Millions of HIV-infected women and children in low-income countries would die because bureaucracies and self-interested research would withhold treatment with known effective ARVs (Ammann 2016).

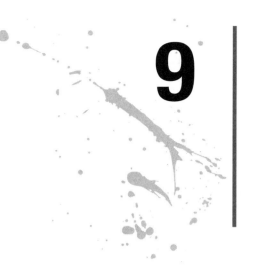

A Priority at Last

Pediatric HIV/AIDS

9

THINKING DIFFERENTLY

The HIV/AIDS epidemic revolutionized how international public health crises were approached, including prioritizing areas of research and then finding the funds to conduct that research. Previously, many foundations had been formed in response to a public health crisis or to find answers to the prevention and treatment of specific diseases. None of those diseases, however, had carried the same degree of urgency as the AIDS epidemic, which was threatening worldwide stability and taking the lives of millions with no signs of slowing. When the Pediatric AIDS Foundation, renamed the Elizabeth Glaser Pediatric AIDS Foundation (EGPAF) after Elizabeth's death, was founded in 1988, it hoped to set research priorities and fund outstanding scientists who were using entirely new approaches, unencumbered with an ever-increasing bureaucracy that was beginning to dominate academic research and, in some eyes, was leading to research for the sake of research, quickly losing sight of the urgency of stopping the epidemic.

From my very first meeting with Dr. Michael Gottlieb and Elizabeth Glaser, I realized that there lay before us an opportunity to utilize the best of scientific and research principles while discarding the many obstacles that had haunted research projects during the past decades and had often slowed discoveries rather than accelerating them. From the beginning, we knew that things had to be done quickly and innovatively. Elizabeth and I had spoken about somehow supporting a series of think tanks that could approach pediatric AIDS from three critical research perspectives—what is known, what needs to be known, and how can it be done—and get answers to those questions, not only from people engaged in the field of AIDS, but also from scientists with expertise in other areas of research (Ammann 1994). On another front, I was very much aware of the difficulties faced by young investigators who go into academic research careers, uncertain of funding and lacking well-defined and secure career pathways. A new pool of young scientists was needed to take on areas of pediatric AIDS research, not only as a challenge, but also as a means of providing solutions to one of the world's greatest infectious disease epidemics. With more than twenty years of clinical research experience myself, I realized how important it was to recruit young researchers who had innovative ideas and provide them with the necessary funds and independence to pursue the most pressing scientific issues surrounding HIV. During my academic career and years at Genentech, a rapidly expanding biotechnology company, I had met an extraordinary number of brilliant basic scientists and clinical researchers who had made major advances in the study of viruses, immunology, cancer research, therapeutics, and other areas, many of which were related to the research priorities for pediatric AIDS. Few of them had a background in pediatrics, yet we needed to call on these individuals to help provide answers to pediatric AIDS.

This willingness to take chances and to invest in young scientists was an incredible strength of the Pediatric AIDS Foundation. Accordingly, through the foundation and the SAC, I was able to establish scholar awards that provided two years of salary support for promising young scientists, short-term scientific awards for individuals to address "hot topics" without having to make major changes in their career, and importantly, student intern awards to allow the up-and-coming cadre of medical students, interns, and residents to see what they could accomplish in pediatric AIDS research.

THINK TANKS: A TIME TO THINK, A TIME TO ACT

My academic career officially began when I started my fellowship in pediatric immunology at the University of Minnesota in Minneapolis in 1968 under the tutelage of internationally recognized immunologist Dr. Robert Good. It was at this time that I was introduced to the standard academic tradition of presenting research at national conferences. University professors spend a lot of time preparing their research results and data for presentation to large groups of experts who are, for the most part, similarly trained and in the same specialty. I soon found myself dismayed by the routine and seemingly unnecessary practices that had become enshrined into the presentations, which perhaps even diminished the potential for learning and the exchange of ideas.

Scientific presentations at national and international meetings are meant to convey the results of research to a broad audience. Traditionally, presentations are confined to ten minutes, with five minutes allocated at the end for discussion and questions. Almost all presentations use projected slides to summarize the data. As soon as the first slide is projected, all eyes in the audience focus on the overhead screen, rather than on the speaker, who typically is also staring up at the screen while quickly scrolling through the slides. As the lights dim, the dark room and the lack of eye contact create a soporific effect, causing many in the audience who might have traveled long distances to an international meeting to stop paying attention or doze off completely. Even for those who do pay attention, there is not enough time allotted to present everything on a single slide, let alone an entire presentation's worth, so speakers typically resort to presenting at a rate of one or more slides per minute while speaking too quickly to be understood or echoing repetitively, "skip that slide, skip that slide, skip that slide," etc. As most speakers go past their time limit in a valiant attempt to present a year's worth of research in ten minutes, there often is no time remaining for questions.

In most instances, the audiences listening to the presentations are made up exclusively of experts in the same scientific specialty, resulting in a distinct phenomenon of "group thinking," with very little exploration of new ideas "outside the box." On the rare occasion when there is time for questions, they seem to focus on the immediate topic at hand, with no interchange of perspectives from other specialties. In the case of the pediatric AIDS epidemic, it was clear that such group thinking would not be effective. In order to understand the evolution of HIV infection in a population of infants and children—who were infected in a unique manner and in whom the disease progressed much more rapidly than had been observed in adults—it would be critical to generate new ideas, new ways of thinking about the epidemic, and new ideas for research. And a new way of gathering scientific experts together and discussing the magnitude of the HIV/AIDS epidemic was essential.

THE THINK TANKS BEGIN

As one of my conditions when I began working with the Pediatric AIDS Foundation in 1988, I insisted that it was critical for the scientific and medical community to rethink the way that information was shared and discussed. I asked permission to start a series of "Think Tanks," which would deviate significantly from the traditional methods of presenting scientific evidence, developing research objectives, and establishing research priorities.[1] With support and funding from the Pediatric AIDS Foundation and working with Phil Pizzo, I organized the first Pediatric AIDS Think Tank at the NCI in Bethesda, Maryland, in December 1988. This first Think Tank, which was focused on discussing and identifying the most critical research priorities for the pediatric AIDS epidemic, would lay the groundwork for the Think Tanks that followed (EGPAF 2016a). During the next eight years, with the assistance of Natasha Martin, I organized thirty-two Think Tanks, sometimes as many as four per year. More than 350 scientists from around the world would ultimately participate, including both basic and clinical researchers as well as Nobel Prize winners such as David Baltimore and Howard Temin. Experts included geneticists, immunologists, molecular biologists, statisticians, epidemiologists, obstetricians, pediatricians, pharmacologists, and representatives from the fields of internal medicine, infectious disease, oncology, academia, the pharmaceutical industry, the CDC, and the NIH.[2] Organizing the Think Tanks, communicating with the scientists, and arranging the logistics of the meetings was at times a daunting task that was carried out by an able staff without whom the number, quality, and impact of the Think Tanks would not have occurred.[3]

The philosophy behind the Think Tanks was best summed up in the statement included in the invitation sent to each Think Tank participant:

> Science has expanded into hundreds of disciplines with a complex array
> of highly diversified fields of study. Although this has enormous benefits in
> expanding knowledge, a disadvantage is the lack of "cross fertilization" of ideas.
> Often, scientists gather only with individuals from their own subspecialties
> where they speak a highly technical language. Critical scientific advances may
> be missed simply because the right individual from a different field is absent
> from the discussion. New discoveries often require new ideas. To have these
> new ideas, scientists must put behind them rigid ideas of thinking and problem
> solving. A Think Tank brings together scientists from diverse disciplines, seques-
> ters them in an environment conducive to exchange of ideas rather than data,
> presents problems rather than formulas, and looks for innovative solutions.
> The Think Tank fundamentally consists of three questions: 1) What do we

know 2) What do we need to know 3) How can we do it? The "What do we know" component brings the knowledge base to a common ground that can be understood by all participants. The next step, "What do we need to know," is the result of intense discussion and multidisciplinary exchange of facts, data, and ideas. It is the result of a thorough dissection of all aspects of the problem under consideration. The final step, "How can we do it," is the solution-oriented component. It calls upon the diverse experience in problem solving of each individual as they apply their expertise to the issue under consideration. Thus, an HIV vaccine Think Tank takes the previous experience of immunologists, microbiologists, biochemists, and molecular virologists, and extracts from them what is known about successful vaccine development. They consider what information is missing and who are the parties that should band together to develop a successful vaccine. Finally they identify who and how research can go forward until a successful vaccine is found.

In accordance with this statement, I established a set of three basic rules that would govern all of the Think Tanks. First, the subject for discussion would always be divided into the aforementioned three major topics. The final topic—How can we do it?—was particularly important, as this was where the attendees would set action items for follow-up, ensuring that a Think Tank wouldn't simply conclude with plans for additional meetings but with concrete plans to actively find answers to the questions that had been raised. Second, the use of slides or overheads was strictly prohibited. Unsurprisingly, this caused great apprehension among presenters who had rarely given a scientific presentation without the use of slides. I was steadfast in this rule—even when presenters begged to use just one or two slides, the answer was always a firm "No." Third, it was required that individuals invited to a Think Tank represent a different biomedical discipline or area of expertise. "Group thinking" was a great pitfall to be avoided, and by bringing in not only the brightest minds on the cutting edge of AIDS research but also creative minds from other disciplines and specialties, ideas were encouraged from participants whose experience might bring a completely new perspective to some of the most difficult questions raised. This requirement also tended to cause apprehension, as individuals who were asked to speak on a topic often nervously told me that they were not experts in the field of AIDS. My answer was always the same: "We're asking you to participate because of your expertise, your ability to perform good science, and your ability to think outside of the box." Thus, each Think Tank would consist of highly select scientists, researchers, and physicians from the best organizations, such as the NIH, the CDC, the pharmaceutical-biotech industry, university centers, and research institutions and other foundations, that would all gather for two to three days to pool their expertise and focus on specific research priorities.

The Think Tanks were held at a number of locations across the United States and Europe that offered facilities conducive to interactions among small groups with few outside diversions: the Endicott House in Massachusetts; the Pocantico Conference Center on the Rockefeller Estate in New York; the Kroc Estate outside of Santa Barbara, California; the Pembrook House in Oxford, England; and locations in Spoleto and Siena, Italy. My favorite location was always Ted Field's family ranch along the coast of

Santa Barbara. While at first glance it may have seemed an unlikely location for scientific discussion, the natural atmosphere disarmed the formality that often surrounds academic meetings and promoted informal discussion and the exchange of ideas.

The Think Tanks covered a variety of diverse and important topics. Early in the epidemic, the most important questions focused on how to prevent transmission of HIV from mothers to their infants. Other topics included how and when to treat children for HIV, which animal models could be used for HIV research, gene therapy and the possibility of establishing a stem cell repository, acceleration of pediatric drug evaluation and approval, and identifying the factors associated with the increasing numbers of HIV-infected children who were surviving into their teenage years.

Each Think Tank, which would go on for two-and-a-half days, was limited to a maximum of thirty to forty participants in order to optimize conversation and interchange between individuals, not just during the formal discussions but also during the meals and into the late evening. Each individual's responsibility was to provide new ideas and direction. At the Field's ranch, meetings were held in a theater-like room with large, comfortable swivel chairs so that attendees could easily turn to face whoever was speaking. The room remained brightly lit. Within each major category of discussion, subtopics were presented by various individuals, with a rapporteur and two discussion leaders in charge of keeping the discussion on track, directing questions to the presenters, and summarizing the presentations. Between meetings, attendees continued their discussion and work priorities, whether over the catered meals or late into the night. The final morning of the Think Tank would prove to be critical, as this was when all that had been discussed was summarized to answer the final question—How can we do it?

A few weeks after the conclusion of each Think Tank, the rapporteurs, Natasha, and I would put together a summary that was sent to all Think Tank participants, the founders of the Pediatric AIDS Foundation, and its Health Advisory Committee for review. I would then summarize the research priorities that had been identified in a request for application (RFA), which was sent to a broad base of highly regarded research investigators—national and international, young and old—who could respond with research proposals. Importantly, knowing who some of the best HIV researchers were, I made certain that the RFA reached them as well. Following a screening process, the scientists who had submitted potentially successful proposals were asked to submit a full grant application that was then reviewed to determine whether it should be eligible for funding. This process was conducted surprisingly efficiently, as it typically took fewer than three months from the Think Tank to funding the research projects.

The Think Tanks ultimately proved to be a crucial forum for experts from around the world to discuss the most urgent issues in the pediatric AIDS epidemic. No matter what discipline they came from, all Think Tank attendees recognized that they had the ability to contribute to the advancement of pediatric AIDS research. It was clear that without their participation, pediatric AIDS research would not advance quickly enough to meet the escalating crisis of the epidemic and would continue to lag far behind HIV research in adults. The Think Tanks, along with Elizabeth Glaser's tireless effort to raise funds for targeted research projects, were crucial in initiating research into pediatric AIDS and would ultimately result in an understanding of how the effects of HIV in children differed from that of adults and in the acceleration of solutions to both prevent perinatal HIV transmission and treat HIV in infants. The Think Tanks also provided a credible platform from which to advocate for early HIV treatment in pregnant women and infants.

The Think Tank method was a pioneering process for identifying research priorities and long-term research goals. It changed the traditionally passive approach of distributing RFAs with generalized goals for research to an unknown audience of scientists to a more active one of distributing RFAs to scientists with known expertise and competence in specific areas of research that could be adapted to answer some of the most critical questions in the pediatric AIDS epidemic. Importantly, it also reduced the time for identifying research priorities for funding from more than a year to a matter of months.

GROUNDBREAKING THINK TANKS

Two especially important Think Tanks were The Role of Immunity in Maternal/Infant HIV Transmission, held in March 1990, and Interaction of HIV, the Fetal Immune System, and the Placenta, held in September 1991. Both were conducted at Ted Field's ranch. One of the very highest priorities in bringing the pediatric AIDS epidemic to a halt was to prevent the transmission of HIV from infected mothers to their infants. The scientific community remained perplexed as to why only 30 percent of infants born to HIV-infected mothers contracted the virus during pregnancy and childbirth ("Report of a Consensus Workshop" 1992; Lambert et al. 1997). It was believed that an understanding of how 70 percent of infants escaped infection might prompt solutions to prevent all infants from becoming infected. Thus, the initial focus of the two Think Tanks was on the interaction of HIV, the placenta, and the fetal immune system.

By 1990, the relative risk of transmitting HIV by different routes of exposure was well documented. Transmission of HIV from contaminated blood transfusions carried the highest risk, followed by anal sex between two homosexual partners (with the receptive partner being at greater risk). Breastfeeding also held a high risk of transmitting HIV, yet only 30 to 40 percent of infants who breastfed from an HIV-positive mother—even for extensive periods of time—contracted the virus. In the case of heterosexual intercourse, the female partner carried a greater risk of acquiring HIV from an infected partner than did the male. In all these scenarios, what was puzzling was the fact that HIV transmission did not occur in every instance. The 1990/1991 Think Tanks attempted to shed some light on this discrepancy by focusing on mother-to-infant HIV transmission.

While there were many experts present at the Think Tanks, the key individual turned out to be Ruth Ruprecht from the Dana Farber Cancer Institute in Massachusetts. Ruprecht had been studying a transgenic mouse model of retroviral transmission, which had suggested that it was possible to block mother-to-child transmission of a retrovirus using ZDV, the newly approved ARV for the treatment of HIV infection (Ruprecht et al. 1990; Sharpe et al. 1988; Sharpe, Jaenisch, and Ruprecht 1987). The results of Ruprecht's study would shift the entire direction of the 1991 Think Tank.

WHAT TREATMENT WAS AVAILABLE, AND WAS IT SAFE?

In 1991 there were only a few viable treatments that could be safely evaluated for their potential to prevent mother-to-child transmission of HIV. Each was discussed in depth, along with a distinct rationale for further evaluation. First, Merlin Robb, a pediatrician at the Walter Reed Army Institute in Rockville, Maryland, discussed the possibility of developing an HIV vaccine that would either enhance the immunity of an HIV-infected pregnant woman or protect her infant from contracting the virus (Barouch 2013). The rationale for the development and use of such a vaccine was based on the theoretical possibility that the induction of antibodies from a vaccine might be more potent in preventing HIV than the antibodies that were transmitted to the infant via the mother's placenta. However, a viable HIV-vaccine candidate seemed a remote possibility that would likely take years, if not decades, to develop. The conclusion turned out to be correct; even at the time of this book's writing in 2016, no vaccine for HIV has been discovered that is capable of conclusively preventing HIV infection.

Robb was followed by Jack Lambert from the Infectious Disease Division at the University of Rochester Medical Center. Lambert discussed a second potential solution: hyperimmune HIV immunoglobulin G (HIVIG), a preparation of high antibody concentration derived from the blood of chronically HIV-infected donors (Stiehm et al. 2000). There were clear risks to evaluating a blood product obtained from HIV-infected individuals, even though the HIV was felt to be thoroughly inactivated. But there was evidence from studies of other infectious diseases suggesting that concentrated passive antibody preparations could prevent infection. For example, a hyperimmune varicella (chickenpox) antibody preparation was used to prevent varicella in individuals who had been exposed to the virus and might otherwise be particularly susceptible to uncontrolled infection. It was also known that hepatitis B immunoglobulin (HBIG) could prevent hepatitis B infection in infants born to infected mothers (Stiehm 1991).

Unlike the use of a vaccine-induced antibody, which might take weeks to months to develop, one theoretical advantage of passive antibody was that it would provide exposed individuals with an immediate source of concentrated antibody. Since concentrated antibody preparations were known to prevent viral infections, it was argued that the administration of HIVIG to HIV-infected pregnant women and their infants might prevent HIV transmission. However, questions quickly arose. Why would an HIV antibody preparation prevent infection when it was known that antibodies to HIV, present in HIV-infected women and transferred in high concentrations to their infants, failed to protect 30 percent of infants from HIV infection? Further, why would concentrated antibody preparations obtained from chronically HIV-infected individuals be protective when they failed to control infection in the individual donors? Could administration of antibody actually facilitate HIV infection? And would the concentrated antibody preparations contain antibodies that could also protect against the various HIV subtypes that were known to exist?

Third, Anne-Marie Duliege, a pediatrician from France who had been working with me at Genentech, discussed a highly experimental new product called CD4-IgG. The CD4-IgG molecule had been inspired by Dan Capon, a research scientist at Genentech who had become intrigued with the idea of developing a recombinant DNA molecule that could block the entry of HIV into a cell. At the time, it was believed that HIV could only enter an immune cell through attachment of the viral gp120 of the virus to the host cell's CD4 receptor, facilitating the infection and destruction of the cell. CD4-IgG was an engineered recombinant molecule with a CD4 receptor attached to a portion of immunoglobulin G molecule, giving it a long lifespan in the bloodstream. In vitro, it was proven that this molecule could prevent HIV from infecting immune cells. However, CD4-IgG had not yet been administered to pregnant women or infants, and thus carried unknown risks. Moreover, in later years scientists would learn that HIV had several other means of infecting immune cells other than the CD4 receptor (Chamow et al. 1992).

Finally, Yvonne Bryson, a pediatric infectious disease specialist from the University of California in Los Angeles, discussed ZDV. In 1987, ZDV had been proven to decrease morbidity and mortality in adult HIV patients by interfering with a critical enzyme known as reverse transcriptase, but by 1991, it had still not been tested on pregnant women, infants, or children (Fischl, Richman, Grieco, et al. 1987). However, Ruprecht's mouse model provided evidence suggesting that the ARV might be effective in preventing HIV transmission in humans. Moreover, compared to the other therapeutic models that had been discussed, ZDV was the most readily available. Based on Bryson's discussion and Ruprecht's animal-model evidence, a consensus was reached that ZDV was the therapeutic approach with the greatest potential for preventing perinatal HIV transmission. The focus of the Think Tank quickly shifted from understanding why only 30 percent of infants born to HIV-positive mothers became infected to whether it would be possible to use ZDV to prevent the transmission of HIV to all infants. The caveat, since it would need to be administered to HIV-infected pregnant women, of course, lay in whether ZDV would prove safe for the pregnant mother and the developing fetus.

OBSTACLES AHEAD

The obstacles to moving forward with studying ZDV in pregnant women and infants were significant and challenging. First, ZDV was known to cause toxicity in animals and was associated with the appearance of malignancies when administered in very high doses to mice (Lee et al. 1991). One action item from the Think Tank was a request for further studies on the potential toxicity, teratogenicity, and carcinogenicity of ZDV in animal models before proceeding with human studies. Second, the correct dose of ZDV for an infant could not simply be extrapolated mathematically from the adult dose, but would require pharmacokinetic studies in infants. Nevertheless, despite these obstacles, the Think Tank ended with great optimism that among the multiple possibilities for preventing mother-to-child HIV, there was one option immediately available that had already shown efficacy in controlling HIV disease progression in adults and could potentially end the pediatric AIDS epidemic. A year of planning followed the Think Tank and culminated in the NIH sponsoring a clinical trial of ZDV in pregnant women and infants which, in 1994, proved that ZDV could prevent 60 percent of HIV infections in infants exposed to HIV during pregnancy and delivery (Connor et al. 1994). The design, implementation, and clinical research study result was a milestone in the HIV/AIDS epidemic. For the first time, it was shown that an ARV could prevent HIV transmission. The study paved the way for future studies of ARVs for post-exposure prophylaxis (PEP) in health-care workers accidentally exposed to HIV, prevention of transmission between HIV discordant sexual couples, and treatment as prevention—studies that revolutionized the thinking on using treatment worldwide to prevent the spread of the HIV/AIDS epidemic (J. Cohen 2011; El-Sadr et al. 2006; Lundgren et al. 2015).

A THINK TANK ON STIGMA AND NEGLECTED PSYCHOSOCIAL ASPECTS OF CHILDREN WITH HIV/AIDS

As the HIV/AIDS epidemic expanded, new aspects of an HIV diagnosis's impact on a child emerged, not all of which required basic research studies. HIV was not simply a virus that affected the immune system but also one that was associated with severe stigma and social discrimination among both adults and children. In many instances, HIV-infected children, particularly vulnerable members of the population unable to defend themselves against hatred and bias, seemed deliberately targeted for discrimination. Thus in 1993, the first Think Tank focusing on psychosocial priorities for "long term survivors"—children born with HIV who survived into their teenage years without ARV treatment—was held at the Loews Summit Hotel in New York City (Chen et al. 1997; Martin et al. 1996; Nielsen et al. 1997).

The phenomenon of "long-term survivors" had been identified in the early 1990s, but what had not yet been addressed was how to deal with the psychosocial effects of an HIV diagnosis that was specific to those children. The disruption in a child's life that resulted from an HIV diagnosis could not be underestimated. The physical problems that stemmed from being born with HIV, including neurological abnormalities and significant growth failure, consigned an infant to a future dominated by frequent clinic visits and extended hospital stays. Most children with HIV contracted the virus from their mothers, meaning that their primary caregivers, at best, were ill and undergoing treatment themselves or, at worst, had succumbed to AIDS. The goal of the 1993 Think Tank, which was attended by a highly selective group of psychologists, sociologists, nurses, and social workers, was to identify what was currently known or being studied regarding psychosocial issues facing long-term survivors, what resources were needed to further study those issues, how to determine the top priorities for future studies, and how to deal with the unique issues of stigma. These issues had been neglected for years on the pessimistic basis that, without ART, HIV-infected infants would not survive to their teenage years.

The participants recognized that there was a high degree of stigma and secrecy surrounding an HIV diagnosis, and if it were disclosed, HIV-positive children were often treated as pariahs. Unlike the poster children for other diseases, who generated plentiful community support and funding, HIV-infected children often suffered in isolation and silence. By the 1990s, much of the discrimination and ostracism that had once been directed toward the gay community and HIV-infected adults had subsided, thanks to the establishment of anti-discrimination laws and the support of prominent HIV-infected celebrities such as Rock Hudson, Arthur Ashe, and Magic Johnson. Tragically, this discrimination soon turned toward HIV-infected children, who had neither an ability to defend themselves nor well-known advocates to represent them in the media.

One of the most publicized cases of such discrimination was that of Ryan White. In 1984, twelve-year-old Ryan had been diagnosed with HIV, having contracted the virus during treatment for hemophilia. Immediately following his diagnosis, Ryan was expelled from his Indiana middle school. Ryan's doctors, with the support of Indiana State Commissioner Woodrow Myers, tried to explain to the school board that Ryan posed no threat to other students, but they were plunged into a lengthy legal battle as parents and teachers alike rallied against his re-admittance. At the time, people were so fearful and uninformed about HIV that a number of families on Ryan's paperboy route cancelled their subscriptions, fearing that HIV could be transmitted through shared contact with a newspaper (HRSA 2015; "HIV: Science and Stigma" 2014).

In 1986, the *NEJM* published a study on more than one hundred individuals who had been living in close contact with HIV-infected individuals (Friedland et al. 1986). The study concluded that there was zero risk of transmission through sharing of food, sleeping in the same bed, sharing toothbrushes, razors, clothing, and combs, or through hugging and kissing. In response to the medical evidence, the school board reluctantly gave Ryan permission to go back to school but required him to eat with disposable utensils, use a separate bathroom, and refrain from participating in physical education classes (Bogart et al. 2008). Even with all the restrictions in place, more than half of the four hundred students stayed home on the first day of Ryan's return. Sadly, that return was short-lived, as the White family soon decided to relocate after a bullet was fired through their living room window.

Ryan's story gained prominent media coverage, and Ryan soon became a different kind of poster boy and spokesperson, educating the public on the truth about HIV so as to end the stigma and discrimination against HIV-infected individuals. A number of celebrities took a stand alongside Ryan, including Elton John, Michael Jackson, Greg Louganis, President Ronald Reagan and Nancy Reagan, and Surgeon General C. Everett Koop. When Ryan died on April 8, 1990, just one month before his high school graduation, more than fifteen hundred people attended his standing-room-only funeral in Indianapolis. On August 18 of that year, Congress enacted the Ryan White Care Act, which would ultimately become the most significant provider of health services for HIV-infected men, women, and children in the United States (HRSA 2015).

Ryan White was not the only child to face such severe discrimination. In 1987, one week after HIV-positive brothers Ricky, Robert, and Randy Ray won a legal battle to attend public school in Arcadia, Florida, their house was burned to the ground. It soon became clear that there was an increasing number of HIV-infected children surviving into their teenage years and encountering psychosocial issues that the medical community had never before faced ("HIV: Science and Stigma" 2014).

For the Psychosocial Think Tank, the stories of discrimination and stigma clearly fell into the category of "What Do We Need to Know?" To many, however, the issues seemed almost overwhelming. One problem was that when children were diagnosed with HIV, dozens of people in their communities were directly or indirectly involved in addressing the psychosocial effects of the diagnosis, so it was difficult to develop one cohesive solution to provide all the necessary support. Within a child's school, for example, what programs needed to be developed to educate school administrators, teachers, and students? Within the community, what roles would various individuals play to ensure that appropriate health-care services were provided? Moreover, while there was considerable knowledge on the psychosocial care of children with HIV at larger medical centers that had more experience with HIV patients, an HIV-positive child residing in a less populous area might be the only child in a school, a hospital, or even an entire community who was affected, limiting the resources available.

Despite the difficulty of questions to be addressed, a number of important conclusions came out of the workshop. First, it was determined that the number of children in the United States who had been orphaned as a result of HIV desperately needed to be documented. This statistic was not readily available, meaning that many public health groups and legislators failed to realize the epidemic's full impact on children. While 70 percent of infants born to HIV-infected mothers escaped infection, many of them still faced a high rate of orphanhood if their HIV-infected parents died from AIDS. And in many cases, even if the child had escaped HIV infection, the community would presume that the child was infected. In the mid-1990s it was estimated that there were more than one hundred thousand children in the United States who had been orphaned by HIV. Worldwide, the numbers were even greater, and by 2012 the WHO estimated that there were more than fifteen million orphans as a consequence of AIDS, with fifteen hundred newly orphaned children every day, each requiring unique psychosocial, financial, and educational support (USAID 2015). This parallel epidemic of orphaned children seemed lost in the focus on the larger AIDS epidemic, and even with all the progress in HIV prevention and treatment accomplished by 2016, the orphan epidemic remains comparatively ignored.

Second, it was determined that there were numerous fundamental but unresolved issues surrounding how to tell children about their HIV diagnosis. When a child was diagnosed with HIV, who should be informed? Only the parents or other community members as well? What about school administrators, nurses, and teachers? Perhaps a more important question was when should the child be informed of the HIV infection? Most Think Tank attendees felt it was essential to disclose an HIV diagnosis to a child to help explain why it was important to take medications and visit clinics frequently. However, at what age should children be told? And how could their illness best be explained? In-depth psychosocial studies were necessary to answer these questions. Historically, very little research had been done on psychosocial issues facing children with other diseases such as leukemia or muscular dystrophy, so to a certain extent, the HIV researchers at the Think Tank pioneered the need for such studies not only in HIV but also in other chronic illnesses affecting children (Jansen and Ammann 1994).

By the end of the Think Tank, four major clinical research categories were defined as top priorities: resilience and coping; coping with an HIV diagnosis in a school environment; family considerations; and methodologies for performing studies in children. The conclusions of the workshop were published in a document that ended with the statement: "Although the hope is that HIV infection in infants can be prevented in the future by means of prenatal screening and treatment of HIV-infected pregnant women, it is likely that we will continue to see HIV-infected children, many of whom will be long-term survivors. For these new children as well as those who already are long-term survivors, we must address their unique psychological and social needs" (Jansen and Ammann 1994).

SETTING ACHIEVABLE GOALS

In 1994, the results of the NIH-sponsored ACTG 076 ZDV clinical study demonstrated that ZDV could reduce the transmission of HIV from mothers to children by 60 percent. As additional ARVs were introduced and combination antiretroviral therapy (cART) was implemented, the rate of children infected with HIV in the United States plummeted from two thousand new infections each year to fewer than one hundred over the course of the next decade. (Sperling et al. 1996; Garcia et al. 1999; Stoto, Almario, and McCormick 1999; Rogers, Taylor, and Nesheim 2010; Frederick et al. 2012). However, the same impact was not seen in low-income countries, where it was estimated that as many as sixteen hundred infants were being infected with HIV each day.

I felt strongly that it was essential to maintain the momentum of successful research results that came from the ACTG 076 trial. It was time for another crucial Think Tank. An advantage of the Think Tanks was that we used a streamlined approach to assembling expert scientists from different fields of research. We had no restrictions on who could be invited, which allowed us to quickly assemble and conduct Think Tanks and rapidly fund the research priorities that were identified. Spurred on by the enthusiasm to improve on the results of the ACTG 076 ZDV study, a Think Tank was held on September 8, 1995, to discuss initiating early therapy, including the use of combination ARVs for HIV-infected mothers and their infants. In attendance were representatives of the NIH, pediatric infectious-disease specialists, pharmacologists, pharmaceutical-company representatives who were involved in developing some of the newest and most potent antiviral drugs, and thought leaders such as David Ho, from the Aaron Diamond AIDS Research Center, and Catherine Wilfert, an infectious-disease pediatrician from Duke University Medical Center. The Think Tank was held at the Endicott House in Deedham, Massachusetts, in an atmosphere significantly removed from stuffy academic halls, industry-dominated conference rooms, or cramped government meeting rooms, lending itself to focused discussion on the critical matters at hand. The informal atmosphere did not, however, dampen the Think Tank participants' enthusiasm and eagerness to more aggressively move ahead with HIV prevention strategies. The vision before everyone's eyes was a quick end to the pediatric AIDS epidemic.

The 1995 Think Tank was one of the shorter ones, lasting just one-and-a-half days. Nonetheless, it stood out because it conveyed a new sense of urgency. The first session addressed important questions surrounding the scientific rationale for performing studies on HIV-infected mothers and children and what pediatric trials might look like if treatment were to be started earlier. While these discussions seemed obvious in hindsight, at the time there were still many individuals who believed that ARVs were too toxic to be used in pregnant women, that early ART might cause patients to develop resistance to the drugs, or even that treatment should be delayed until HIV infection had advanced to AIDS. I found these excuses to be absurd—they had never before been invoked for the prevention and treatment of any other infectious disease. Once an effective treatment became available, physicians were obligated to use the drugs to halt infection. If side effects of the drug were present, the drug continued to be used until safer drugs became available. The key was that the patient survived the infection. It would be considered unethical and medical malpractice to deliberately withhold known effective treatment for any disease until the disease had advanced to an untreatable point.

It seemed that calls for delaying treatment were coming from organizations that were not themselves responsible for the care and welfare of HIV-infected individuals, especially WHO, which promoted "standard of care" guidelines that recommended delaying treatment until HIV had advanced to AIDS, to the point where the disease was no longer reversible. These policies played into the hands of some countries' ministries of health, who failed to make individuals' health a priority. The guidelines were also adopted by NIH-supported pediatric clinical researchers who, with the increasing avail-ability of funding and a shortage of research subjects in the United States, used them to justify conducting unethical research and evaluation of inferior treatment approaches in poor countries. Ultimately, the fallacious reasoning would cost millions of lives as a con-sequence of unnecessarily withholding effective treatment over the almost two decades before these theoretical obstacles were removed (Ammann 2003, 2005, 2009, 2016).

The rapporteur for the 1995 Think Tank's first session was David Ho, who became the primary leader in promoting early and aggressive treatment of HIV, proving that treatment could halt disease progression as well as HIV transmission. His mantra was "Hit hard. Hit early" (Ho 1995). Katherine Luzuriaga, a pediatric immunologist from the University of Massachusetts, co-led the session, and she too acknowledged that more aggressive early treatment was necessary to make progress in preventing HIV—taking into account safety and toxicity issues, of course, but nevertheless moving forward more quickly.

The rapporteur for the second session was Kathy Wilfert from Duke University, who two years previously had been the primary individual campaigning for a clinical trial of ZDV in pregnant women to prevent perinatal HIV transmission. Wilfert argued passionately that a more aggressive approach to HIV prevention was required for the pediatric epidemic to be controlled, and she put forward study designs that could move early treatment from a theoretical approach to a reality. Phil Pizzo supported Wilfert's suggestions. Pizzo treated HIV-infected children as well as children with cancer, and he knew that one of the major advances in controlling childhood cancer had been to ini-tiate early treatment with combinations of drugs that were directed at different targets. Why would treatment of HIV not benefit from similar approaches? It was not difficult to extrapolate from his experience and understand the potential of cART in controlling the larger and more deadly HIV/AIDS epidemic.

On the morning of the Think Tank's second day, there was considerable optimism that the four goals that I had presented as a challenge on the previous day could be achieved and that they could bring an end to the pediatric AIDS epidemic. The goals were to reduce HIV transmission from mothers to infants to less than 2 percent; increase the five-year survival rate of HIV-infected infants by greater than 90 percent; control HIV replication so that HIV viral levels would be undetectable; and develop an eco-nomically viable approach to HIV prevention and treatment for low-income countries. Presenting those goals to the outside world, however, would hinge on having a sound scientific rationale based on clinical research results. I summarized the data from recent studies that supported the contention that early initiation of cART would control both the transmission and progression of HIV. The array of potentially effective new ARVs was increasing. Whereas in the past there had only been a single class of ARVs—RT inhibitors—that when used as monotherapy were only partially effective and resulted in the emergence of viral resistance, the new PIs acted by a different mechanism, were much more powerful, and were showing amazing promise in adult clinical trials. There was no valid scientific reason to believe that they would not be as effective in both the treatment of HIV-infected pregnant women and children and the prevention of peri-natal HIV transmission ("Abbott Protease Inhibitor" 1995; "Protease Inhibitor" 1995).

Encouraging data was also coming from Ho's laboratory at the Aaron Diamond AIDS Research Center. Even though viral replication occurred at about one billion viral particles per day, with half of an individual's viral load being replenished every six hours, it was becoming clear that drugs such as PIs could render the virus progeny ineffective (Ho et al. 1995). Research studies also showed that the majority of pediatric AIDS infections began with a relatively homogenous virus population that persisted for several months, and in this time period, before multiple HIV mutations occurred, treatment was much more likely to be effective.

Think Tank participants repeatedly pointed out that cART would be necessary to control HIV replication and reach the goal of preventing more than 98 percent of HIV infections in infants. ZDV, lamivudine, nevirapine (NVP), stavudine, and new PIs like ritonavir (RTV) were all becoming available, and early study results using a combination of drugs showed that they were far more effective than single drugs (monotherapy) (Del Rio and Hernandez-Tepichin 1996; Moyle and Gazzard 1996). The obstacles lay in making appropriate formulations available for infants and children and determining proper pediatric drug doses. To address these issues, I invited representatives from the major pharmaceutical companies involved in developing ARVs—Merck, Abbott, Boehringer Ingelheim, Bristol-Myers Squibb, Glaxo Wellcome, and Hoffmann-La Roche—to the Think Tank. They needed to hear the unique needs of the pediatric population, and their input and advice was necessary. Most importantly, it was also essential for them to understand the dire necessity of defining safety, dosing, and formulation issues for infants enrolled in pediatric clinical trials (Thaul 2012).

The Think Tank concluded with the realistic considerations that new, controlled clinical trials of therapeutic interventions to reduce perinatal HIV transmission might no longer be possible in the United States. The ACTG 076 ZDV study had been relatively small, consisting of only 477 pregnant women and their infants, as it had been designed to compare treatment with ZDV to a placebo at a time when there had been no known effective treatment to prevent HIV transmission. New studies were needed to evaluate whether cART was indeed superior to monotherapy and to determine whether these drugs could also prevent HIV transmission through breastfeeding, which was essential in low-income countries. It was deemed unethical to conduct further placebo-controlled trials, which meant that larger numbers of HIV-infected mothers and infants would be required than were available in the United States to reach a definitive conclusion. All the Think Tank participants agreed that future studies would likely have to be conducted in low-income countries, where there were thousands of HIV-infected pregnant women and where prevention measures were desperately needed. During the years that followed, the ethical issues of conducting research studies on vulnerable women and children loomed large, as there were no guarantees that the research subjects, or any of the individuals in low-income countries where studies were performed, would ultimately receive any drugs that were shown to be successful. Questions were raised surrounding justice, equity, and whether international codes for performing research in vulnerable populations would be violated (Alfano 2013; Varmus and Satcher 1997; Nuffield Council on Bioethics Working Group 2016).

While the enthusiasm was strong, it was tempered by frustration over increased delays, and my fear of ever lengthening delays in implementing the highly active combination antiretroviral therapy (HAART) to halt the pediatric AIDS epidemic was subsequently realized. The obstacles did not come from expected sources but from within the very pediatric research community that had previously demanded that all HIV-infected women and children have immediate access to ART and had committed itself to rapidly ending HIV infection in infants worldwide. (The obstacles that emerged and the reasons for them will be discussed in detail in Part Three).

There was one glimmer of optimism: the beginnings of large increases in funding and resources directed toward pediatric AIDS research and clinical investigations, which added to the hope that had dominated the Think Tanks—a major change in the trajectory of the pediatric AIDS epidemic could be accomplished by bringing together the brightest and most talented individuals in an environment of innovative thinking and collaboration, supplying them with sufficient funding, and promoting the cause by a committed group of advocates for HIV-infected women and children.

CHECKING ON PROGRESS

Three years and nine Think Tanks had passed since the Early Intervention Think Tank in 1995, and it was time to check on the progress and to analyze what more needed to be done. A Think Tank was scheduled in 1998, once again at the Endicott Center in Deedham, Massachusetts. On this occasion, the topic was the seemingly unachievable goal of HIV eradication. During the previous three years, new and ever more potent ARVs had been approved, and it was well established that a combination of those drugs could control viral replication and reduce the amount of virus in the blood to undetectable levels. The potent drug combination was referred to as Highly Active Antiretroviral Therapy (HAART), and the promising results of HAART studies were stimulating researchers to go beyond bringing HIV to undetectable levels to pursuing the bold vision of eradicating HIV from "hiding places" in the body, as the brain, lymph nodes, and other organs were known to be reservoirs of the latent virus ("New Trials" 1995; Carpenter et al. 1996; Ho 1995, 1996b).

The 1998 Think Tank was sponsored by amfAR, where I had just recently accepted a position as president. The principles of previous Think Tanks remained in place, so it was not surprising that Jon Cohen, a writer for the medical journal *Science*, began his article by saying, "Arthur Ammann, head of the American Foundation for AIDS Research, placed a small placard next to a slide projector sitting in the back of the lecture hall at a small scientific meeting he co-organized two weeks previously. 'Don't even think about it,' the plaque warned the three dozen scientists who attended the weekend gathering in this quaint Massachusetts town." Cohen speculated that the sign was not simply a warning against using slides during the discussion, but perhaps expressed a more philosophical sentiment, reflecting that just three years earlier people didn't believe that the eradication of HIV was a possibility (J. Cohen 1998).

Discussion of the possibilities and obstacles to eradicating HIV was intense. Once again Ho set the stage with the bold question, "Is eradication possible?" Much of the discussion surrounded where exactly the virus could hide. Ho believed that the most likely location, and the one most vulnerable to treatment, was the lymphocytes themselves, which were known to carry the virus. Suzanne Crowe, from Australia's MacFarlane Burnett Center for Research, revealed that she continued to find HIV in macrophages, even in patients who had undetectable levels of virus in their bloodstream. Martin Markowitz, an expert physician working with the Aaron Diamond AIDS Research

Center, speculated that latent HIV-infected cells might be flushed out of the body by stimulating them with a variety of hormonal agents. Abul Abbas, a Harvard immunologist, suggested that cells harboring the virus in other locations might be stimulated to become active and therefore potential targets for treatment by various hormones called "interleukins." When it was suggested that a combination of HAART and stimulation of the immune system by a vaccine might have the potential to eliminate the virus by synergizing drugs and immunity, John Coffin, a retrovirologist from Tufts University, sprang into action. He provoked some of the most heated discussion at the Think Tank, bluntly stating, "You're not going to eradicate the virus with an immune response." Amid the intense debate, we ultimately reached the conclusion that HIV eradication was indeed possible, current research supported the possibility, and it could be achieved through persistent research efforts (see Chapter 29).

10

A Living Legacy

Elizabeth Glaser Scientist Awards

INVESTING IN PEOPLE, NOT BUILDINGS

In 1994, despite her initial hesitation and discomfort, Elizabeth finally agreed to my repeated suggestion that her legacy take the form of an award named after her to assist young and promising researchers studying HIV/AIDS. It had also taken great effort to convince the foundation's board of directors to commit to funding a scientist as well as laboratory support for a full five years, which was the proposed length for each award. When I crunched the figures and presented them to the board, it was clear that the program would be costly. The board initially decided to provide five outstanding scientists with an Elizabeth Glaser Scientist Award. These individuals would receive an award each year for five years, totaling twenty-five awards. To accomplish this, funding was required in advance as a long-term commitment to each investigator. The annual cost of the program was $650,000, with a total of $17 million required for a five-year period. If fully approved, it would be the largest funding requirement that the foundation had made up to that point.

As the board discussed what would be provided with the Elizabeth Glaser Scientist Awards, I drew on what I had experienced in research conducted at academic institutions to convince them to provide sufficient support to make a real impact. Too often talented young investigators received a faculty appointment without funds to continue the successful research for which they had been recruited. In addition, young scientists needed to spend their time on research and not on time-consuming grant writing, especially since many of those grants would never be funded because they did not fit the research priorities of larger funding organizations such as the NIH.

The first advertisements for the Elizabeth Glaser Scientist Award appeared in various medical and scientific journals in May 1995, and the first awards were given later that year ("The Elizabeth Glaser Scientist Award Announcement" 1995). By 1996, the foundation had not only successfully identified major pediatric AIDS research priorities but had also begun obtaining the millions of dollars of research funding specifically for pediatric AIDS. This was the first time since the epidemic began in 1981 that either had been achieved. I was continuously amazed at the foundation's capability to make the right contacts, whether they were in New York with *People Magazine* or with first lady Hillary Clinton or in California with the entertainment industry at large. The most popular of the fundraisers by far was the June 7, 1992, "A Time for Heroes" gala, an annual, almost old-fashioned picnic event, except that rather than a group of friends or a single family, it was an extended family of sorts, all of whom had an interest in conquering the pediatric AIDS epidemic. The picnic was made possible not only because of personal contacts, but also because of foundation volunteers who recruited an astounding number of well-known people to donate their time. Children played games while their parents interacted with high-profile personalities, and at the end of the day each family was able to choose a famous person with whom to have a Polaroid photo taken as a keepsake. The volunteers came from the sports community, the entertainment industry, and politics. They included Billy Crystal, Richard Dreyfuss, Alan Alda, Barbra Streisand, Jimmy Connors, Martin Short, Henry Winkler, Tracy Austin, Dorothy Hamill, Paula Abdul, Elton John, C. Everett Koop, former president Ronald Reagan and first lady Nancy Reagan, John Glenn, and Sandy Koufax, to name a few. Over the years, many more celebrities participated in the picnic and raised millions of dollars for AIDS research that otherwise would not have been available.

To both encourage and evaluate scientists, the Elizabeth Glaser Scientist Award Review Board was established. Senior individuals with successful careers in immunology, virology, infectious diseases, molecular virology and biology, and clinical research staffed the board; their energy and enthusiasm were extraordinary. Board members felt as if they were developing a cadre of scientists who could make a difference in the pediatric AIDS epidemic. Knowing they could only accept five scientists, the board wanted to select those with not only great promise but also the same dedication Elizabeth had shown in her quest for answers to the AIDS epidemic. Indeed, many of the scientists who were chosen quickly contributed to advancing the understanding of pediatric AIDS pathogenesis, which was essential for ending the epidemic. A few of the early Elizabeth Glaser Scientists are highlighted below, and a review of the medical and scientific literature confirms their ongoing contributions.[1]

ELIZABETH GLASER SCIENTISTS: SOME EXAMPLES

Mike (Joseph) McCune, MD, PhD, was a frequent attendee at the Think Tank series and was chosen not only for his scientific knowledge but also for his ability to think outside the box. It is difficult to summarize his many accomplishments, but when he was considered for one of the first Elizabeth Glaser Scientist Awards there was little question that he would honor Elizabeth and all that she represented. I particularly admired Mike because he was provocative, dug deeply into the scientific issues, and came up with innovative solutions. His early work focused on the use of the SCID-hu mouse model, a sort of mouse/human chimera that he used to evaluate human viral pathogenesis and human stem-cell maturation. He used another chimeric mouse model for preclinical antiviral drug evaluation. Mike and his team worked with more than fifty biotech/pharmaceutical companies to identify and prioritize lead antiretroviral compounds. While pursuing his postdoctoral studies with Dr. Irving Weissman at Stanford, Mike realized that HIV could destroy key cells in the thymus, an organ that is vital to the development of the immune system. He catalyzed the hypothesis that HIV disease progression is in part related to defects in TDL production. In testament to his broad thinking skills, Mike established two biotechnology companies

(SyStemix and Progenesys) along with Drs. Weissman, Nobel Prize winner David Baltimore, and Leroy Hood to move better therapies for HIV disease into a clinical setting. But Mike's heart was in basic research, and he wanted to devote his full-time activity to both HIV prevention and eradication.

In 1995, McCunne took his first full-time academic position so that he could extend observations made in the SCID-hu mouse model to testable hypotheses in HIV-infected patients. It was at this point that he received an Elizabeth Glaser Scientist Award. He focused primarily on the effects of HIV on organs of central hematopoiesis (e.g., the bone marrow and thymus). Mike's research revealed HIV's effects on TDL differentiation and proliferation in the bone marrow and the thymus and represented a major lesion underlying the loss of the critically important CD4+ TDL in the course of HIV progression. The research also demonstrated that TDL production in the thymus could be reactivated as needed. Although the studies were all carried out in a mouse model of human hematopoiesis, the results were pertinent to both the blood-forming system of the human fetus and neonate and to events that occur in adults as well.

McCune is an example of what I had talked to Elizabeth about when I first suggested to her that an Elizabeth Glaser Scientist Award should be established. Investing in a person could take research far beyond what investing in a building could do. During the time of his award, Mike established the "Center for Creative Therapies" at San Francisco General Hospital. The center created core laboratories in immunology and virology to develop, optimize, and provide key assays for a variety of clinical studies on HIV and other disorders. It also caused the hospital to become the premier institution worldwide for translational HIV research. Importantly, it also became a hub for new young scientists who were recruited to conduct research.

As Elizabeth and I had hoped, the initial support provided by the Elizabeth Glaser Scientist Award allowed individuals such as Mike McCune to continue their research beyond the five years of support. McCune's research turned to the question of differential immune responses against HIV, based on the hypothesis that some, if not all, pro-inflammatory immune responses to infection are associated with pathologic outcomes of HIV transmission and disease. His ongoing inquiry into the pathogenesis of HIV infection led to a series of studies funded by both the NIH and the Bill and Melinda Gates Foundation. These studies hoped to create an HIV vaccine and to develop therapies that might lead to HIV's eradication.

In 2005, while continuing in an advisory capacity with EGPAF, McCune received $123 million in NIH funding to create the Clinical and Translational Science Institute with the mission of finding how improved treatments could be brought more quickly from laboratory "bench" research to the community. Mike recruited more than two hundred UCSF Medical Center faculty members to participate in this effort. Characteristically, McCune is a good listener and entertained suggestions whether they came from activists or scientists. It is not surprising that he would later represent the leadership of the Martin Delaney AIDS Research Enterprise to Defeat HIV (DARE). Delaney, now deceased, was a well-respected San Francisco HIV activist and persistent voice in pushing the agenda to cure pediatric and adult HIV. I had interacted with him many times when we both advocated for rapid approval of ART for infants and children. Today, McCune remains focused on research for an HIV cure.

Richard Koup, MD, recalls describing his pediatric AIDS research to Elizabeth in 1989. "That's all very nice," she told him, "but how will it help my son?" With those words, Koup realized that while he saw HIV as a scientific curiosity, for Elizabeth it was a personal battle that would not conform to the typically slow advances of scientific discovery. She made him, then a young scientist just embarking on his career, re-evaluate his priorities and his approach to HIV and AIDS. At the time, Koup was working in the University of Massachusetts Medical Center Department of Pediatrics with John Sullivan, one of the early pioneers in pediatric AIDS research, who gave him the opportunity to observe the effects of HIV on children first hand. It was there that Koup did the first test-tube studies on NVP, the ARV that later revolutionized the international prevention of mother-to-child HIV transmission, when studies in Uganda showed that a single dose given to mother and infant could prevent 50 percent of HIV infections in HIV-exposed infants (Guay et al. 1999).

Subsequently, Koup moved to the Aaron Diamond AIDS Research Center in New York. He worked on the Ariel Project, named for Elizabeth's daughter who died of AIDS. Koup was also named one of the first Elizabeth Glaser Scientists, which was, in his own words, a truly great honor. The award allowed him to study individuals who never became infected with HIV despite multiple exposures and to discover the major co-receptor for HIV as well as a natural genetic mutation in that co-receptor, the latter of which renders certain individuals almost completely resistant to HIV infection. The pharmaceutical industry was quick to realize the importance of this finding and rapidly developed ARVs that targeted the interaction of HIV with its co-receptor, adding to the therapeutic options for both children and adults (Paxton, Kang, and Koup 1998).

Koup continued his dedication to the foundation, as did many of the Elizabeth Glaser Scientists, often working with it directly to establish research priorities. He worked in an advisory capacity with Katherine Luzuriaga, another Elizabeth Glaser Scientist, co-chairing the Scientific Advisory Board of the Elizabeth Glaser Scientist program. In the tradition of the original Think Tanks, begun in 1988 and continuing with the Pediatric AIDS Foundation, Koup felt that one of the program highlights was the annual meeting of awardees, where basic scientists and international leaders dedicated to pediatric AIDS research would gather to review data and brainstorm new research opportunities. Koup believes that, "When you receive an award from the Elizabeth Glaser Pediatric AIDS Foundation, you become part of a family, and the love you receive helps drive your commitment to succeed."

For the last eleven years, Koup has been Chief of the Immunology Laboratory at the Vaccine Research Center (VRC) at the NIH, where he continues to work on scientific projects relevant to the goals of EGPAF. The finding of which he is most proud is the discovery that HIV negatively affects the thymus (the school that educates TDL). Because the thymus is much more active in children than it is in adults, HIV's effect on the thymus is also much more profound in children. In addition, Koup showed that HIV preferentially infects and depletes certain pathogen-specific CD4 TDL, leading to a targeted loss of immunity to certain organisms. One of those is HIV itself—so the virus is able to cripple the immune response against itself. Another is Tuberculosis (TB), thereby helping to explain the co-evolving epidemics of TB and HIV in much of the world, as HIV specifically depletes the immune response to TB.

Koup's ongoing work at the VRC has been highly rewarding for him. A dedicated team of scientists isolated broadly neutralizing antibodies that may be able to block transmission of HIV. In addition, the vaccines currently being tested in adults are being considered as therapeutic agents in HIV-infected children and adolescents as one arm of a cure strategy. Most significantly, if a vaccine can be made that protects adults from becoming infected with HIV, it could ultimately lead to the elimination of pediatric AIDS. Koup believes if HIV infection in women of childbearing age can be eliminated through immunization, pediatric AIDS can also be eliminated. Koup has never forgotten those first words Elizabeth said to him, and while his research may not have helped Elizabeth's son directly, he hopes that what he has accomplished with the love and support of the EGPAF family has had some small impact on this devastating disease.

John Moore, PhD, now a tenured professor of microbiology and immunology at Weill Cornell Medical College in New York, was one of the first PhD recipients of an Elizabeth Glaser Scientist Award. Although the research funding itself was a valuable resource for his laboratory's work on HIV entry via co-receptors, he believes that there were many other less tangible, but perhaps even more important, benefits of receiving the award. Some of these became apparent only years later in hindsight. Perhaps the most substantive gain for an early- to mid-career scientist (in the mid-90s Moore was around forty) was the chance to get to know, as Moore says, "A pretty sharp group of people of around the same age and with broadly similar interests." He explains, "Networking is one of those terms that is hard to define with any precision, but one knows it when experiencing it." The Elizabeth Glaser Scientist awardees are a network for Moore to this day, and Moore also suggests that another relevant term for this award-winner network is "friendship." Thrown together in the annual meetings' social settings, often at the superb White Oak facility in Florida, Moore and others have had the opportunity to get to know people who were previously just names on an author list, and in this way they have formed friendships, many of which have lasted years.

An additional point that Moore feels deserves emphasis is the awareness the Elizabeth Glaser Scientist Award gave him (and presumably others) of just what can be achieved by a group of dedicated volunteers when they put their hearts and souls into a task. The foundation appeared to Moore and to its beneficiaries as a seamless entity, with everything running like clockwork.

One of the gifts Moore received from being an Elizabeth Glaser Scientist awardee was a copy of Elizabeth's book, *In the Absence of Angels*. A book like that brings home the lesson, Moore says, that scientists may too often forget—behind the test tubes and computer printouts there are real people suffering from a deadly infection.

The Ariel Project

The Best, the Brightest, and the Committed

11

A CHILD NOT TO BE FORGOTTEN: THE ARIEL PROJECT

It would be difficult to decide which of the thirty-two Think Tanks, conducted from 1990 to 1998, had the greatest impact on the pediatric AIDS epidemic. The Think Tanks brought together the world's most accomplished scientists and provided them with an opportunity to express their ideas and identify needed areas of research as well as obstacles that prevented progress in halting the pediatric AIDS epidemic. Participants realized that, by collaborating rather than working independently, they could have a greater impact on the worldwide epidemic that by 1998 had infected over four million infants and children with the fatal virus. But it would be incorrect to think of the Think Tanks simply as identifying scientific priorities and research projects alone; they also helped keep the pediatric AIDS epidemic at the forefront of political agendas and in the media spotlight and helped further research into solutions by making sure that pediatric AIDS wouldn't be subsumed into the much larger adult epidemic. The Think Tanks emphasized that, without solving some of the issues involving HIV infection of infants and children, the epidemic would expand into an entirely new generation of HIV-infected children reaching sexual maturity and giving birth to HIV-infected infants.

During her all-too-short life of leadership, Elizabeth Glaser served the crucial role of advocating for and obtaining more funding for the Think Tanks and the research priorities that they identified. She felt what would honor Jake and Ariel the most would be to find answers to perinatal HIV transmission and treatment for children. The Think Tank that perhaps most fulfilled her desires was one that changed not only the direction of the pediatric AIDS research agenda but also how clinical research should be performed. This highly influential Think Tank defined how research success could be achieved through cooperation and collaboration rather than independent and often haphazard approaches to major public health problems. The February 1992 Think Tank identified the initial priorities for prevention of HIV transmission from mothers to infants and for halting the progression of HIV infection in infants who were already infected. At this Think Tank, researchers from multiple disciplines unanimously agreed that studies should focus on the immunologic and virologic factors that might be associated with transmission of the virus. Halting transmission was the key to ending the pediatric AIDS epidemic. Attendees agreed that these studies offered the best hope for ascertaining how

HIV transmission from mother to infant occurred and how it could be prevented. The scope of the investigations went far beyond previous approaches for performing research. A distinct process was implemented that brought together the key researchers with a single goal to work as a consortium. Importantly, it needed to be organized and funded.

In discussions with Elizabeth, I suggested that a major new project focused on perinatal HIV transmission should be put in place and called "The Ariel Project," named after Elizabeth's daughter. Elizabeth agreed. Throughout the project, Ariel remained a symbol of encouragement to move the research agenda forward quickly in hopes of preventing the virus from affecting millions of infants and children like her. The Think Tank that eventually gave birth to the Ariel Project began early on a Saturday morning, February 22, 1992 (Van Dyke et al. 1999). The excitement was palpable. Elizabeth was present and fully anticipated that for the first time some of the best scientists in the entire world—each of whom had focused on different aspects of the HIV/AIDS epidemic—were now gathered to devote their combined efforts to answering the question of how to prevent HIV transmission from mothers to infants.

The scientists came from around the world and included Mike McCune from UCSF, who was particularly interested in the fetal immune system and how the virus interfered with the developing immune system; William Borkowsky from New York University, who provided an overview of the perinatal HIV infection; Miles Cloyd from the New York Blood Bank, who addressed how the virus seemed to affect individuals differently and how there seemed to be a variation in the susceptibility to HIV infection; Irvin Chen from the University of California at Los Angeles, who reviewed data on the variation of individual viruses, which would hopefully offer some insight into whether or not specific HIV species might selectively infect infants; Bette Korber from the Los Alamos Research Laboratory, who had been looking at sequences of HIV from around the world; Jim Mullins from Stanford University, who studied how the feline AIDS virus and the simian immunodeficiency virus behaved differently in different animal species; Jaap Goudsmit from Amsterdam, who had defined the risk factors associated with HIV transmission and disease progression; and Bruce Walker from the Massachusetts Institute of Technology, who had focused on the role of cytotoxic T-lymphocytes (CTL), which could kill off viral infected cells, and how this might pertain to HIV infection.

Other scientists pointed out that we needed to understand where a reservoir of HIV might exist within body organs other than lymphocytes and macrophages and whether the virus simply crossed the placenta and infected infants or whether the virus grew in the vaginal canal and could be transmitted during the birth process. David Ho and Richard Koup from the Aaron Diamond Research Center focused on the need to culture the virus and compare the viruses isolated from the blood, vagina, and gastric aspirates. They pointed out the importance of culturing HIV under varying circumstances and looking at the levels of neutralizing antibody to HIV present in the mother and the infant. Steve Wolinsky from Northwestern University in Chicago suggested that the key to understanding perinatal HIV transmission was the ability to ascertain at what point infants became infected with HIV. His expertise was the polymerase chain reaction (PCR) for early detection of HIV.

Early on Sunday morning, February 23, 1992, following the previous day's detailed scientific discussions, I called for a meeting of the Pediatric AIDS Foundation founders and staff to outline the steps the scientists had identified as necessary for eventually eliminating perinatal HIV transmission: a unifying hypothesis; an international working group to coordinate the research efforts; a process for getting the incredibly gifted researchers to work collaboratively on a singular issue; a repository for storing and distributing blood samples; built-in quality controls for all research studies; a centralized data and statistical analysis site; and an independent advisory group to oversee the progress and relevance of the research. Finally, the project needed adequate funding to attract the best research scientists and allow them to focus on the priorities that had been identified. While the Pediatric AIDS Foundation was already attracting significant funding, the Ariel Project—perhaps because of its advocacy, cohesiveness, and distinctive focus—had the potential to attract even more. Indeed, in the weeks that followed the announcement of the Ariel Project, Magic Johnson, who himself was infected with HIV, committed a large amount of money to support the project, which ensured that the research could move forward quickly.

Later on Sunday morning, the scientists reconvened; the excitement and enthusiasm from the foundation was contagious. The scientists were asked to submit a written grant proposal upon return to their respective institutions. The proposal would define the specific aims related to virologic and immunologic variables that might influence HIV transmission from infected mothers to infants as well as identify which scientists would best be able to carry out the research. Their assignment continued the central theme of the Think Tanks—What do we know, What do we need to know, and How can we do it?

SELECTING THE BEST

Pivotal investigators were identified: David Ho from the Aaron Diamond Research Center; Irvin Chen from the University of Los Angeles; James Mullins from Stanford University; Steve Wolinsky from Northwestern University, Bruce Walker from Massachusetts General Hospital; and Betty Korber from Los Alamos National Laboratory. However, it was anticipated that the Ariel Project would not be limited to these investigators—they would recruit additional scientists once the project was under way. Importantly, the project was identified as a distinct program within the Pediatric AIDS Foundation but administered separately as a consortium of scientists and support groups. I agreed to spearhead the project to be certain that it remained targeted and mission oriented and maintained the primary goal of defining how to prevent perinatal HIV transmission.

To ensure that all investigators had access to precious blood samples, a central repository was established and, for the first time in an HIV clinical research project, blood samples, vaginal secretions, and placental tissue were identified by bar code to avoid any confusion as well as to track which samples were sent to individual laboratories. Quality control was essential for conducting a multi-site, multi-investigator clinical research study. I had considerable experience with quality control while at Genentech and realized that biotechnology companies paid much greater attention to quality control than most academic researchers. The same high standards would be placed on the Ariel Project investigators. Two individuals played a central role in ensuring that the project moved forward in a timely manner and that the conduct of laboratory studies and recording of data was of the highest standard: Natasha Martin and Shelia Clapp.

I had worked closely with Natasha Martin while at the University of California. She was my chief medical technician and distinguished herself as bright, energetic, and a strong leader. She was the ideal person to work alongside me to organize the project, visit the investigators, review the data, and serve as the key individual to review laboratory research protocols and the details of laboratory studies. Sheila Clapp, who had worked with me at Genentech, knew the intricacies of quality control. She was experienced at working with investigators, even those who might be resistant to implementing quality controls, and was skilled at making certain that researchers adhered to the highest principles of research. Clapp developed specialized reporting forms that were used by all investigators for data entry and uniformity of reporting to facilitate analyzing the data for significance.

Each investigator had his or her own task to complete but agreed to share preliminary and final data with other laboratories. David Ho's laboratory was responsible for quantitative viral cultures, identifying the type of viruses that were isolated as well as maternal- and infant-derived HIV-neutralizing antibodies. Bruce Walker had the difficult task of performing CTL studies and determining whether or not TDL immunity played a role in HIV transmission. Irvin Chen was responsible for quantitative RNA and DNA measurements of the virus and relating these to HIV transmission. Jim Mullins focused on the viral diversity to assess the timing and source of the transmitted virus, and Steve Wolinsky focused on the early diagnosis of HIV in infants using PCR as well as viral sequencing and genetic tree analysis for variations of the virus.

But there was more to the Ariel Project than just ensuring that there was excellence in basic and clinical research. In order to perform the clinical research, HIV-infected mothers and their infants were needed to participate so that clinical data and precious blood samples could be accumulated and analyzed for neutralizing antibodies, virus isolation, sequencing and genotyping, antibody dependent cellular cytotoxicity (ADCC), and levels of HIV in the blood of mothers and infants at different points in time—all necessary for sound scientific conclusions. A nationwide search was undertaken to identify the most productive clinical research sites that were run by dedicated physicians who managed large cohorts of HIV-infected mothers and infants (Van Dyke et al. 1999). These sites and their leaders were scattered across the United States and included Arlene Bardeguez at the New Jersey Medical School in Newark, who was working alongside Jim Oleske, the pediatrician who had identified some of the first children with AIDS; Celine Hanson at Texas Children's Hospital in Houston, working alongside William Shearer, who had been engaged in the HIV/AIDS epidemic since it was recognized in Texas; Russell Van Dyke at Tulane University School of Medicine in New Orleans, who had extensive experience in infectious disease and HIV; and Susan Widmayer at the Children's Diagnostic and Treatment Center in Fort Lauderdale, Florida, where she was in charge of a clinical program serving the local community. Finally, there was Andrew Wiznia at the Bronx-Lebanon Hospital Center in the Bronx, New York, who was courageously caring for HIV-infected women and children under some of the most adverse circumstances in the United States. He often remarked, "One need not go to a developing country to see the problems of a developing country. They need only to visit the Bronx."

Diversity among the clinical sites was essential to be certain that there was representation of different populations derived from various ethnic, social, and economic groups.

But it also required incredible organization of shipping and storing biologic samples, a job which fell into the capable hands of Martin and Clapp. To be confident that all the data accrued was accurate, Clapp worked closely with all the investigators of the Ariel Project. She visited each and every investigator site and made certain that the clinical and laboratory data was accurately entered into the database. Having worked with both the pharmaceutical industry and academic institutions, she was meticulous and exacting as data accumulated. No entered data was erased, and each change in a data point had to be crossed out and initialized with the correct information entered. Accurate data was important to establish the statistical analyses and interpretations that followed and the profound impact that results might have on the conclusions derived from the research studies.

I strongly supported the "meticulous and exacting" approach to ensuring the accuracy of the data that was entered. On more than one occasion when reviewing clinical research results on other projects, I found that investigators had selected data to support preconceived conclusions and had dismissed data that did not. I wasn't going to let that happen on the Ariel Project. If necessary, I would travel to a research laboratory and ask to examine the raw data myself to be certain that there was no manipulation of information. In one instance, I stood beside a research technician and carefully went through every laboratory test result, asking why some were included and some were excluded. When no satisfactory explanation was provided, I refused to accept the investigator's conclusions. We had to be certain that every research study in the Arial Project could be relied on. Lives were at stake.

ARIEL PROJECT ACCOMPLISHMENTS

As I reflect on the achievements of the Ariel Project and its investigators, I realize that there were many immediate as well as long-term accomplishments. Perhaps the most immediate was the realization that, in all the time since AIDS was first described in 1981, an undertaking such as the Ariel Project had never been attempted. The Ariel Project brought together key players in one room where all were free to discuss their ideas and dreams—scientists from diverse disciplines, program managers, government and pharmaceutical company representatives, individuals from regulatory agencies, and individuals with experience in conducting clinical trials and statistically analyzing clinical research results. They all exchanged their ideas and concluded with the single mission to prevent HIV transmission from mothers to infants. Visible during the entire Think Tank was Elizabeth Glaser and the memory of Ariel, the project's namesake. It was a tangible presence that fostered the participants' dedication.

Within a year the project was up and running and already returning results (Van Dyke et al. 1999). The immediate availability and sharing of research allowed conclusions to be evaluated quickly. Importantly, it also allowed the scientists to discard further time-consuming and expensive research on elements that were not related to HIV transmission. Although researchers often become "wedded" to the research processes they develop, the oversight of an independent scientific advisory group provided the credibility and authority for discontinuing research studies that failed to show any association with perinatal HIV transmission, saving both time and money.

But of all the variables that had been selected and studied as possibly contributing to perinatal HIV transmission, the level of HIV in the blood of the mother (viral load) stood as the most important—the higher the level of virus in the HIV-infected pregnant woman's blood, the more likely the infant would be HIV-infected. This was such an important finding that three different methods were used to measure the virus, including viral RNA and DNA. Here, then, was a specific target—referred to as "end point"— that could be used as an indicator for perinatal HIV transmission, rather than using the HIV infection of the infant as the end point, which would require months of continued laboratory testing and follow-up. Using a laboratory end point that could be performed prior to birth could obviate the need for large, prolonged, and expensive clinical studies to reach a conclusion on the effectiveness of a new ARV or combination of ARVs to prevent perinatal HIV transmission. It could also have profound effects on reducing the number of HIV-infected pregnant women needed for research, reducing both the number of those placed at risk for disease progression as well as the number of infants at risk for HIV infection. Even more important, it could accelerate the entire process of going from new drug discovery to implementation, making life-saving treatment available sooner. Subsequent to the Ariel Project's findings, other researchers all reported viral load as the most critical association with perinatal HIV transmission.[1]

The consistent results demonstrating an association of viral load and perinatal HIV transmission had significant implications for future studies of prevention of mother-to-child HIV transmission. One important study concluded: "Among pregnant women and their infants, all treated with zidovudine, the maternal plasma HIV-1 RNA level was the best predictor of the risk of perinatal transmission of HIV-1"(Sperling et al. 1996). Similar findings from additional studies should have resulted in the immediate implementation of HAART to bring the pediatric HIV epidemic under control ("Report of the NIH Panel" 1998; "FDA Community Meeting" 1997; Contopoulos-Ioannidis and Ioannidis 1998; Lambert et al. 1997; Garcia et al. 1999). There was no need for additional large, expensive, and prolonged clinical research in low-income countries, which placed hundreds of thousands of patients at risk and depleted much-needed resource funding. The conclusions, however, were largely ignored by the pediatric clinical researchers responsible for the design of future clinical trials of prevention of mother-to-child HIV transmission in low-income countries. A single, conclusive, large clinical research study could have been conducted evaluating HAART and viral load in HIV-infected pregnant women and their infants, bringing life-saving treatment to them decades earlier than what occurred as a result of WHO's recommendations to withhold treatment and clinical research studies that offered only partial and inferior treatment.

Too Urgent to Wait

The American Foundation for AIDS Research

12

THE ENTERTAINMENT INDUSTRY ACCELERATES THE HIV/AIDS RESEARCH AGENDA

Even though HIV had been discovered as the cause of AIDS only two years after AIDS was first described in 1981, and a test to diagnose HIV infection was approved in 1985, there was still not much known about how HIV entered the human body and caused destruction of the immune system. In addition, much more needed to be known about HIV's molecular virology if new, safe, and effective treatment was to be discovered. The number of new HIV infections was increasing every month, and there was concern that AIDS would become a major worldwide epidemic. Too many of the unknowns were frightening—it was clear that HIV was a unique virus, new to the world, and that it destroyed the infected person's immune system by mechanisms that were entirely unique. Research was essential for almost everything that the virus touched, and there were loud and persistent calls for looking into every aspect—epidemiology, virology, pathogenesis, treatment, prevention, vaccine development, drug development, and treatments for the complications of AIDS. By 1984, state and federal governments slowly began to realize the growing magnitude of HIV, which could no longer be relegated to a small population of young, gay men but was clearly and rapidly spreading to other populations. Bureaucracies, in a pattern that would continue throughout the HIV epidemic, steadfastly refused to respond to the emerging epidemic quickly and in a meaningful way. It was as if the bureaucracies that controlled prevention and treatment priorities hoped that HIV would simply go away on its own. But it didn't.

Frustrated with the slow pace of research and the lack of substantial research funding, three individuals, each with distinct talents and capabilities and each with their own spheres of influence, began to take matters into their own hands. They believed that the only way to make significant progress in this new epidemic would be to bypass government health agencies and form a nonprofit foundation specifically dedicated to focusing on the highest priority issues related to the prevention and treatment of AIDS. The personalities and backgrounds of these individuals were dramatically distinct, and yet their individual passions and expertise resulted in the world's first successful foundation for fostering AIDS research. The three individuals were Elizabeth Taylor, Mathilde Krim, and Michael Gottlieb (amfAR 2012b; Ammann 2006).

In the early 1980s, Elizabeth Taylor realized that this new disease called acquired immunodeficiency syndrome was prematurely taking the lives of many people she knew personally in the entertainment industry, and through them, she learned firsthand some of the incredible discrimination against many gay individuals who had AIDS. Taylor felt that someone with her visibility and ability to raise funds should be doing something to help them and to provide answers to the plaguing questions of why treatment was unavailable. One of her first fundraising projects, the AIDS Project Los Angeles Commitment to Life Dinner, was held in January 1985. Even as the event plans were being made, it was clear that AIDS was quickly spreading throughout the entertainment industry and elsewhere. It soon became personal to Taylor when, in July 1985, she learned that her friend and costar Rock Hudson was dying of AIDS. She saw the physical difference between the handsome costar she once knew and the disease-ravaged friend he became (amfAR 2012b).[1]

During this time, Taylor spoke often with Dr. Michael Gottlieb (Hudson's physician) and learned more about the disease and what needed to be done to address it. As a fund-raising dinner, Commitment to Life was a success: 2,500 packed into the Bonaventure Hotel in Los Angeles for the event. As with so many of the fundraising dinners supported by the entertainment industry, those attending the Commitment to Life Dinner were highly recognized and willing to participate in advocacy, despite the stigma associated with AIDS. Although millions of dollars were raised for research that evening, it was too late for Rock Hudson—he died from AIDS less than two weeks later.

Hudson became an example of the desperation that AIDS patients felt as they experienced repeated infections and watched their bodies waste to a mere fraction of what they had been before—desperation so great that in the absence of any available treatment in the United States, those with the financial ability were willing to try anything to reverse the disease. Hudson had flown to Paris in July of that year for an experimental treatment providing only a glimmer of hope for bringing HIV under control. The treatment, called HPA-23, had not been thoroughly tested in HIV-infected patients. Ultimately, it did not work to reverse the ravages of HIV in his body, nor did it work subsequently in other patients. Rock Hudson returned to the United States on a privately chartered 747 jet, at a cost of $300,000. Even access to and the ability to pay for an experimental medicine were unable to reverse Hudson's progression to death on October 2, 1985, at age fifty-nine.[2]

While Taylor and Gottlieb were moving the AIDS research agenda forward on the West Coast, Mathilde Krim was actively pushing the advocacy and research agenda forward in New York. Krim, who had received her training at the University of Geneva in Switzerland, had moved to New York and joined the research staff of Cornell University Medical School. She was married to Arthur B. Krim, a New York attorney who was head of United Artists and founder of Orion Pictures. Both Mathilde and Arthur Krim were politically active and had interacted with Presidents Kennedy and Johnson. This provided them with influence within political circles, which would later become important in Mathilde's role in persuading the US government to fully support AIDS research. In 1983, Dr. Krim and others formed the New York-based AIDS Medical Foundation, which supported scientific and medical research on AIDS, distributing its first funding for research grants in 1984. The AIDS Medical Foundation was also active in distributing accurate information to the legislature regarding how HIV was spread, as well as about the need to reduce the AIDS stigma.

It didn't take long for Krim, Taylor, and Gottlieb to realize that merging the National AIDS Research Foundation with the AIDS Medical Foundation could result in a powerful synergy in the combination of Taylor's fundraising and media strength, Krim's politically powerful influence, and Gottlieb's scientific credibility. In September 1985, an announcement was made that the National AIDS Research Foundation on the West Coast and the AIDS Medical Foundation on the East Coast would merge to form the American Foundation for AIDS Research (amfAR), with Elizabeth Taylor as the founding national chairperson and Krim and Gottlieb as the founding co-chairs. AmfAR moved quickly to accelerate the HIV research agenda. Armed with highly influential and motivated founders, access to people of influence, and the capability to raise significant funds for AIDS research, rapid progress could be made in developing a research and advocacy agenda (amfAR 2012a). Although amfAR's initial emphasis was not pediatric AIDS research or prevention of perinatal HIV transmission, it went on to play one of the most critical roles in defining the early priorities for pediatric AIDS research and advocacy for women and children with AIDS. Its early support of preliminary studies to prevent HIV transmission was one of the most important contributions.

One of the individuals appointed to the amfAR board of directors was Helen Kushnick, whose influence in the entertainment industry was increasing with her and her husband Jerry's successful cultivation of rising star Jay Leno. They initially discovered Leno as a standup comedian, and with the help of increasing visibility and associated income, the demand for his comedy quickly increased. The Kushnicks aggressively marketed Leno, who was eventually selected to take over Johnny Carson's position on *The Tonight Show*.[3]

I had first gotten to know the Kushnicks because of the blood transfusions given to their son at Cedars-Sinai Medical Center in Los Angeles that resulted in his acquiring HIV. This tragedy led to the Kushnicks forcefully advocating to increase the safety of blood transfusions (see Chapter 4). At one of the amfAR board meetings, Helen Kushnick suggested that I be appointed to the SAC as an expert on pediatric AIDS and therefore someone who could help direct amfAR in research specific to that area. Kushnick emphasized that this was an area even more neglected than AIDS research in general. In 1986, I agreed to accept the position, which initially meant that I would be involved not only in establishing priorities and advocating for pediatric AIDS research but also in reviewing the grants covering all aspects of AIDS research that were now flowing into amfAR at an increasingly rapid rate. I received the list of committee members on the SAC and recognized many of them, but I also saw the names of individuals whom I had only heard of peripherally but who were already well known in the area of AIDS research. It initially seemed intimidating because so many on the SAC were experts in areas outside of my field of immunology, but I realized that my contribution was in both pediatrics and immunology, and I would learn much as I reviewed other areas of research.

Once amfAR received a grant application, staff members, some located in New York and some in Los Angeles, would take care of all the logistics of grant review, including helping with hotels, meals, and airline reservations. The staff made certain that the grant review process itself (which was always an in-person meeting) went smoothly. In fact, the dedication of the amfAR staff in all areas was quite extraordinary. It was not a nine-to-five job for them. Many were themselves advocates for AIDS awareness, and many were young gay men who realized the importance of performing research if the epidemic was ever to come under control through prevention and treatment. Their commitment was quite astounding, and I remember the long days and weekends that they worked to put grant review meetings together. Some, who were themselves infected with HIV, attended the grant review sessions they helped to organize even though they were suffering from advanced AIDS. I recall in particular Jay Theodore, who was responsible for all of the general amfAR grants, and Bernie Dempsey, who was responsible for the pediatric AIDS grants. They worked in tandem, one on the East Coast and one on the West Coast, to ensure that the amfAR research agenda moved forward rapidly with expert scientific review. On occasion, I would visit amfAR's Los Angeles office and find Jay Theodore lying on a cot, too weak to fully function but still putting together the grants for review. Theodore died from AIDS in 1993.

No financial compensation was provided to the grant reviewers, but the education and discovery process itself was more than enough compensation for spending long hours reviewing the grants, coming together to discuss how they should be ranked, and deciding whether they should be funded. In most cases, a week before the biannual grant meetings, a Federal Express box or boxes of grants would come to my office. The numbers varied but were usually in the range of thirty to fifty. Each grant had a primary and secondary reviewer and a tertiary reviewer who could act as a tiebreaker. However, members of the SAC were expected to read all the grants, and the primary and secondary reviewers were to provide a written evaluation of the grant that would be presented at the meeting.

The grant review meetings themselves were held in fairly upscale hotels, which either donated the rooms or provided them at a steep discount through amfAR's contacts. Meetings at the Four Seasons hotels were frequent, and the hotel staff, knowing the dedication of the reviewers, provided them with special attention. The scientific review process would begin early in the morning with all of the scientists gathering around a group of tables arranged in a square with an opening in the center. Between fifteen and twenty scientists from all over the country, and in some cases from Europe, were present. The scientists individually reviewed each grant and then opened it up for discussion. The discussions were always intense, with the scientists intent on fully understanding the significance of the proposed research and conscious of the possibility that many of the grant applicants could advance the field of HIV/AIDS treatment and prevention. Following each presentation the grants were scored anonymously, and then the scientists would go on to review the next grant. Importantly, the merits of each grant were determined on the basis of the quality and importance of the science and not on an individual's position on the academic ladder. After each grant was reviewed, in a rather unceremonious procedure, the scientists would lift the reviewed grant into the air and adroitly throw it into the middle of the room. By late afternoon, the grants were haphazardly stacked from the floor to the tops of the tables, producing a vivid image of the work that had been accomplished.

GETTING SERIOUS ABOUT GRANT REVIEWS

My negative experience with the casual nature with which one of my grants had been treated by the University of California when the epidemic was first recognized caused me to take the grant reviews very seriously and delve deeply into each grant to search out its potential. I felt especially sympathetic to young investigators with new ideas who had preliminary data and were willing to take a risk in their research careers. The grant review process was an extraordinary learning process and an education in itself, well worth the investment that I put into reading and reviewing them, as they taught me even more about HIV, the pathogenesis of infection, and the spread of HIV throughout the world. Through reading the grants and participating in the discussion, I learned about the structure of the virus, how it infected a cell, how it replicated, and how it destroyed the immune system. There were also other areas that were important, such as the epidemiology of HIV, how the virus spread throughout the world, different viral subtypes, behaviors that contributed to increased risks of HIV infection, and new and emerging targets for drug development. I realized that I was learning things that had not yet been published and that maintaining confidentiality was essential, yet it was exciting to realize that I was witnessing the cusp of new discoveries. Many scientists whose grants were reviewed were destined to make major breakthroughs, and the HIV/ AIDS epidemic became their chosen career.

In 1988, I was asked if I would accept the position of chair of amfAR's Science Policy Committee, responsible not only for the scientific direction of pediatric AIDS research but also of amfAR's SAC. I was also asked if I would agree to join amfAR's board of directors. I considered these requests to be compliments, and the positions as privileges, as they provided increased opportunities to learn about all aspects of science that related to HIV, see how science worked, determine what successful research was, and examine how to accelerate the research that could solve problems. I also learned some fundraising skills and became familiar with the vast network of individuals needed to make a foundation successful, not only in supporting research but also in increasing visibility and thereby influencing public policy decisions in science, sociology, and economics. With enthusiasm, I immersed myself as much as I could in the grant review process, realizing that I was being exposed to discoveries and opportunities that many individuals would never have in their lifetime.

Because of its dedication and focus, amfAR was successful in its mission to bring the AIDS research agenda to the forefront on an international level. But it is not surprising that not everything went smoothly. Although the scientists who reviewed the grants and advised the foundation worked together collaboratively with very little difficulty, there were bumps in the road for amfAR, to be expected when working with high visibility, high maintenance, politically influential, and economically endowed individuals. Tensions sometimes ran high as egos were bent out of shape over things that were seemingly unimportant for the foundation's mission. Much of the responsibility for smoothing things out fell to Mathilde Krim. I was impressed with Krim's tenacity, integrity, and dedication even under difficult circumstances. Many people failed to realize how compassionate she was and how hard she worked to find solutions to not only the scientific challenges of HIV but also the political and social issues surrounding it, including discrimination against people with AIDS. I remember several meetings at which Krim was booed by the very individuals she was trying to help because she could not satisfy all of their demands (which were many). They failed to realize that she had dedicated her life to HIV and to helping those who were infected. In spite of these hurtful episodes, Krim continued to work at obtaining funds to support research and increase access to the treatment that was so desperately needed by HIV-infected individuals.

In 1995, on World AIDS Day, I was honored by amfAR with an award for distinction in scientific leadership. During the awards ceremony, held at the United Nations (UN), amfAR announced that since its founding in 1985, it had awarded more than $79 million in grants to more than 1,600 research teams worldwide. It had come a long way since it was first founded—its national and international influence would continue to affect the course of the HIV/AIDS epidemic worldwide (amfAR 2012a).

My last formal association with amfAR was from 1997 to 1998, when I accepted a one-year term as president to assist with critical transitions in research priorities. I gained an extensive amount of knowledge and experience from my years at amfAR that served me well in helping to establish another new foundation—the Pediatric AIDS Foundation—under the championship of Elizabeth Glaser and, once again, with the assistance of Michael Gottlieb.

AMFAR'S MANY ACCOMPLISHMENTS

Within a year of inaugurating amfAR, the foundation stepped up its advocacy role primarily thanks to Mathilde Krim's efforts. Along with the board of directors and the SAC, Krim realized that the AIDS epidemic was not just in need of scientific discovery for treatment of HIV infection but also in need of defending against the widespread discrimination and stigma associated with AIDS. Krim and Elizabeth Taylor made an incredibly impressive duo in their testimony before Congress. While Krim was not one of the best public speakers, she always spoke with compassion, authority, understanding, and first-hand experience. Taylor, of course, could hold any audience captive. Almost any time she appeared before Congress there was an immediate overflow audience in the congressional testimony room.

In 1986, both Krim and Taylor appeared before Congress to emphasize the need for clinical research to be conducted in the community setting. AIDS activists had long argued that they were excluded from many of the decisions as to what communities should be involved and which types of clinical research should be performed regarding AIDS. Although in 1986 there was only one ARV candidate (ZDV) that looked promising for the treatment of HIV infection, the activist community felt that they should not wait until research studies were completed before gaining access to clinical research trials. Krim and Taylor provided testimony that this was a compassionate approach to treatment. They further emphasized that those affected by AIDS needed to obtain faster access to promising new drugs. As my interaction with amfAR increased, I saw the organization develop a multipronged approach to the ever-expanding AIDS epidemic. It was not just looking for priority research targets and finding funding to support the research, but it was also addressing the issues that Krim had seen from the very first year when she became involved with patients suffering from AIDS and Kaposi's sarcoma. Krim abandoned her own research career to devote her full attention to some of these problems (Ammann 2006). She often held meetings with New York City officials, including Mayor Koch, reminding them that the city had an ethical responsibility to care for the increasing numbers of AIDS patients who were being discriminated against in various medical facilities. The AIDS epidemic raised a myriad of complex economic, legal, political, ethical, and social issues, and amfAR began to call upon experts in all of these fields to define what needed to be done to address some of these problems.

I was impressed with amfAR's political influence. During my years with the foundation, I noted that it was instrumental in the introduction and passage of key items of federal legislation, ensuring that HIV was not excluded from legislative renewal, including the Hope Act of 1988, the Ryan White Comprehensive AIDS Resource Emergency (CARE) of 1990, the Americans with Disabilities Act of 1990, and the NIH's Revitalization Act of 1993. Through the foundation's influence, Congress passed the first AIDS drug-assistance program, which provided financial help to cover the high cost of ARVs for patients throughout the United States. Over the years, as a consequence of amfAR's aggressive legislative efforts, activists and advocates saw the amount of funding increase significantly, not only for AIDS research but also for the care of AIDS-infected patients.

However, not all of amfAR's political efforts were successful, and unfortunately, some of the failed efforts related to the pediatric AIDS epidemic. In 1998, Krim and I visited the offices of John Coburn, a congressional representative from Oklahoma who was also a physician and obstetrician holding conservative views regarding the AIDS epidemic. A bill was coming before Congress that would uphold the ban on US funding of needle-exchange programs. By 1999, it was well documented that providing clean needles and syringes to drug addicts could significantly reduce HIV transmission. I had a particular interest in overturning this bill, not only because it resulted in the HIV infection of so many young adults, but also because it was one of the major sources of HIV infection of young women who, when they became pregnant, would transmit HIV to their infants. In fact, the very earliest children with AIDS, described by Oleske and Rubenstein in New York and Newark, had in common a history of intravenous drug abuse by their mothers (CDC 1982b). Providing clean needles and syringes could help young drug addicts avoid HIV transmission and could thereby significantly reduce HIV transmission infection not only in the addicts themselves but also in infants. I naïvely thought this would be an easy persuasion. As a pediatrician, I had spoken with many obstetricians throughout the epidemic who were sympathetic to how pregnant women had become infected with HIV and how it affected their infants. But Coburn was absolutely resistant. I even asked Coburn what he did in his medical office with needles that were used for injection or drawing blood, to which Coburn replied that they were disposed of in special containers so that they could not be reused by drug addicts. At that point I looked at Coburn and asked, "Why then wouldn't you provide clean needles to drug addicts?" There was no reply.

One of amfAR's advantages was that it was not dependent on government funding to conduct research in certain subjects. Realizing that even someone as powerful as Donna Shalala, the secretary of HHS, would be unable to overturn Congress's decision to ban federal funds for needle-exchange programs, amfAR decided to provide the funds for both researching needle-exchange programs and implementing them.

During my year as president of amfAR, I was tasked with helping them define their strategic approaches to clinical research and overall programs. Living in California since 1971, I did not want to move to New York City, so with Krim's and the board's agreement, I lived in Manhattan for one week out of each month, travelling on Friday from San Francisco to Manhattan and returning one week later on Sunday evening. During the week I would meet with all of the amfAR staff, working more directly with them than I had in previous years. During this time, I realized that the staff's dedication to overcoming the AIDS epidemic continued in spite of funding problems. By 1999, public interest in the AIDS epidemic began to wane. Many individuals were beginning to think that foundations such as amfAR might not need as much funding as in previous years, as US government funding for all aspects of HIV/AIDS was increasing. This, of course, was an unfortunate interpretation; the significant advances in treatment, increased life expectancy of HIV-infected individuals, and decrease in perinatal HIV transmission in the United States did not mean the HIV/AIDS epidemic was over. But with decreasing and limited money available, not everything of importance could be funded, and some difficult decisions needed to be made. One of amfAR's strengths had always been that it could shift from research that was no longer of high priority to newer research targets as advances were made. One thing that tested me during my year as president was that certain programs could no longer be funded, and I was the one who had to tell clinical research groups that their funding would be cut. It turned out to be a difficult and intense year, but one that increased my knowledge of how foundations interact with advocacy and political organizations under trying circumstances to most benefit individuals who are affected by a specific disease.

In spite of my position as amfAR president, I too experienced the impact of decreased funding on research and implementation priorities. I had the opportunity to present the newest results on preventing perinatal HIV transmission to the entire board at one of their New York City meetings. The NIH-sponsored HIV Network for Prevention Trials (HIVNET) 012 study in Uganda had demonstrated that a single dose of the drug NVP, given to the mother at the time of labor and delivery and to the infant after birth, could prevent 50 percent of perinatal HIV transmissions (Guay et al. 1999). I pointed out that in the United States, with the use of cART, the pediatric AIDS epidemic had plummeted from approximately two thousand new infections in infants each year to less than one hundred; the number of infants infected worldwide in low-income countries was greater than six hundred thousand per year, and if similar results could be achieved with single dose of NVP, three million infant lives could be saved over ten years ("Call to Action" 2005). The board of directors declined to pursue the advance in perinatal HIV transmission with financial support. Their response gave me pause in continuing my involvement with HIV foundations in the United States that were focused on the domestic HIV/AIDS epidemic and stimulated me to think about alternatives.

I continued to meet with Krim one day out of each week while I was in New York as I thought about the board's cool reaction to preventing perinatal HIV infection in developing countries. I would leave amfAR's downtown Manhattan offices, grab a taxi, and go to Krim's weekday home on Sixty-Third Street in Manhattan, only blocks from Central Park. It was a wonderful old brownstone that reflected New York sophistication and wealth. I would enter the home, take the elevator with its brass doors up to the second floor, and meet Krim for an informal sit-down lunch. During that time, we discussed everything from the history of the AIDS epidemic to the extraordinary progress that had been made, even though at many times it had seemed like progress would never occur. After lunch, Krim would pull out a cigarette, insert it into a long cigarette holder, and sit smoking while we continued our discussion. By 1998, Krim and I had been engaged in the HIV/AIDS epidemic for almost twenty years. I had a profound respect for Dr. Krim and all that she had accomplished, and it was clear that she, like me, would not abandon the HIV/AIDS epidemic. We had put too much of ourselves into it and could not rest until much more had been accomplished. While she needed to continue in her role as amFAR chairperson, I felt that I needed to step down as president to form a new foundation that would specifically address the prevention of HIV transmission from infected mothers to their infants.

What about the Rest of the World?

The First Conference on Global Strategies for the Prevention of HIV Transmission from Mothers to Infants

THE GREATER WORLDWIDE EPIDEMIC

The 1994 discovery from the ACTG 076 clinical study that ZDV, when administered to HIV-infected pregnant women and their infants, could reduce HIV transmission by 60 percent precipitated an urgent call for quickly implementing the discovery (Connor et al. 1994). Recognizing that ZDV had the potential to eradicate perinatal HIV transmission in the United States drove the urgency. For the first time since the beginning of the HIV/AIDS epidemic in 1981, prevention of HIV transmission moved beyond mere speculation into a reality. The surprise was that prevention was now possible not with a vaccine, but with a readily available and FDA-approved ARV that was also being used to treat infection. Based on the initial successful use of ZDV for the prevention of prenatal transmission, some researchers and clinicians began to conjecture that the worldwide pediatric AIDS epidemic could also be brought under control and, perhaps, HIV infection of infants and children could even be eradicated (Ammann 1994; "Call to Action" 2005). Importantly, it was concluded that cART, through the lowering of viral load, could also reduce HIV transmission between sexual partners, a hypothesis that proved to be correct and was first documented in 2008 and confirmed in 2011 (M. S. Cohen et al. 2011; Vernazza et al. 2008).

Each year the results were more encouraging as early diagnosis of HIV infection in pregnant women became more common and ZDV was offered to both the HIV-infected mother and her infant. The number of infants born with HIV infections began to plummet within years of implementation of the ACTG 076 protocol, decreasing from more than two thousand infections each year in the United States in 1994 to fewer than five hundred in 1997 to fewer than two hundred fifty by 1998. The decrease, however, was not entirely attributed to ZDV, as more potent ARVs such as the PIs were added to treat HIV infection in pregnant women. With the use of HAART, the number of newly infected infants declined even more drastically, dropping to fewer than one hundred infected infants each year in the entire United States by 2000. Soon, some medical centers no longer saw any HIV-infected infants. In 2015, along with a CDC report of a 20 percent decline in new HIV infections in the United States, Susan Buchbinder from the

San Francisco Public Health Department reported that there were no new HIV-infected infants in the city in the previous decade (CDC 2015).[1]

Unfortunately for infants born to HIV-infected mothers in poor countries, the potential for HAART to prevent perinatal HIV transmission was not immediately embraced by all of those engaged in HIV prevention. Rather than rapidly implementing HAART, which had caused the steep decline in new infections in the United States, ministries of health, global funders, and clinicians in low-income countries followed WHO treatment guidelines, which did not include treating all HIV-infected individuals (WHO 2002). NIH-supported research studies, seemingly indifferent to the plight of HIV-infected pregnant women and their infants, failed to deploy HAART, choosing instead to compare inferior treatment regimens to newer ones in painstakingly stepwise fashion that denied effective ART to HIV-infected pregnant women (Ammann, Gough, and Caplan 2012; Lallemant et al. 2000; Mofenson 2009; Onyango-Makumbi et al. 2011; Thistle et al. 2007; Wade et al. 1998).

The CDC surveillance studies of perinatal HIV transmission and studies in HIV-infected adults utilizing HAART documented three extremely important observations that should have immediately accelerated efforts to bring HAART treatment to low-income countries to help prevent perinatal HIV transmission ("Perinatal HIV Down" 1997; Townsend et al. 2014). First, a significant decline in perinatal HIV transmission was observed one year before the results of the ACTG 076 ZDV clinical trial were available and official USPHS guidelines were released in 1995 for the prevention of perinatal HIV transmission. This could not be attributed to fewer HIV-infected pregnant women being diagnosed, as the number of HIV-infected women was increasing each year. The most likely explanation was that it reflected individual physician judgment to protect their patients from the ravages of HIV by treating all HIV-infected individuals—men, women, and HIV-infected pregnant women equally—with the most advanced treatment available. Obstetricians were not waiting for research studies to prove that pregnant women needed to be treated with ZDV (or later, HAART). Nor did they need to wait for the delayed government guidelines to get caught up on the most advanced treatment options before deciding what was best for their patients.

Second, the most dramatic decline in perinatal HIV transmission coincided with the increased use of HAART in HIV-infected adults. This occurred prior to the release of "official" guidelines. Once again physicians caring for HIV-infected pregnant women were practicing good medicine and applying research advances to benefit their patients directly—just as a physician today, caring for any patient with a treatable disease, would prescribe treatment at the time of diagnosis rather than negligently delaying treatment until the disease has advanced to an incurable stage. Third, there were definitive studies performed in pregnant women that correlated decreased HIV transmission with reduction in viral load, especially when HAART was administered (Dickover et al. 1996; Sperling et al. 1996; Thea et al. 1997; Ioannidis and Contopoulos-Ioannidis 1999; Ioannidis et al. 2014). Here was an ARV regimen's proven "surrogate" marker for efficacy, which obviated the need of using an end point of fatal HIV infection to prove efficacy (Deyton 1996; Katzenstein et al. 1996; Novitsky and Essex 2012). Had it been used in research studies on perinatal transmission, it would have documented the immediate need for HAART treatment for all HIV-infected pregnant women and their infants without resorting to end points of life-threatening progression to AIDS and death.

There were some initial reasons why prevention of perinatal HIV transmission was not moving forward more quickly in low-income countries. The infrastructure for HIV testing of pregnant women was severely deficient, as was the number of health-care workers required to administer ZDV to pregnant women, especially the intravenous doses. In addition, the cost of ZDV for the regimen that was proven to be most effective was too costly for most poor countries ("New Drugs Emerge, but Who Will Pay the Bill?" 1996). An additional factor complicating the implementation of the US ZDV regimen was the issue of breastfeeding. By 1990, it was known that breastfeeding accounted for an additional 30 percent of HIV transmissions (Bobat et al. 1997; Fowler and Newell 2002; Slater, Stringer, and Stringer 2010). While breastfeeding could be safely discontinued by HIV-infected women in developed countries, it was necessary in low-income countries to prevent infants' deaths from infectious diarrhea and respiratory illnesses.

It was not that the problems could not be solved. Many predicted that a shorter course of ARVs and perhaps other less expensive but equally effective antiretroviral treatments might become available. Certainly the cost of administering ARVs could be significantly reduced if the duration of treatment were shorter. But it seemed that the theoretical obstacles were beginning to overtake action. Once again, I was frustrated by the slow pace of progress in addressing the larger problem that was looming: a pediatric AIDS epidemic during the decades that followed that would add millions of HIV-infected infants and tens of millions of HIV-related orphans to HIV's toll unless immediate action was taken.

THE FIRST CONFERENCE ON GLOBAL STRATEGIES FOR THE PREVENTION OF HIV TRANSMISSION FROM MOTHERS TO INFANTS

While the HIV/AIDS epidemic in infants was slowing in the United States, it was expanding at an alarming rate in low-income countries. Clinical research studies showed the dramatic impact of cART on HIV-related morbidity and mortality as well as on prevention of perinatal HIV transmission ("Report of the NIH Panel" 1998; Havlir and Lange 1998; Gulick 1998; Ho 1996a). But these results were not being applied rapidly in regions of the world where the HIV epidemic was out of control.

I had learned from my previous experience with HIV activism and advocacy that without media and political attention, the HIV epidemic's visibility, especially when it was located in poor countries thousands of miles from the United States, would diminish. In 1997, I began plans for an international conference named Global Strategies for the Prevention of HIV Transmission from Mothers to Infants. The purpose of the conference was to engage in a political and scientific dialogue focused specifically on prevention of mother-to-child HIV transmission, especially in disadvantaged countries where treatment options were limited and HIV was a raging epidemic. It was held in Washington, DC, to gain the attention of government decision makers. A special effort was made to provide travel grants so that representatives from developing countries could attend. Having a mix of attendees in one location ensured that everyone would hear the same information. I was joined in my efforts by the American Society for Microbiology, the NIH Office of AIDS Research, the American Foundation for AIDS Research, and several other organizations to co-sponsor the first ever international conference focused solely on developing ways to prevent mother-to-child HIV transmission.

It took more than six months to plan the conference and raise attendance funds for participants from low-income countries. Leading up to the conference, I heard the frustration of individuals working in low-income countries as they observed the dramatic progress in preventing HIV infection of infants in the United States and Europe but lacked the opportunity and resources to replicate those successes in their own countries. It was urgent that the right mix of people attended the conference—not just scientists but also key individuals who could influence health policy, drug development, and funding for implementation of research results. It was essential that the conference bring attendees up-to-date about HIV prevention, address what needed to be known, and define how HIV prevention could be rapidly implemented in low-income countries.

The conference was held September 3–6, 1997. It was a crucial meeting and, as with most large conferences where speakers need to travel long distances, there was concern that some speakers might not show up. Before the conference began, I received a phone call indicating that one of the opening speakers was caught in bad weather in Canada and would not be able to make it for the opening ceremonies. Plans were immediately put in place to identify an alternate speaker. The real surprise, however, came when I woke up on the morning of September 1 to learn that Princess Diana had been killed in a car accident in the Pont de l'Alma tunnel in Paris, France. Although this occurred days before the conference was to begin, the tragedy had the potential to affect the speakers' and delegates' travel plans and to diminish the conference's much-needed media attention. Fortunately, by the time the conference started, most people attending had either heard the news of Diana's death before they left their own country or were made aware of it as they travelled from distant countries to Washington, DC.

The opening ceremony began with acknowledgment of the tragic death of a single person, Princess Diana, but also with an overwhelming sense of the tragic deaths of thousands of infants each year from a preventable infection. Dr. Helene Gayle, director of the CDC's National Center for HIV, STD, and TB Prevention, opened the conference and highlighted the importance of the ACTG 076 ZDV HIV-prevention regimen, stating, "It shows if you put into place the right approach and the right strategies, you can really make a difference. In many ways this is a part of the epidemic where we should be hopeful about our ability to make a difference, not only in this country, but worldwide with the right strategy and interventions."

I felt that it was necessary to place a realistic perspective on the conference's purpose, and so I followed Gayle's comments by stating, "The fact that we have treatment in this country that is very successful does not mean that the epidemic is over worldwide. Industrialized nations have a moral and ethical obligation to develop ways to prevent and treat HIV and AIDS in developing countries as well. The challenge is in figuring out how to accomplish this in ways that are practicable, affordable, and realistic for the various countries that are involved in major epidemics. The goal of this conference is to bring together people involved in this effort, provide updates on the latest progress, and discuss directions to take in the future."

During the conference, one of the major obstacles to implementation of prevention measures was the potential expense. The drug regimen that had been used for the ACTG 076 ZDV protocol—estimated to be between $5,000 and $7,000—was far beyond the financial means of health-care providers in most poor countries ("New Drugs Emerge"

1996). It was important that the major pharmaceutical companies' representatives hear that drug costs were keeping hundreds of thousands of infants from being protected from HIV infection. Administering ZDV was also difficult; at that time it was recommended that ZDV be administered five times a day beginning at fourteen weeks of pregnancy, with an intravenous administration given throughout labor. The infant had to receive oral ZDV four times a day for six weeks (Conner et al. 1994). The complexity and the cost of the administration of ZDV made it seem impossible for this type of treatment, although lifesaving, to be administered in countries where more than 60 percent of pregnant women did not visit a clinic for prenatal care until the third trimester, or where women delivered their babies at home, often with no health-care workers present. Yet in spite of frustration, there was considerable optimism that the combined efforts of the scientific community, clinical researchers, and policymakers could identify and solve some of the major obstacles to saving the lives of infants and children from the consequences of HIV in poor countries.

The reality of the AIDS epidemic was highlighted by a number of speakers. By 1997, there were thirty million people worldwide living with HIV infection, including twelve million women and one million children. An estimated twelve million adults and three million children had died since the epidemic began. By 1996, half of the new HIV infections occurred in women, most of whom were of childbearing age (UNAIDS and WHO 1998). Certainty set in: unless something radical was done, the HIV/AIDS epidemic would continue to escalate, resulting in millions more HIV-infected women and infants. Some form of ART was needed that could be easily administered in a setting of diminished infrastructure and which poor countries could afford. ARV cost had to be drastically reduced.

An important issue at the conference was a discussion on how to best prevent HIV infection of women at the outset. Primary HIV prevention was acknowledged as the best way to ultimately end the pediatric AIDS epidemic. Most women in low-income countries had no choice as to whether or not they would become HIV-infected. Decisions on sexual intercourse were dominated by men, and whether a lethal infection such as HIV would be transmitted during intercourse was not a consideration. Everyone at the conference knew that the percentage of HIV infection in women had increased from less than 5 percent in 1983 to more than 50 percent by 1996. The impact of increased HIV infection in women, especially of childbearing age, would be extraordinary—in most cultures in poor countries, women are the primary caregivers and often the primary wage earners. If they were HIV-infected and developed AIDS, they would be immobilized and unable to care for themselves and their families. A vast secondary epidemic of orphans would result with the loss of one or more parents.

During the conference, I repeatedly pointed out that in the past the public-health control of STIs had included contact tracing. I suggested that we return to this approach to prevent the spread of HIV to vulnerable women. In 1997, it was well known that sexual partners often transmitted HIV, along with other STIs such as gonorrhea and syphilis, to their sexual partners. The woman's vulnerability to HIV increased when other STIs were present, and while contact tracing was often conducted for syphilis and gonorrhea, it was not conducted in the HIV/AIDS epidemic due to fear that it might increase stigma and discrimination. Instead, a somewhat hypocritical approach was proposed—the use of safe sexual practices was emphasized, even though most women in poor countries were powerless to demand that their sexual partners follow safe sexual practices such as using condoms.

Few at the conferences were willing to advocate for contact tracing as a means to reduce primary HIV infection. I was disappointed. It seemed inconsistent to advocate for the protection of women from physical and sexual violence while at the same time denying them the protection of contact tracing to prevent their acquiring fatal HIV infection. In addition, failing to warn a woman that she had been exposed to HIV from a sexual partner was discriminatory in itself, as it could, and often did, result in HIV infection against her will. In my view, the failure to conduct contact tracing was a failure in public-health policy that would ensure perpetuation of the HIV/AIDS epidemic (Adler and Johnson 1988; Ammann 2015c). It was also a lost opportunity to demand that the international community devise means for protecting women from physical and sexual violence, cofactors known to be associated with HIV transmission (Dunkle et al. 2004; Townsend et al. 2011).

Critically important presentations and discussions at the conference addressed the virologic and immunologic aspects of perinatal HIV transmission. It was agreed that HIV transmission from mother to infant was linked to viral load in the mother and that reduction in viral load correlated with reduced HIV transmission. The discussion encompassed whether cART (the administration of more than one antiviral drug working by different mechanisms) might be a more effective way to reduce HIV transmission, as several studies had shown that cART dramatically reduced viral load in adults (Carpenter et al. 1996; Ho 1996a). Use of HAART for prevention of mother-to-child HIV transmission was identified as an important area of research, especially for low-income countries where more effective means of reducing perinatal HIV transmission during pregnancy and breastfeeding were necessary. Unfortunately, the repeated urging by clinicians and advocates to move forward quickly with administrating HAART to HIV-infected pregnant women was subsequently ignored in spite of the consensus reached at the conference. WHO and NIH research took a dreadful and lethal detour, withholding effective ART and conducting studies for decades that used the end points of advancement to AIDS and death.

Ensuring That Voices from Low-Income Countries Are Heard

14

ADDRESSING OBSTACLES

I had attended many international conferences dealing with global health problems that failed to provide adequate representation from the most affected people, so for the 1997 Global Strategies for the Prevention of HIV Transmission from Mothers to Infants conference, I deliberately invited more than half of the participants from low-income countries to be certain that they were well-represented and had an opportunity to present their views. Raising the funds to help health-care professionals from low-income countries attend was a major undertaking. In addition, throughout my years of attending conferences I had learned that individuals from low-income countries were too often passive participants rather than active contributors. Their concerns and views, however, needed to be heard, and so a workshop was conducted on relevant practical and ethical aspects of conducting international studies in low-income countries. Of concern to health-care professionals from these countries was what they called "helicopter research," resources brought into a country for clinical research that were subsequently removed or abandoned when the study was completed, without leaving any sustaining infrastructure. There was also concern that the clinical research studies would be designed without their input, dictating what would be of benefit to the clinical researchers but not of benefit to the country's residents. They suggested that there be a mutually agreed upon design with consensus among wealthy countries' public health officials, government policy makers, pharmaceutical companies, clinical researchers, and funders of the study. Concern about the availability of drugs once a trial was completed was a major and sometimes volatile concern to many individuals from low-income countries. They had unfortunately experienced situations where clinical research had proven to be successful, but the new treatment was not made available to either the research study participants or to the population of their country as a whole.

Issues on the ethics of research, especially in relation to equity and justice, emerged throughout the conference. Both the CDC and the NIH had come under criticism for sponsoring international clinical trials that used placebos as a comparator arm when studying perinatal HIV transmission (discussed in more detail in Chapter 25) (Angell 1997; Lurie and Wolfe 1997; Korschun 1999). The ACTG 076 on ZDV to reduce perinatal HIV transmission was an example of a study that had been stopped early so that women and their infants who had received placebos could be given ZDV, the proven regimen. Knowing this, there were several individuals who felt that the CDC and NIH should not conduct additional research trials in low-income countries using a placebo-controlled study design. Edward Mbidde, from the Uganda Cancer Institute in Kampala, Uganda, countered these arguments, stating that the difficulty was not that low-income countries didn't want to use ZDV; they needed other options because they could not afford the ZDV. He explained, "The whole idea now is to say, what would be the best regimen for our people? What would be practical and applicable in our countries?" Dr. Mofenson, Associate Branch Chief of Clinical Research at NIH, stated, "We need to study regimens in developing countries that we can in the end leave with them, that they can potentially use." Under these circumstances, a better approach would be a trial comparing the ZDV regimen to alternative regimens that might be equally effective but less costly without requiring a placebo-controlled study. (Just how contorted this argument became and who would benefit from this approach to clinical research is further discussed in Chapter 25.)

Some of the obstacles related to implementation of effective prevention and treatment concerned the role of pharmaceutical companies and their interaction with clinical researchers. I called together a small group of individuals from specific pharmaceutical companies and regulatory and international organizations, as well as clinical researchers from various countries and key representatives from selected NGOs. These included Bristol-Myers Squibb, Merck, and Glaxo Wellcome, as well as the FDA, the Joint UN Program on HIV/AIDS (UNAIDS), and the IAS. Researchers who were engaged in conducting or planning studies on the prevention of perinatal HIV transmission came from the United States, Thailand, Brazil, India, and Italy; individuals representing the planned HIVNET 012 NVP study in Uganda and the SAINT study (ZDV vs. lamivudine) in South Africa were also present (Guay et al. 1999; Moodley et al. 2003).

Several interesting debates ensued during these meetings. The FDA was concerned about safety, especially teratogenesis. Pharmaceutical industry representatives were concerned about profitability in low-income countries if drugs proved successful, and pressure was placed on the companies to drastically reduce drug prices or even provide free drugs. One US-based NGO suggested that studies of perinatal HIV transmission were unethical since mothers were treated primarily for the benefit of their infants. Regardless of the issues debated, the pressure was on to make pediatric HIV/AIDS prevention and treatment highly visible so that it could no longer be ignored by the media or governments.

GIVING CREDIT TO LEADERSHIP

In planning the conference, I felt that it was important to take time to recognize the important leadership of individuals who had the foresight and scientific abilities as well as the dedication to advance clinical research for prevention of perinatal HIV transmission. Therefore, "Therapeutic Intervention Special Recognition" awards were presented at the conference. The heroes who could not attend were acknowledged first—the mothers and their infants who participated in the research studies. Their willingness to risk their lives and the lives of their infants in a study with an unknown outcome would ultimately benefit millions of women and children. Specific individuals who were involved in the design of the ACTG 076 ZDV study were recognized for their important contributions (Connor et al. 1994). Recipients of the award were the following: James Balsley, chief of the Pediatric Medicine Branch of the Division of AIDS at NIH; Edward Connor, founding vice chairman of the Pediatric Research Committee of the ACTG; Lynne Mofenson, associate branch chief for clinical research in the Adolescent and Maternal AIDS Branch at the NIH; Rhoda Sperling, professor of obstetrics and gynecology and reproductive sciences at Mount Sinai School of Medicine; and Catherine Wilfert, emeritus professor of pediatrics at Duke University Medical Center.

I was especially pleased to provide a recognition award to Cathy Wilfert. Not everyone at the conference realized how difficult the path to approving the first study of ZDV had been. In April 1987, Cathy Wilfert, C. Everett Koop, and I attended the Surgeon General's Workshop on Children with HIV Infection and Their Families at Philadelphia Children's Hospital, where Wilfert proposed using ZDV for prevention of perinatal HIV transmission. Wilfert's advocacy was based on Ruprecht's study in mice (Sharpe et al. 1988). Wilfert's tenacity and passion for reducing perinatal HIV transmission was apparent—she insisted that a clinical study of ZDV in HIV-infected pregnant women was necessary. In 1994 the study called ACTG 076 reported the first ever decrease in HIV transmission when using ZDV in infected pregnant women. On June 6, 1994, HHS convened a workshop in Bethesda, Maryland, to develop guidelines for the use of ZDV in HIV-infected pregnant women. The guidelines, with significant input from Wilfert, were published on August 5, 1994 (US Public Health Service Task Force 1994).

While no new preventive treatments to reduce perinatal HIV transmission were presented at the conference, the aggregation and collaboration of equal numbers of individuals from low-income countries with international scientists and influential political figures provided the much-needed impetus for moving forward with an agenda that directly addressed the urgent needs of low-income countries to attack an epidemic that was clearly out of control. The success of the ACTG 076 study in the United States and Europe provided hope for conference participants that perhaps research was turning toward the vaster problem of perinatal HIV infection in low-income countries—what types of treatment should be made available, priorities for health care, drug pricing, protection of research subjects, and the availability of experimental treatments once they are proven to be efficacious for the country's population as a whole. The conference was the beginning of a discussion and debate about what was most important to ending the pediatric AIDS epidemic in low-income countries. It allowed the entire subject of perinatal HIV transmission to take a more prominent and rightful place within the broader discussion of the global HIV/AIDS epidemic.

GLOBAL STRATEGIES FOR HIV PREVENTION

Delays in the availability of the new ARVs for the treatment of HIV meant that without treatment, progression from HIV infection to irreversible AIDS was inevitable. I had personally experienced the impact of these delays, not only with my own patients, but also in the life of Elizabeth Glaser, with whom I had closely worked while with the Pediatric AIDS Foundation. Elizabeth fought bravely for her own access to ARVs, but also for infants' and children's access. Elizabeth had been treated only with ZDV. While single-drug therapy, referred to as monotherapy, slowed HIV disease progression, it did not control the multiplication of HIV, and resistance to the drug eventually developed. Just months before Elizabeth died, the first potent new class of ARV, a PI, became available (HHS 1995).[1] But the drug came too late for Elizabeth, and she gradually succumbed to dissemination of the virus. Her loss was major, not just for her immediate family and friends, but also for the entire world of pediatric AIDS advocacy.

It was not only the loss of Elizabeth's advocacy that affected the visibility of pediatric AIDS and the prevention of perinatal HIV transmission. I sensed that the impact of the successful treatment of HIV by ARVs in the United States and the dramatic decline in perinatal HIV transmission was diminishing the sense of urgency over the much larger and overwhelming HIV/AIDS epidemic in low-income countries. The numbers were telling—fewer than two hundred newly infected infants in one year in the United States but more than 600,000 each year in the developing world.

I had always heard physicians and scientists say that the purpose of their discoveries was to benefit all humanity, yet I observed that the discovery of new potent ARVs to prevent and treat HIV infection was not being made available to individuals in poor countries. Although I had testified before congressional committees, the FDA, a multitude of foundations, and other organizations about the needs of HIV-infected women and children in the United States, the HIV/AIDS epidemic outside the US borders was being overlooked. Advocacy for ending the international pediatric HIV/AIDS epidemic was beginning to wane, even as newer discoveries were increasing the possibility for more effective treatments with the potential of saving not thousands but hundreds of thousands of lives each year. I knew that we needed to provide the same degree of advocacy for the seemingly invisible women and children in low-income countries as we were for those in the United States.

A unique opportunity lay before me. During the seven years that I had worked at Genentech, I had accumulated stock options that had become extremely valuable. Armed with these stock options and not needing a salary, I began establishing a nonprofit foundation called Global Strategies for HIV Prevention, formed in 1998 with me as president, my wife as secretary-treasurer, and Natasha Martin as international program director. I had known Martin since the mid-1970s when I was an assistant professor at the UCSF Medical Center, and she was one of the most important technicians in my laboratory. Ready to take on any challenge and always enthusiastic about new endeavors, she worked with me throughout the early days of immunology and into the early discovery of AIDS in infants and children. When I directed the pediatric research programs for the Pediatric AIDS Foundation, I recruited Natasha to help me establish high-quality research programs that investigated priorities for understanding HIV infection in infants and children.

My wife, Marilyn, had been a teacher during our early married life. She was skilled in communications and eager to learn about the epidemic's impact and to communicate with researchers and clinicians in the United States and in developing countries. As secretary-treasurer, she attended many national and international meetings and had a good knowledge of individual investigators. In fact, when Marilyn developed breast cancer in 2001, many of the compassionate voices of concern came from individuals around the world whom she had met at the various meetings.

During the initial phase of the foundation, all of the planning meetings were held in the living room of our San Rafael home. No one received a salary, and there was no need to pay rent for office space, so the operational costs were minimal, and any funds raised were devoted to moving forward the implementation agenda for HIV prevention. It was during these meetings at our home that the second and third international conferences on Global Strategies for the Prevention of HIV Transmission from Mothers to Infants were planned and executed. Our home-office fax machine was programmed to run almost continuously to communicate with individuals in different time zones. In the absence of e-mail for those in low-income countries, fax was a primary means of communicating not only clinical research results but also invitations to the international conferences.

Initially, one of the most important tasks was to raise funds for the second international conference, which would be held in Montreal, Canada, a city chosen because of its international flavor and because it was much more affordable than the location of our first conference: Washington, DC, in 1997. In addition, I felt that the meeting could not be successful unless there were scholarships available for the hardworking and dedicated individuals in low-income countries who lacked funds for international travel. In retrospect, it was quite extraordinary what three individuals, all volunteers, could accomplish in a short period of time when unencumbered by bureaucratic rules and regulations.

A Call to Action

15

The Second Conference on Global Strategies for the Prevention of HIV Transmission from Mothers to Infants

ORGANIZING A PIVOTAL INTERNATIONAL CONFERENCE ON HIV PREVENTION

Thanks to the success of the first international conference on perinatal HIV transmission in 1997, there were unanimous pleas from clinicians around the world for a second conference that would present up-to-date information on progress being made in prevention of mother-to-child HIV transmission, as well as a call for workshops that would extend HIV-prevention education to health-care workers throughout the world. Of critical need was a less expensive means of providing ART to prevent perinatal HIV transmission in low-income countries (Soderlund et al. 1993; Holmes et al. 2010).

Planning for the next conference began almost immediately after the first conference in Washington, DC. Major issues were determining the location and cost, increasing the number of scholarships, and identifying the list of speakers and workshop leaders who would ensure the conference's success. Although an annual conference was desirable, we decided that holding the conference every other year would allow for better organization and sufficient time to raise the needed funds.

There were many potential funding sources, most of which would require personal contact. My wife, Marilyn, worked tirelessly as a volunteer on fundraising, directly calling government agencies, foundations, and nonprofit health organizations. Included in the calls were pharmaceutical companies that had produced diagnostic tests and ARVs now on the market or that were currently developing new drugs. She also wrote letters to the heads of pharmaceutical companies, cajoling them into providing conference funding. One of the difficulties with getting pharmaceutical-company donations was that the global HIV-infected community, comprised of mainly women and children, was unable to develop the same level of activism and attention that had occurred with HIV-infected young men in the United States. The market for ARVs, all of which were under patent protection, was considerable in wealthy countries, and pharmaceutical companies viewed the US and European drug markets as highly profitable and ultimately able to cover the costs not only of current drug research and development but also of new research to discover additional ARVs. Because the HIV/AIDS epidemic in women and children was primarily in developing countries where patented drugs were not affordable, pharmaceutical companies did not consider this population as an emerging market.

Pharmaceutical companies were also reluctant to donate drugs to affected populations in poor countries or to even support an international meeting on prevention and treatment, fearing that high visibility would result in demands by activists and advocates to reduce drug prices in poor countries and to allow the drugs to be produced without patent protection, thus eroding their global market.

I was familiar with many of the arguments against the development and use of ARVs in low-income countries. My previous work at Genentech allowed me to participate in many of the nonpublic discussions suggesting that if drugs were successful in a population where they were unaffordable, there would soon be public pressure and advocacy to reduce drug prices. This had occurred in the United States when the new PIs became available and Abbott Laboratories sought to charge excessive amounts for the life-saving drugs. However, in spite of a reluctance from some pharmaceutical companies, others did contribute to the conference, but in amounts significantly lower than those donated to international conferences addressing the HIV/AIDS epidemic in adults in the United States.

Mark Wainberg (from McGill University in Montreal) and I co-chaired the Montreal conference and agreed to assist the organizing committee in making the conference a success. Wainberg was president of the IAS, and his networking contributed greatly to obtaining the necessary experts who would discuss critical components of HIV prevention. His enthusiasm and encouragement did not wane at any time throughout the planning or duration of the conference. The planning committee and I developed the invitation list, but there were certain individuals who made it known in advance that they wanted to attend the conference. These individuals wanted to attend, not necessarily because they had something to contribute, but because they realized that the conference might increase their own visibility. These people were primarily those associated with governments, especially from the health ministries of low-income countries. My initial naïve interpretation was that they wanted to attend to learn about preventing HIV transmission and treating infected mothers and infants in their own countries. I soon learned, however, that their motivation was more related to political opportunity and potential media attention. Their unwillingness to financially support the conference and to move the HIV prevention and treatment agenda forward in their own countries was disheartening.

On July 14, 1999, two months before the conference and as the plans were being finalized, the NIH and the Ugandan Ministry of Health announced the striking results of the HIVNET 012 clinical study using a single dose of NVP to prevent perinatal HIV transmission (Guay et al. 1999). The study was still in its planning phase during the 1997 Washington, DC, conference but moved quickly during the following years. The study compared the antiretroviral drug NVP with short-course ZDV in HIV-infected mothers and their infants. Announcing the study results set the stage for extraordinary optimism and the hope that at last a low-cost solution to HIV prevention had been discovered that could be used in low-income countries.

When the Montreal conference began, the study was officially published in the international medical journal *Lancet* under the title "Intrapartum and Neonatal Single-Dose Nevirapine Compared with Zidovudine for Prevention of Mother-to-Child Transmission of HIV-1 in Kampala, Uganda: HIVNET 012 Randomized Trial" (Guay et al. 1999). It reported that a single dose of the drug NVP, given to the mother at the time of labor and delivery, and a single dose given to the infant shortly after birth, could reduce HIV transmission by 50 percent, even if the mother continued to breastfeed. At that time, the cost for two doses of NVP was less than four dollars. This was a major breakthrough for countries that wanted to quickly implement ART to prevent HIV transmission. And while the reduced transmission of 50 percent was not as great as the 60 percent reduction achieved by ZDV in the 1994 study, it was still dramatic, and the cost difference of four dollars compared to more than $1,000 for the ZDV regimen was dramatic as well. NVP had many additional advantages: it was stable at room temperature, which meant that it could be distributed to rural areas that lacked refrigeration, and it could be hidden anywhere in the home if a woman wanted to keep her diagnosis of HIV infection confidential. Some innovative women even sewed the drug into their dresses. Thus, single-dose NVP could be administered without openly identifying a woman as HIV-infected, something that often resulted in stigma and discrimination.

Although single-dose NVP had a fairly straightforward administration of just two doses of the drug, one to the mother and another to the infant, there were many unanswered questions associated with the study. Would resistance to the drug develop since it was only a single drug given for a short period of time? Would administration of the drug for a second pregnancy work if the same drug were used for the first pregnancy? What would be the drug's effect if breastfeeding were continued for long periods of time? Now these questions could be addressed directly, both by experts studying the prevention of HIV transmission as well as those who would be implementing the new regimen in their countries.

CALL TO ACTION

The results of the NVP HIVNET 012 clinical trial to prevent perinatal HIV transmission fulfilled the hope, first expressed at the Washington, DC, conference in 1997, that a simple, inexpensive treatment would soon be available for prevention of mother-to-child HIV transmission. Now, only two years later, here was an alternative, much less expensive approach to bringing the HIV/AIDS epidemic in infants and children under control. But it would need funding, and to keep the agenda moving, the funding would need to come quickly. Everyone at the conference knew that sufficient funding from governments could take years to obtain. But where else would the funds come from?

I had learned of the NVP study results several months before they were officially announced and realized that the Global Strategies for the Prevention of HIV Transmission from Mothers to Infants international conference would be the perfect venue for attracting media and political attention. Immediate action was necessary—I was intent on not allowing the results on the HIVNET 012 study to be buried in the medical literature or to sit unimplemented on policymakers' desks. A July 14, 1999, NIH press release regarding the NVP study further spurred me to do more than just announce the results at the conference. Both HHS Secretary Donna Shalala and National Institute of Allergy and Infectious Diseases (NIAID) Director Anthony Fauci were quoted as enthusiastically endorsing the results as a significant advance in the prevention of HIV transmission from mothers to infants in low-income countries. The press release provided attribution to the investigators and to the pharmaceutical companies who manufactured the drugs that were used in the study, but it did not contain any statement or details regarding how the study results would be implemented (NIAID 1999). Fearing once again that research results, although conducted with NIH funding and under their direction, would not be implemented by the NIH because of restrictions on research versus implementation, I began to contact key individuals to see if by the time of the September meeting in Montreal a clear "Call to Action" could be presented, coupled with a funding commitment that would directly benefit health-care delivery sites engaged in diagnosing and caring for HIV-infected pregnant women. With the low cost of the drug and of HIV testing, it was essential that funding go directly to clinicians engaged in the care of HIV-infected pregnant women, rather than to government bureaucracies that could keep much of the funding for themselves or introduce obstacles that could prevent life-saving treatment from reaching the clinical sites caring for HIV-infected pregnant women.

One of the individuals I contacted about the Call to Action was Chuck Hirsch, whom I had known for many years and who had been engaged with several nonprofit organizations directed toward helping women and children, both in the AIDS epidemic and with other major health-care issues. Chuck had worked with the Michael Jackson Foundation, Steven Spielberg, the Pediatric AIDS Foundation, and the Gates Foundation. Of all of his contacts, the Gates Foundation seemed to offer the most potential for obtaining immediate funding to implement the NVP study results. After several email exchanges during the month of July, Chuck and I decided to move forward, contacting the foundations that would most likely respond to our requests. We constructed definitive plans to announce this Call to Action at the Montreal conference, coupled with a pledge of financial commitment for as much money as could be garnered by the conference's September 1, 1999, opening session. By July 22, I had put together a preliminary Call to Action directed at potential donors, challenging them to participate in raising at least $3 million to prevent perinatal HIV transmission.[1] With an estimated two million HIV-infected pregnant women giving birth each year, this amount of money would be enough to provide NVP to 500,000 pregnant women and, with continued efficacy and reduction in price, perhaps all HIV-infected women and their infants.

The Call to Action was announced at the opening ceremony of the conference on Global Strategies for the Prevention of HIV Transmission from Mothers to Infants to jumpstart the implementation of single-dose NVP. Catherine Wilfert and I put together a list of potential donors, hoping that $3 million was a realistic goal. We identified the Gates Foundation, which had expressed interest in providing funding for HIV in low-income countries, amfAR, and the IAS. The UN Children's Fund (UNICEF), WHO, and several US government agencies were included, although it was unlikely that they would or could respond in a timely manner. I realized that time was short; there were only nine days left before the conference's opening ceremony. Few organizations would be sufficiently streamlined to get the necessary approvals from their boards in time to respond. Nevertheless, a degree of optimism was present, and enthusiasm followed each email and phone call to an individual who might be able to commit to the Call to Action.

By the beginning of the conference on September 1, there were three donors who had recognized the value of immediately committing funds—each could bypass the restrictions that plague large international organizations, foundations, and their overly cautious boards of directors. Of all of the foundations and international organizations that were contacted, only Global Strategies for HIV Prevention, the IAS, and EGPAF pledged donations, altogether totaling more than $1 million.

Along with the donations, a sign-on was developed to allow all of those attending the conference to support the Call to Action for immediate implementation of HIV prevention strategies for women and infants. The sign-on was accompanied by a statement developed with the help of Tim Westmorland, who had worked with the Pediatric AIDS Foundation and with me over many years of the HIV/AIDS epidemic. Tim was a longtime aide to Congressman Henry Waxman and had gained considerable experience in the legislative process. He was a master of writing; the final Call to Action was crafted as a three-page document. It began with a review of the slow progress that had been made in HIV prevention in low-income countries and then introduced the dramatic change anticipated with single-dose NVP at the cost of less than four dollars per treatment. (Later, the cost of the drug was reduced to less than one dollar.) The Call to Action was inclusive, calling upon the public, governments, pharmaceutical companies, religious groups, charities, foundations, and non-government organizations to support preventing perinatal HIV infection. It pointed out that an investment of only $12 million could prevent more than 600,000 HIV infections in infants each year, something that had seemed impossible only two years earlier.

The final Call to Action was completed just twenty-four hours before the conference. Plans were made to have it available for all conference participants to sign after the opening ceremony and throughout the remainder of the conference. The implications of the failure to respond quickly were clearly outlined—a delay of a couple of days would mean that as many as 2,400 infants could become infected. A delay of a year would mean that more than 600,000 infants might become infected and die from HIV. Before the opening ceremony, only a few individuals knew that there would be an announcement regarding the Call to Action or the amount of funding that had been procured to jump start the implementation of single-dose NVP for perinatal HIV prevention. An announcement at the beginning of the meeting was critical for setting the stage and instilling hope that prevention of perinatal HIV transmission might finally be affordable for even the poorest countries.

A potential wrinkle in the presentation of the Call to Action occurred the morning of the opening ceremony. I received a phone call from the Office of AIDS Research (OAR), an internal NIH group that had been established during the HIV/AIDS epidemic and given the responsibility for overseeing the direction of much of the research funded by the NIH. They wanted to meet with me before breakfast to discuss a "serious matter." Individuals from the OAR had heard about the Call to Action announcement, and they expressed concern that this would not be politically acceptable at the conference. Taken aback by their seemingly insensitive interference in the need to implement life-saving measures for preventing perinatal HIV transmission, I asked why they felt they had the right to try to prevent the presentation of the Call to Action. They responded that because the OAR had contributed to funding some of the meeting's costs, the conference should not engage in what they viewed as political activity. They wanted me to cancel the announcement about the Call to Action and the funding that had been raised. Here was a government agency established to facilitate advances in HIV/AIDS that was attempting to derail progress. Of course, I refused to comply and pointed out that the purpose of the conference was to advance the implementation of clinical research that had been funded by the NIH, the very organization they represented, and that this was not about some political agenda but about a public health agenda that would save hundreds of thousands of infants' lives.

During the opening ceremony, I called Mark Wainberg to the platform, followed by Catherine Wilfert. I asked them to join in announcing the $1 million that had already been committed to the Call to Action—not quite the hoped for $3 million, but certainly a great start. Following the announcement, there were loud cheers from the entire audience of almost one thousand. What followed was certainly unusual for any of the normally subdued international conferences: Samite, a Ugandan musician, led the entire audience in singing songs of hope for women and children, and the singing culminated in attendees dancing in the auditorium's aisles.

Given the ACTG 076 study's success in preventing perinatal HIV transmission and its application in developed countries, it was not surprising that the breakthrough HIVNET 012 study would fan the flames of enthusiasm among all presenters, regardless of the topic. The conference was packed, not only with health-care workers and individuals whose expertise covered every component of the HIV/AIDS epidemic, but also with representatives from international organizations, non-government organizations, scientists, and clinical researchers, who were now eager to participate in ending the pediatric HIV/AIDS epidemic. Clinical research abstracts were submitted from a diversity of countries—Thailand, China, Poland, Kenya, South Africa, Mozambique, Uganda, Bangladesh, Spain, Sweden, Germany, Italy, England, Brazil, Canada, Latvia, and tens of other countries scattered across the world—all of whom were desirous of ending the pediatric AIDS epidemic. To accommodate all of the presentations and discussions, the conference covered a period of five days with an additional day added to discuss issues related to advances in diagnosing and treating HIV-infected children.

One of the most important outcomes of the conference was related to solidifying the data on how to prevent HIV transmission from infected mothers to their infants. Clinical researchers from different institutions and different countries once again confirmed the strong association of HIV transmission with viral load, and they reasoned that if HAART could reduce viral load, then it should be considered for prevention of perinatal HIV transmission. They did not need to wait for more research studies. Some health-care professionals reported that they had already moved forward quickly and were providing HAART to HIV-infected pregnant women and observing less than 2 percent HIV transmission rates compared to the 35 percent without treatment. One investigator reported not seeing any HIV-infected infants born to HIV-infected mothers when HAART was used. Although PIs were new to the treatment armamentarium, some incorporated a PI in their treatment regimen as they recognized the potency of these new ARVs and their potential for reducing HIV transmission to insignificant levels.

Armed with the success of the ACTG 076 study, the HIVNET 012 study, and the recognition that the more potent the treatment, the greater the reduction in viral load, many of the conference participants pushed the envelope of prevention recommendations. They realized what could be accomplished with more aggressive approaches using HAART. They wanted, as do all health-care providers who care for their patients, to provide the most advanced treatment available. Regrettably, in the years that followed, the results of these early studies were dismissed by influential individuals who insisted that more research studies were required before HAART could be implemented in low-income countries. These actions slowed the momentum to implement research results, which could have saved the lives of hundreds of thousands of women and children each year.

One of the conference workshops was devoted entirely to the issue of breastfeeding and HIV transmission. The data demonstrating breastfeeding significantly contributed to infant HIV infection was sobering. In income-rich countries, breastfeeding could be discontinued and artificial feeding safely utilized. But in poor countries, stopping breastfeeding resulted in increased mortality, not as a result of HIV infection, but because of increased respiratory and gastrointestinal-tract infections in the infants who no longer benefited from the protection afforded by maternal breastfeeding. Grace John from the University of Washington in Seattle and Paolo Miotti from NIH led discussions on the importance of breastfeeding and its relationship to HIV transmission. One of the most interesting and important presentations was that of South African Anna Coutsoudis, who presented her observations that exclusive breastfeeding was associated with a reduced rate of HIV transmission (Bobat et al. 1997). By exclusive breastfeeding, she meant providing only breast milk and no food or additional liquids to an infant. Coutsoudis concluded her presentation by stating, "If confirmed, exclusive breastfeeding may offer HIV-infected women in developing countries an affordable, culturally acceptable, and effective means of reducing transmission of HIV, while maintaining the overwhelming benefits of breastfeeding." Initially controversial at the time of the conference, her observations were subsequently confirmed by several other studies conducted in African countries, demonstrating the benefits of exclusive breastfeeding for at least the first six months of life (Slater, Stringer, and Stringer 2010). Exclusive breastfeeding, however, was a stopgap measure—it did not prevent all HIV transmission; it merely reduced it. In contrast, the use of HAART during breastfeeding, exclusive or not, could reduce perinatal HIV transmission to less than 2 percent (Mofenson 2010; Cooper et al. 2002).

The conference participants did not tire of the presentations or of the discussions. Each morning there was a keynote speaker, followed by specific presentations on specialized topics, and then presentations of recent clinical research results. The afternoon was filled with workshops on specific topics, and workshops were added in the evenings as a result of the HIVNET 012 study and the Call to Action. The evening workshops often lasted until 11:00 p.m. or midnight, as leaders from low-income countries hammered out what could be done to control the epidemic of HIV infection in infants in regions with limited infrastructure and access to health care. Looking back at the conference schedule and the multitude of topics presented, I find it impressive that almost no stone was left unturned in addressing the global issue of HIV transmission to infants and how to end the pediatric HIV/AIDS epidemic. Topics included nutrition, international clinical trials, breastfeeding, factors associated with transmission, the potential of an HIV vaccine, gene therapy, drug toxicity, and adverse drug reactions.

One session was devoted to a relatively new topic, one that triggered intense discussion and controversy. Stephan Blanche and his collaborators from the Hôpital Necker

Enfants Malades, Paris, France, had reported that five infants exposed to ARVs in utero had developed features of mitochondrial disease, which included neurologic abnormalities (Blanche et al. 1997; Blanche et al. 1999). Two of the infants had died. They suggested that ARVs administered during pregnancy might have caused mitochondrial toxicity in the developing fetus. This was initially an alarming observation that, if confirmed, would be a warning that in-depth studies of drug toxicity were needed before the widespread implementation of HAART in pregnant women could occur. A detailed report by Blanche and his collaborators was published in *Lancet* the same month of the conference (Blanche et al. 1999). However, US investigators who had access to much larger numbers of infants from clinical trials of perinatal HIV prevention, and who were aware that Blanche would present his observations at the conference, had retrospectively analyzed large cohorts of infants exposed to ARVs in the United States. Combining information obtained from the CDC, the Pediatric AIDS Clinical Trial Group (PACTG), the Perinatal AIDS Collaborative Transmission Study, and pediatric surveillance reporting, they could not identify any deaths attributed to mitochondrial toxicity (Bulterys et al. 2000; Lindegren et al. 2000). Nevertheless, most acknowledged that this was too important an issue to ignore in spite of the urgency of preventing perinatal HIV transmission (De Mendoza, Blanco, and Soriano 2003; Taylor and Low-Beer 2001). Detailed data collection and continued evaluation of infants exposed to ARVs was recommended, especially since the number of infants exposed to ARVs was increasing significantly in both the United States and in low-income countries, where monitoring safety would be more difficult.

The night before the session focusing on mitochondrial toxicity, I received a call from one of the Blanche team, who expressed concern that they were being "ganged up on" by other clinical research investigators. I had to reassure him that their report was important and could not be ignored. It was essential to determine if mitochondrial toxicity was indeed related to the administration of ARVs and, if so, to carefully monitor exposed infants in other countries. After the conference, follow-up studies and meetings focused solely on mitochondrial toxicity were conducted. Fortunately, in studies of much larger numbers of infants and children, the results of severe mitochondrial toxicity were not confirmed.[2]

MONTREAL RECOGNITION AWARDS

As with the Washington, DC, Global Strategies international conference, the Montreal meeting ended with a special session recognizing specific individuals who had contributed to advancing HIV prevention and treatment in women and children. As conference participants gathered early in the morning of the final day, the excitement of the NVP study had not subsided. All those present looked forward to the special recognition awards. The first awardees were integral to making the NVP perinatal HIV-prevention study successful (Guay et al. 1999). Two of the leaders were from Uganda. Frances Mmiro was a professor of obstetrics and gynecology at Makerere Medical School in Kampala, where the study was conducted. He was the protocol chair and the most senior of the investigators to play a major role in the study's design and implementation. Philippa Mudido Musoke, a junior faculty member at the time, was an essential member of the HIVNET 012 team, and as a team leader ensured rapid patient enrollment, adherence to the research protocol, and ultimately a highly successful clinical research study. It was especially important to recognize the two physicians from Uganda, as this was the first successful clinical study for prevention of HIV transmission from mothers to infants performed in an African country with, of course, hundreds of Ugandan mothers and infants contributing to the study. The organizing committee and I had struggled with how to appropriately recognize the women who participated in the study and placed their own lives and the lives of their infants at risk to benefit others. I verbally acknowledged their importance in the clinical research study, but it seemed inadequate for what they had contributed.

On the US side, there were several important leaders who moved the trial forward. John Sullivan, professor of pediatrics at the University of Massachusetts Medical School, was the first to perform studies using the drug NVP, demonstrating the precipitous decline of the virus following treatment. He initially proposed using NVP to interrupt HIV transmission from mothers to infants, and conducted the first phase one study of the drug in pregnant women and their infants in the United States. Mary Glenn Fowler was the chief of the Maternal Child Transmission Division of HIV at the CDC. She played a major role in the early phase one and phase two studies of NVP, which formed the basis of the clinical trial. Fowler had proposed that the International Perinatal Initiative insure funding for the HIVNET 012 study. Laura Guay was an assistant professor at the Johns Hopkins School of Medicine and had lived in Uganda for eight years. She assumed a leadership role in implementing the clinical trial to ensure prompt enrollment and adherence to the clinical trial design. Brooks Jackson was a professor at Johns Hopkins and had previously participated in other clinical trials for HIV prevention. As US chair of the clinical trial, he assumed a major responsibility for guiding the study through the many scientific, ethical, political, and logistical obstacles.

There were two additional awards. Kenneth Bridbord, a modest individual, was recognized for his leadership role in meeting the education and training needs in the HIV/AIDS epidemic. Bridbord was the director of the International Training and Research Program at the Fogarty International Center, a division of the NIH. He was recognized for his indefatigable advocacy for scholarships and support of clinical investigators in low-income countries. When he stepped up to the platform to receive his award, he looked at the audience, expressed his gratitude, and asked how many people in the audience had received a full or partial scholarship from the Fogarty International Center. It seemed that more than one-fourth of those present raised their hands, an indication of the program's success in spite of the limited funding it had received.

The final award went to Countess Albina du Boisrouvray in recognition for her advocacy and her personal response to the HIV/AIDS orphans crisis. She was the founding president of the François-Xavier Bagnoud Foundation, which, although initiated with family wealth, had raised more than $100 million over ten years' time to provide for innovative worldwide programs in pediatric HIV/AIDS and the promotion of children's rights. The foundation was formed in memory of her son, who at the time of his death was on a humanitarian mission delivering emergency health-care supplies by helicopter in Africa.

Following the Countess's award acceptance, someone in the audience stood up and shouted that there were more important problems to solve in the HIV/AIDS epidemic than orphaned children and that rather than devoting large amounts of resources to infants and children, the focus should be on HIV-infected adults. As if she had heard that criticism before, the Countess calmly answered, "I see it this way: I believe that the beauty of a mosaic is derived from the whole. If you go close to a mosaic you will see individual pieces that contribute to the whole. We each have a piece that we contribute. Supporting the orphans and vulnerable children is my piece of the mosaic." There was silence in the entire auditorium—it was a fitting way to end one of the most exciting conferences in the HIV/AIDS epidemic.

Throughout the conference there were interviews, press meetings, and the long-awaited media attention. At last, I felt that this convergence of research study results, dedicated and vocal health-care professionals, and appropriate recognition of the importance of perinatal HIV transmission could bring worldwide attention to preventing HIV transmission from mothers to infants. Perhaps now, prevention of infant infection and death from HIV could be accomplished in even the world's poorest countries, and perhaps we could even see an end to the pediatric AIDS epidemic.

The meeting concluded on September 6, with the organizers exhausted but encouraged as they reflected on the importance of the information that had been presented and the thorough discussion of the many issues that surrounded maternal HIV transmission to infants. The few episodes of controversy failed to dampen the optimism and hope that pervaded the conference. The overwhelming number of advances in prevention and treatment that were presented, coupled with the Call to Action, created a level of enthusiasm that provided meeting participants with the confidence to return to their countries of origin and begin implementing efficient and low-cost intervention that could save hundreds of thousands of infants each year. But there was still more to be done. Without additional funding, implementation of perinatal HIV prevention strategies would falter.

GATES FOUNDATION TO THE RESCUE

One of the critical follow-up tasks once the conference was over was ensuring that the momentum we had gained would not be lost. When I originally contacted the Gates Foundation regarding the Call to Action, I was told they did not feel they could commit to participating. However, several months later the Gates Foundation did entertain a joint proposal from Global Strategies and the Pediatric AIDS Foundation regarding how to implement expansion of perinatal HIV prevention measures. Wilfert and I put together a mere twelve-page proposal to present to the Gates Foundation, explaining the rationale as well as the process of implementation. Armed with the proposal, Wilfert, David Kessler (former head of the FDA and now chairman of the Pediatric AIDS Foundation), Susie Zeegen (cofounder of the Pediatric AIDS Foundation), and I went to Seattle to present our case. Our request was for $15 million, a sum that seemed large at that time considering how little money had previously gone toward implementing these life-saving clinical research results. It did not take long for the Gates Foundation to respond; within weeks, I received a letter stating that they would grant the full $15 million. After writing lengthy grants of a hundred or more pages with complex regulations and guidelines, Wilfert and I felt that submitting a twelve-page report and getting $15 million in return was in the category of miraculous.

Optimism and hope now abounded. But there were obstacles that emerged over the years that followed—obstacles that prevented the pediatric HIV/AIDS epidemic from coming to an end and which came from surprising sources. Although hundreds of thousands of infants would be spared HIV infection during the next ten years, delays, confusion, and issues of power, control, money, and unnecessary complexities conspired to prevent full implementation of the most advanced HIV preventive measures, which could have ended the pediatric HIV/AIDS epidemic. Over the next decades, ARVs increased in potency, and combinations of ARVs were used to reduce viral load to almost undetectable levels. The prices of the drugs also plummeted. Nonetheless, the delays in implementation tragically allowed perinatal HIV transmission to continue with the unnecessary loss of health and life at catastrophic numbers. At the time of this writing in 2016, 300,000 infants still become infected each year, not because there is no treatment to prevent HIV transmission, but because of delays in protecting women from acquiring HIV infection and in implementing HAART for those already infected.

Now Just Go and Do It

16

The Third Conference on Global Strategies for the Prevention of HIV Transmission from Mothers to Infants

WHERE IS THE BEST PLACE TO MEET?

Selecting the site for the third international conference was difficult. Although there were many cities in developing countries that were eager to host the conference for prestige purposes, the conference organizers and I wanted the chosen location to make a clear statement about why it was important to move forward rapidly with the treatment and prevention agenda. South Africa seemed like a logical choice initially, but it was home to the emerging HIV denialism of President Thabo Mvuyelwa Mbeki, who was beginning to associate with US denialists such as Peter Duesberg at the University of California in Berkeley, even while accepting funds from the United States and international organizations to attack the HIV/AIDS epidemic. Although other countries had shown leadership in addressing HIV—including Thailand, Botswana, Kenya, and Brazil—it seemed that Uganda was the logical choice since it had been the site of so much of the research that had moved the prevention of mother-to-child HIV transmission forward.

But the choice of Uganda was also problematic because of Ugandan political history and past atrocities. It had only recently emerged from the terrible dictatorship of its previous leader, Milton Obote, and there was uncertainty as to the infrastructure and resources that a developing country would have available (Tumushabe 2006). Raising funds was also a challenging issue. A conference on prevention of perinatal HIV transmission was not as high on the funding priority list for international donors and pharmaceutical companies as the vastly larger IAS meetings that were held in large and mostly modern metropolitan areas.

A location at the "heart of the epidemic" where progress had been demonstrated was attractive—the organizing committee agreed that Kampala, Uganda, should receive serious consideration. It took several visits to Kampala to be certain that it was an appropriate conference venue. Lucy Felicissimo, who had assisted me in planning the Montreal conference, and Natasha Martin, who had worked with me to organize many other workshops and conferences, had a good sense of what was needed down to the finest details. On the first visit to Kampala, we learned there was only one conference center large enough for the more than one thousand participants and the satellite workshops we planned to have. Nothing could be taken for granted. When the conference center was first evaluated, we had to be certain that the air conditioning was in working condition, that there was an appropriate number of chairs, that the projection and acoustics would be adequate for all conference delegates to see and hear clearly, and that there would be enough independent meeting rooms for the breakout workshops. All these seemed to be present except for one: there were an inadequate number of chairs for the more than one thousand delegates. As a non-governmental organization, Global Strategies could bypass the many obstacles that often interfered with overcoming trivial matters, such as the stipulation to "buy American" when funded by US government grants. Our team agreed to go to the local market, buy whatever chairs were available, and donate them to the conference center.

In order to encourage local participation and promote the ownership of the conference by the Ugandan health-care community, as much as possible was done using the local economy rather than bringing in prepared materials. Several months before the conference began, conference organizers sought out local sources for printing conference materials, schedules, abstracts, and posters. Natasha also toured the marketplace to find someone who could make conference bags for each of the participants. In most conferences, the bags were either gaudy, inexpensive plastic bags made in countries offering the lowest manufacturing price, or high-end bags prominently displaying the sponsor's name rather than reflecting local culture. Natasha found a local husband-and-wife team who were willing to make one thousand bags out of a colorful local cloth, fully lined and bearing the insignia "Third International Conference for the Prevention of Mother to Child HIV Transmission." In the years that followed, I frequently saw the bags in airports and at other meetings, bringing back incredible memories of a conference that moved the prevention agenda forward.

Where the more than one thousand conference participants would stay was another difficult issue. Several hotels in Kampala were being upgraded but were not within walking distance or a short drive from the conference center. The Sheraton hotel was the most comfortable but also the most expensive. Adjacent to the conference center was the Nile Hotel, which was convenient for those who needed to be near the conference center, such as the conference organizers and the speakers. Unknown to me at the time, the hotel had "ghosts" of a gruesome past. Many people had frightful memories of that hotel. In the mid-1980s, the hotel had been used by Obote for interrogation and torture, but in the two years that had passed since the history of rebel activity and dictatorship in Uganda, things had changed.[1]

In 1986, following negotiations and a pledge to improve respect for human rights, decrease tribal rivalry, and conduct fair elections, Yoweri Kaguta Museveni became president of Uganda. Soon after his election, he had to confront a rapidly increasing HIV/AIDS epidemic. First identified in Uganda in 1982 in a fishing village on the western shores of Lake Victoria, HIV spread rapidly, and by 1998 an estimated 1.9 million Ugandans were living with HIV/AIDS. While Museveni certainly did know about the HIV/AIDS epidemic in his country during his early presidency, his concern for halting the spread of HIV/AIDS is said to have come about in an unusual manner.

Various versions of the story exist, but Museveni is said to have stated that he was not aware how extensive the HIV problem was until 1986, after he sent sixty military personnel to Cuba. Fidel Castro had a policy of mandatory HIV testing, so each of the Ugandan soldiers was tested for HIV. Eighteen of the sixty soldiers were positive. Castro allegedly took Museveni aside and told him that he had a "big problem." Many interpret Museveni's subsequent concern about HIV to have been more about the threat to his military power base than concern for his constituents. Nevertheless, he quickly established a government AIDS Control Program to address the issue of HIV (Murphy et al. 2006; Tumushabe 2006).

Uganda's government demonstrated early leadership in addressing the HIV/AIDS epidemic. It established prevention of mother-to-child HIV transmission services and was the first African country to open a voluntary counseling and testing center. The Ugandan government, faith-based groups, NGOs, schools, and workplaces launched a broad-based campaign termed the ABC program (Abstinence, Be faithful, Condoms), that was praised for successfully reducing new HIV infections. (In later years, some would question whether the numbers were as good as reported (Parikh 2007; Allen et al. 2011; Okware et al. 2005; Hearst et al. 2012). Given the national leadership that Uganda was demonstrating in a region that was in the heart of the HIV/AIDS epidemic, it seemed to the conference-organizing committee to be an ideal location for furthering the HIV-prevention agenda.

This was the first of the three Global Strategies conferences to be held in an income-poor country, an essential step toward shifting greater responsibility for HIV prevention and care to the governments and health-care workers in low-income countries. It could not be a simple handover, but instead needed to be a process that equipped the countries with the knowledge and assistance to move forward in locations where the epidemic far outstripped available resources.

The conference was held from September 9 to 13, 2001. By that time, new HIV infections in infants in the United States and Europe had plummeted due to implementation of HAART. Two years had elapsed since it was first reported that a single dose of NVP had resulted in a 50 percent reduction in HIV transmission. Although NVP provided what had been hoped for since the very first conference in 1997—a low-cost and easily administered antiretroviral strategy—implementation in developing countries was not moving as quickly as it should have been. All too frequently, HIV-infected mothers and infants were left out of public-health priorities regarding the HIV/AIDS epidemic.

The conference was memorable for a number of reasons, some of which were anticipated and some of which were not under the control of the conference organizers. Of all the complications and unexpected events, the most extreme by far occurred in the middle of the conference. I was sitting in my hotel room planning for the next sessions when Lucy Felicissimo, the conference planner, knocked on the door and said, "You had better turn on the television." Each channel was filled with the vivid pictures of the September 11 terrorist attack, which played over and over again throughout the day. Although I had the unfortunate task of announcing the tragedy to the conference participants, many had already learned about it; it was indeed a somber conference opening the next morning. There were decisions to be made about how to proceed, so I called together the conference organizers. Clearly there would be problems with conference delegates and participants returning to their own countries, and the question of whether it was appropriate to finish the conference arose. It turned out that there were not many other options. Airports rapidly closed, and it was almost impossible for the majority of the participants to find alternative transportation to their home countries in the next twenty-four hours. When I asked some of the conference organizers for their suggestions and comments, I was moved by Professor Mmiro, who pleaded for understanding and compassion for those who were affected by the terrorist attack, and by conference participants from outside the United States, who acknowledged that terrorism was not confined to their own countries but could occur even in the richest country in the world.

After September 11, the conference continued, much more subdued, with conference-goers now even more focused on the importance of individual lives and on saving the lives of infants and women who were living obscurely in remote regions of the world and seemingly ignored by public-health programs. It was all the more fitting, then, that a new Call to Action was initiated at the conference and signed by more than eight hundred individuals from fifty-two different countries. The Call to Action broadened the global challenge and called for countrywide implementation of HIV treatment and prevention. For the first time, a Call to Action for treatment of HIV-infected mothers and children was issued, reflecting the conference delegates' consensus that it was no longer ethical to withhold treatment from HIV-infected women by providing ARVs to the mothers solely for the benefit of their infants (Rosenfield and Figdor 2001). ARVs need to be given to the HIV-infected mothers for their own health as well. In spite of the consensus expressed in the Call to Action, WHO, national ministries of health, and US government-supported research grants would turn a deaf ear and continue to recommend treatment regimens that would neither control HIV progression to AIDS nor dramatically reduce perinatal HIV transmission.

PREVENTION OF MOTHER-TO-CHILD HIV TRANSMISSION PLUS

The champion for treating HIV-infected pregnant women with ART just as health-care professionals were treating all HIV-infected men and women was Dean Allan Rosenfield (Myer et al. 2005; Rosenfield and Figdor 2001). He was a longtime advocate for women's and infants' health. Rosenfield was an obstetrician by training but had assumed the deanship of the Mailman School of Public Health at Columbia University in New York City. Throughout the conference and in special sessions, he pointed out that it was not ethical to neglect the treatment of mothers and focus solely on infants. He proposed a new terminology: "prevention of mother-to-child HIV transmission plus," which was meant to call attention to the fact that one should not view the mother simply as a vehicle for bearing an infant—the international health community also needed to focus on the health of the mother.

Rosenfield was correct—adding prevention of mother-to-child HIV transmission plus to the advocacy issues addressed at the international conference was appropriate. In fact, it was recognized that preserving the health of the mother would also preserve her ability to care for her children and provide the financial support that families were often totally dependent on. Prevention of mother-to-child HIV transmission plus became one of the slogans carried back to the United States after the conference. But it did not remain a mere slogan; it was put into action by Rosenfield and Wafaa El-Sadr, a professor at Columbia who was aggressive in bringing standard of care to HIV-infected women at Harlem Hospital in New York City. El-Sadr attended the conference and presented the case for prevention of mother-to-child HIV transmission plus. Her presentation to the conference delegates provided a compassionate and scientifically well-reasoned approach to why HIV-infected women did not deserve to be excluded from treatment. Taking the lead in demonstrating more could and was being done to address the care and prevention of HIV-infected women and children, Rosenfield and the Rockefeller Foundation announced that they were jointly spearheading an initiative to obtain $100 million to move forward with the prevention of mother-to-child HIV transmission plus program. At the time of the conference, they had already obtained commitments for $60 million.

By all standards, the conference was again viewed as an immense success. More than one thousand individuals from developed and developing countries gathered and formed concrete plans for prevention. Eight health ministers or their representatives attended the conference, and more than 150 individuals from forty-four countries were selected for scholarships. With more than 75 percent of the delegates from developing countries, the conference placed the emphasis where it was most needed—where the epidemic was accelerating at an unacceptable rate. Conference organizers were sensitive to the lack of infrastructure in many of the delivery sites where conference delegates practiced medicine. Many delegates from low-income countries felt that distributing information to their coworkers in the traditional paper format was difficult. This, of course, was 2001, and the Internet and portable memory devices were just becoming more widely available. Global Strategies introduced a new approach to distributing information, used for the first time at the Uganda conference. All of the conference presentations, the abstracts, guidelines, practice methods, drug availability, and doses were placed on CD-ROM by the dedicated staff at UCSF's Center for HIV Information (CHI). These could be copied and provided not only to conference participants but also to their coworkers in their country of origin. More than five thousand pages of HIV information were thereby distributed to assist in education and training.

Involving women in the conference was essential to giving them a greater voice in the epidemic, and indeed some 120 women participated in major portions of the conference as well as in a "Focus on Women" satellite meeting organized by US activists Emily Bass, Angela Garcia, Greg Gonsalves, and Anne-Christine d'Adesky. At the closing ceremony, Faith Spicer Akiki stood up to represent the entire community of women at the conference. She delivered a moving and forceful declaration calling for greater acknowledgement of women and their participation in the HIV/AIDS epidemic. The declaration was subsequently published in the *British Medical Journal* (Akiki 2002). It was the first time HIV-infected women, without academic degrees, had been published in a medical journal and given an international forum in which to voice their concerns.

Given the history of presenting awards at the Global Strategies international conferences, it was appropriate that the tradition should continue, but on this particular occasion, all of the award recipients were from low-income countries whose ministers and ministries of public health had demonstrated that they were committed to moving forward with implementation of the research successes that had proven effective in preventing HIV transmission. Among the countries acknowledged was Brazil, an early leader in recognizing that perinatal HIV testing should be integrated into prenatal care and that "HIV testing is the right of women to protect their babies from AIDS." (França-Junior, Calazans, and Zucchi 2008). By 2001, ZDV was already being provided free of charge in Brazil for all HIV-infected mothers and infants. Brazil also provided infant formula along with safe water so that infants did not need to be breastfed, eliminating the potential for HIV transmission through breastfeeding. Brazil had also shown leadership in challenging pharmaceutical companies to develop pricing structures that would make life-saving drugs available in poor countries (Ford et al. 2007).

A recognition award was also given to the Ministry of Public Health in Thailand, where a study had first been performed demonstrating that an abbreviated course of ZDV in non-breastfeeding mothers could reduce HIV transmission by 50 percent (Mock et al. 1999). Similar to Brazil, Thailand was in the process of implementing a nation-wide education and training program and providing ZDV and formula for HIV-infected mothers and their infants.

The third recognition award went to Botswana, a country with one of the highest rates of HIV infection in Africa. Undaunted, the country health-care leaders encouraged basic and clinical research, and in 1999 they initiated one of the first programs in Africa to directly address HIV prevention from mothers to infants. Their ministry of health also initiated prophylaxis with co-trimoxazole (CTX) to prevent opportunistic infections in HIV-infected individuals. It was noted that Botswana's standard of care contrasted sharply with the regressive treatment recommendations distributed by WHO, which refused to recommend this inexpensive, life-saving, prophylactic approach to preventing secondary infections in HIV-infected individuals despite evidence of its effectiveness. The cost of CTX was less than six dollars for daily treatment of one person for an entire year. By implementing this treatment early, Botswana delayed the progression of HIV to AIDS in thousands of people and subsequently reduced mortality from opportunistic infections and malaria.

The closing session of the 2001 conference was perhaps one of the most important held during any of the three international conferences. The participants had been given extensive knowledge about implementing measures to prevent HIV transmission from mothers to infants and how to treat HIV-infected mothers, and they were convinced of the need to return to their home countries armed with the knowledge, tools, and ability to train additional health-care workers. The moving declaration made by the community women added to the feeling that this was about paying attention to the needs of women and children who had a limited voice in the vast international community but were being affected by HIV in a manner that seemed inequitable and unjust.

A UNIQUE CLOSING CEREMONY

The closing ceremony for the 2001 conference was the most somber that I had participated in during the entire HIV/AIDS epidemic. The dual tragedies—one immediate and resulting in three thousand deaths from terrorist attacks in the United States, the other relentless and far-reaching, causing over four thousand deaths each day from HIV—seemed both worlds apart as well as the same; each focused on the value inherent in individual life.

The chairs of the closing session were Philippa Musoke Mudido and Helene Gayle. Mudido was one of the lead investigators in the HIVNET 012 NVP perinatal HIV prevention clinical study (Guay et al. 1999). She lived daily with the often overwhelming HIV/AIDS epidemic in Uganda, where she worked tirelessly to reduce the number of women who were infected and who, without treatment, could transmit HIV to their infants. Gayle was originally a leader in HIV prevention at the CDC and then at the

Bill and Melinda Gates Foundation, one of the largest non-government providers of funds for international health. Mudido and Gayle introduced the speakers who followed: Suniti Solomon, who had fought well-entrenched government bureaucracies in India and established an NGO that engaged community responses to the HIV/AIDS epidemic; Catherine Wilfert from EGPAF, who presented the exciting progress that the Call to Action had made since the 1999 Global Strategies conference in Montreal; Doreen Mulenga from UNICEF, who presented the realistic challenges and opportunities for future perinatal HIV prevention; and Francis Mmiro, the energetic Ugandan obstetrician who co-chaired the conference with me and championed conducting perinatal HIV-prevention studies in Africa. Given the dramatic events of September 11 that highlighted the value of human life, each speaker, chosen in advance, now had an added and special responsibility, and the momentum to prevent fatal HIV infection took on a new sense of urgency.

As conference co-chair, I had one last opportunity to provide a final challenge to the conference participants. I thought carefully about what I would say and felt it had to be something dramatic. One of the most important messages to impart was that individuals caring for HIV-infected patients needed to lead the charge for change and that they should not be held back from using what was already available to save the lives of women and infants. Those who attended the conference now had all of the information and tools necessary to go into action and establish programs to prevent perinatal HIV infection in their own countries, hospitals, and clinics. But I was well aware that unnecessary obstacles were already emerging that might slow progress. Therefore, I needed to not only present theoretical possibilities but also demonstrate how perinatal HIV prevention programs could be immediately and practically implemented.

I had prepared a PowerPoint picture of a doll that I had wrapped in red tape. It was the first slide that I used when speaking to the over one thousand conference participants at the closing ceremony and was accompanied with a warning that all those at the conference needed to guard against needless and unwarranted obstacles that could prevent clinicians from doing what they considered to be their ethical and moral responsibility—use the most potent ARVs available to prevent and treat HIV infection. They needed to move quickly with what they had learned at the conference. At that point, I paused in my presentation and asked Natasha Martin to open a suitcase filled with NVP that lay on a table in front of the podium. "We can and must act quickly," I said, and then I invited those in the audience who could use NVP for their patients to come and take what they needed. All that was required was that they report back their experiences. Predictably, some in the audience were angered; they had missed the point. Perinatal HIV prevention needed to be implemented rapidly, not just discussed, by cutting thorough the red tape. Perhaps those who were offended were threatened by their own loss of control. Indeed, in the years following the conference, in spite of an ongoing uncontrolled HIV epidemic in their own country, they betrayed their previous commitment to providing the best ART to women and infants by claiming, in spite of the opinion of HIV experts, that treating all women and children was not the right thing to do (Coutsoudis et al. 2013).

Individuals did report back to me—Charles Kilewo at the Muhimbili Medical Center in Dar es Salaam, Tanzania, reported that he had used the NVP to initiate perinatal HIV prevention in his clinic. With government approval, he went on to participate in a large clinical trial using cART that resulted in one of the lowest HIV-transmission rates reported at that time (Leroy et al. 2005). Twins in Malawi received single-dose NVP and were spared from HIV infection. Clinics unable to access ARVs from their governments used their NVP to demonstrate that perinatal HIV prevention could begin with simple and careful approaches to prevention (Institute for Global Health and Infectious Diseases 2015).[2]

The conference ended with optimism and hope, but perhaps somewhat prophetically, for many the journey home to their countries of origin was difficult. The September 11 terrorist attack had closed the United States to entry for everyone, including US citizens, and had complicated air travel everywhere. Getting back to San Francisco for me was only accomplished by trading or buying tickets, no matter what airline, at each airport on the way home, whether in Belgium or England or Canada. Adding to the difficulties, just before the closing ceremony, I received a telephone call that my wife had been hospitalized following complications from breast-cancer treatment, and on the long way home I began to experience pain in my back from a kidney stone. But during the days that it took to return home, there was plenty of time to think about what was next in the struggle to end the pediatric AIDS epidemic.

SAVING THE LIVES OF INFANTS FOR ONE DOLLAR

When I finally reached home, my wife was out of the hospital, and my kidney stone had passed. Waiting for me was an encouraging letter from a former student who had selected Global Strategies for HIV Prevention for a fundraiser. Robert Frascino and his partner Steve Natterstad, both physicians and both talented pianists, were conducting fundraising concerts along with Barbara Nissman, a professional classical pianist. At the conclusion of the concert, an auction was held with "bids" on saving infants' lives from HIV. The auctioneer bellowed out, "Who will bid ten dollars to save ten infant lives, one hundred dollars to save one hundred infant lives, one thousand dollars to save one thousand infant lives?" At the time of the fundraiser, NVP costs had fallen to one dollar for both the mother and infant doses. The funds raised from the benefit concert allowed Global Strategies for HIV Prevention to continue providing HIV testing and single-dose NVP to clinics and hospitals around the world. It also established a long-term relationship with the Frascino Foundation, which continued to provide much-needed financial support for more than a decade for more advanced HIV prevention and treatment.

GLOBAL STRATEGIES' NEXT STEPS: IDENTIFYING THE MOST NEGLECTED

Establishing HIV prevention and treatment programs in low-income countries is admittedly difficult. But establishing them in remote rural and politically unstable areas of the world is even more difficult. Why do it? There are compassionate reasons that motivate us, but I also believe that the spread of HIV (and the Ebola virus and, even more recently, the Zika virus) instruct us that some of the biggest threats to global health originate in these very same regions. Believing that we can eradicate an infectious disease epidemic without paying attention to prevention and treatment in these regions is somewhat naïve. Global Strategies made a deliberate decision to focus on areas often neglected by larger international organizations, realizing their potential to act as reservoirs for the spread of HIV.

As international attention to the HIV/AIDS epidemic increased, there was fortunately a concomitant increase in funding for programs to address HIV prevention and treatment in low-income countries. However, analyzing what was becoming more than a trend, I observed that most of the funding was going to programs affiliated with universities in urban areas with direct access to large international organizations and where trained health-care professionals had the required skills to fill out complex and lengthy grant applications. Often, sophisticated computer programs and access to high-speed Internet were required just to get started on the complex application process. Perhaps most discouraging was that much of the funding had to go through the national government, which happened to take a share of the funds in the process. One could travel just several hours outside a major African city—Nairobi, Kampala, Johannesburg, Durban—and find villages and clinics filled with HIV-infected individuals where diagnosis, prevention, and treatment were not being conducted. How could they access the advances that had been made in HIV prevention and care?

AMPLIFICATION THROUGH EDUCATION AND TRAINING

Back in California, Marilyn, Natasha, and I discussed what should be done following the 2001 international conference in Kampala, Uganda. In spite of pleas from many of the health-care professionals from low-income countries to continue the Global Strategies for the Prevention of HIV Transmission from Mothers to Infants conferences, held every other year, we knew that international conferences had a way of getting larger, more expensive, and losing focus. We decided that the new approach for Global Strategies for HIV Prevention would be to conduct HIV-prevention training and education workshops in neglected rural areas in regions that had strategic importance. At the same time, we would continue our advocacy to keep HIV prevention in women and children at the forefront of health and political agendas. Fully cognizant of the fact that we could not, with our small organization, resolve all of the many issues of a massive HIV/AIDS epidemic, we decided to focus on regions that were not benefiting from the medical advances in HIV that had been effective in slowing the epidemic in income-rich countries. One of the first of these was the Dominican Republic, where we focused specifically on the needs of the Haitians who resided in that country.

A VISION FOR THE HEALTH OF THE PEOPLE
OF THE DOMINICAN REPUBLIC

The Dominican Republic (DR), with a population estimated at just less than nine million people, is located on the island of Hispaniola in the West Indies and is bordered by Haiti. Its government became democratic after the 1961 assassination of dictator Rafael Trujillo. Following the end of Trujillo's regime, the DR experienced economic instability as its economic base shifted from sugar plantations to one driven by tourism.

HIV seroprevalence in the DR was the highest among low-income groups, which included many Haitian immigrants living in rural communities and working in sugarcane plantations. Although the government was aware of this, as is often the case, the DR political leaders responded by creating government commissions and committees instead of directly addressing the epidemic through treatment and prevention. Among the many committees was the Presidential Commission for HIV/AIDS (COPRESIDA), which reported directly to the president and was responsible for coordinating the fight against the epidemic. COPRESIDA was comprised of public, private, and community-based organizations to address HIV on multiple levels—social, economic, and cultural—with an emphasis on prevention of perinatal HIV transmission. Characteristically, many government-initiated endeavors were frequently interrupted by changes in government administration. Almost every election resulted in reassignment of new individuals to government positions, many as political favors rather than based on expertise. What was desperately needed was an individual, independent of the government, who could provide the advocacy and leadership to identify the greatest needs for HIV prevention and treatment and who could work closely with the groups most severely affected by HIV.

Filling this role was Dr. Eddy Perez-Then, an enthusiastic and charismatic pediatrician working at the Hospital Infantil Robert Reid Cabral in Santo Domingo. He had the ability to work with the government as well as the community. Many of those affected by HIV were Haitians who resided in the Bateyes within the DR. The approximately 220 Bateyes were isolated areas attached to the old sugarcane plantations and populated almost exclusively by Haitian migrant workers and/or descendants of Haitian migrant workers. The majority of the Bateyes' population lacked accesses to hospitals/clinics, basic health care, basic hygiene, clean water, and sanitation. As industry in the DR shifted away from sugar cane to tourism, the situation in the Bateyes became increasingly desperate (Perez-Then et al. 2003).

Although the DR is considered an income-poor country, the health care available to its citizens is superior to that of individuals living in the Bateyes, where infant mortality rates are much higher than in the rest of the country, due mainly to lack of prenatal care. Infants and children often suffer from parasitic diseases and malnutrition. Diarrhea remains one of the main causes of infant deaths, most frequently in children under two. Fewer than 30 percent of the children in the Bateyes receive immunizations, which helps explain some of the outbreaks of polio and other preventable diseases that have been seen in the region (Rathe and Moline 2011). Perez-Then had drafted his own plans—sort of an early version of universal health care—for the DR and clearly understood that he needed to work outside the government. That said, he also appreciated the need to include government agencies as he moved forward. He definitely wanted to include the people residing in Bateyes, where HIV seroprevalence was the highest.

In June 2000, Global Strategies began a series of workshops in the DR under the leadership of Eddy Perez-Then. Working with the National Research Center on Maternal and Child Health (CENISMI), Perez-Then had outlined a strategy for improving the health of the individuals who lived in the Bateyes. Under Perez-Then's leadership, tangible progress was seen after each workshop, representing his ability to specifically define the needs of the Haitian population and always including them in group discussions to solicit their ideas. I was often moved by the Haitians' repeated frustration—"We have groups with lots of money coming through the Bateyes all the time talking about what they want to do for us, but years later nothing has changed."

During one of the "breakout" workshop sessions, the participants listed their priorities for action. It was a good lesson on why aid organizations, no matter who they are or how much funding they have, need to listen to what the people identify as their needs. Number one on their list was not HIV, TB, malaria, poverty, or education, although those all appeared somewhere on the priority lists. Number one was provision of identification cards, which the government had promised to those born in the DR but had yet to provide. These cards would give them access to health care, education, and the jobs that they needed.

Perez-Then also understood that HIV was an entry into the health-care system and that integration of HIV into maternal-child health and other diseases was essential. He organized sessions that addressed the issues of TB, HIV, dengue fever, and malaria, all of which were important in reducing maternal and infant mortality and improving overall health. I personally learned the importance of integrating health care. Although I was at a workshop on malaria and TB, and speaking on the subject of HIV, I had neglected to take my malaria prophylaxis. The DR was such a short distance from Miami, about a two-hour airplane flight, that I thought I could get away with skipping the medicine. During one of the workshops, I even took a photograph of a pool of water with hatching mosquito larvae to show to students when I got back to the United States. Two weeks after my return I began to experience shaking chills, severe nausea, and dehydration and required hospitalization—I was infected with malaria. A lesson well learned: "Physician, heal thyself."

While the goal of the workshops was to initiate HIV education and training for the Bateyes, Perez-Then was also committed to using the workshops to improve the health care of all Dominicans. He was masterful at listening to the poorest with the greatest needs and then effectively working with the government. It was a model of action that had great potential, and it worked. Beginning with meager resources and early assistance from Global Strategies, Perez-Then successfully introduced perinatal HIV prevention to the majority of Dominicans, never losing sight of the need to integrate HIV care with maternal child health to reduce maternal and infant mortality overall. The progress made in the DR was an outcome of identifying a committed leader, providing beginning resources, education, and training, and allowing the ownership and expansion of a health program to be in the hands of indigenous leadership. With time, Eddy Perez-Then expanded his vision to become a global health leader and epidemiologist in his own country and beyond (Perez-Then et al. 2003; Lorenzo et al. 2012).

THE IMPORTANCE OF BEGINNING: JOS, NIGERIA

Early in the morning of May 15, 2003, I received a phone call from Cori Stern. She had been on assignment in Nigeria for *National Geographic* when she came across Faith Alive, a clinic in Jos, Nigeria, under the direction of Dr. Chris Isichei and his wife, Mercy, a surgeon. There she found Dr. Isichei dealing with the overwhelming problems of HIV in a region of Nigeria where the estimated HIV seroprevalence was more than 20 percent. The clinic and hospital operated on meager funds and infrastructure—Chris saw HIV-infected patients without charging any fees, working throughout the day into the early morning hours. Their income was derived from Mercy's fees for surgery from those patients who could pay. Stern learned that in spite of the high HIV seroprevalence, especially among pregnant women, there was no program to prevent perinatal HIV transmission. As soon as her plane landed on her return to Los Angeles, she googled

"HIV treatment and pregnancy" and found the Global Strategies website offering a donation program for single-dose NVP and HIV rapid tests.

During a subsequent phone conversation, Cori and I discussed the needs of Faith Alive and concluded that a basic training program was needed on HIV prevention and care that could serve patients in Jos and also reach out into the rural areas where traditional birth attendants (TBAs) were the only resource for delivering infants, more than 25 percent of whom were becoming HIV infected. The question was, could they be trained to provide HIV testing and single-dose NVP? (Later single-dose NVP would be replaced with cART.) It was a somewhat risky proposal. Within the HIV community of clinicians, many felt that birth attendants would not be capable of carrying out perinatal HIV prevention, and training illiterate birth attendants was out of the question. But Chris and I had greater confidence. As a pediatrician, I knew that mothers, perhaps even more than some physicians, knew how to take care of their own infants and children and had no difficulty in administering complex antibiotics for the treatment of pediatric infections. Our plans moved quickly. Between May and August 2003, emails went back and forth between San Francisco, Los Angeles, and Faith Alive. It was decided that Dr. Isichei would come to the United States to organize a workshop on HIV prevention and care, define the required educational needs, and determine who should attend the workshop and how single-dose NVP and HIV rapid tests could be shipped to Nigeria.

Dr. Isichei arrived in California on September 13, 2003. Within days he was sitting in my backyard in San Rafael, California, huddled in a fleece jacket in spite of the warm weather, not yet having become accustomed to the temperature differences between Jos and San Francisco. Seated on a wooden bench, Chris, Cori, and I hammered out a workshop program, identified the presenters, determined how many birth attendants and health-care workers should attend the workshop, where it should be located, how it would be funded, and how the much-needed NVP and HIV rapid tests could be obtained. They were encouraged and optimistic that much could be accomplished through initiating a perinatal HIV-prevention program in a region where HIV infected almost one out of five pregnant women.

Cori was an organizer with multiple contacts throughout the United States, including a cadre of young and energetic individuals who she felt would be interested in traveling to Nigeria, helping with the workshop, and perhaps even raising their own funds for travel and expenses as well as funds to underwrite the workshop. The individuals who responded with surprising enthusiasm were an eclectic mix: a marketing executive, a technical writer, a movie producer, a minister, an interior designer, a furniture designer, a fashion executive, an actor, a travel health specialist, an insurance specialist, a PhD laboratory scientist, a screenwriter, and three energetic women from Bayside Church in Sacramento, which had donated more than $150,000 for prevention of perinatal HIV infection that year. For many of the volunteers, it was their first trip to Africa, and for others, their first trip to an impoverished region of Africa.

In March 2004, twelve volunteers and I landed in Abuja, Nigeria's capital, where we were met by Chris and several vans that would transport everyone to Jos and the people's homes where each volunteer was staying. Even before leaving the airport, the volunteers experienced some of the difficulties in traveling to impoverished areas. One of the vans wouldn't start, and Chris had to negotiate on the spot with the driver of an ancient

Cadillac that didn't look any more promising than the van. At last we were on our way to Jos, but additional difficulties were in store for us. There happened to be an election taking place in the region of Nigeria where the workshop was being conducted, which brought out "bandits" along the highway looking for bribes. These bandits brought vehicles to a halt by placing strips of wood with protruding metal spikes across the road. Chris was adamant about not paying bribes, and at one of the many roadblocks, I looked in the rearview mirror to see a highly animated Dr. Isichei arguing with several bandits who had been plied with enough alcohol to influence their vote (and their judgment). I was worried about Chris, but I became even more concerned when one of the men walked up to my side of the van brandishing a two-by-four board studded with nails. The man knocked on the window, asked me to roll it down, and then asked if we were the volunteers from America who had come to Nigeria to help people with HIV. I looked directly at the man, who seemed to be heavily intoxicated and perhaps even on drugs, and quietly replied, "Yes." The "bandit," clearly having been embarrassed by Chris during the confrontation, then asked, "When you get back to the United States, can you tell them we are good people?" Fortunately, everyone arrived safely in Jos, fatigued and ready to spend a night of rest with a local family.

The opening of the workshop was inspiring. In one room, there were fifty-eight traditional birth attendants, more than originally planned for, but it was difficult to say no to any of them when the need to prevent perinatal HIV transmission was so desperate. Within minutes of the workshop introductions, volunteers were treated to the Nigerian style of opening workshops—words of encouragement, usually from biblical scriptures, singing, and music, with all workshop attendees participating whether Christian, Muslim, or any other religion. The workshop continued for four more days. The participants were attentive and brimming with questions in a mix of Pidgin English, traditional English, and Hausa, and they seemingly did not want the workshop to end. The entire group of birth attendants eagerly listened to animated presentations, participated in play acting, and even practiced getting blood samples from finger sticks to learn how to perform HIV testing. On one occasion, I glanced out to the parking lot and saw a circle of birth attendants, all wearing latex gloves and performing HIV testing under the watchful eyes of Dr. Chip Shepherd, a Global Strategies board member and HIV scientist whom I had known throughout the HIV/AIDS epidemic. I was certain that this was the first time that Shepherd had conducted a classroom in a parking lot.

The workshop ended with the distribution of certificates of attendance, much treasured by the birth attendants, and a "Doc in a Box," containing copies of workshop presentations; instructions for voluntary HIV counseling and testing; information on prevention of perinatal HIV transmission, administration of CTX, and PEP; simplified records for documenting patient results; single-dose NVP tablets and liquid; CTX tablets; screening and confirmatory HIV rapid tests; and training modules that had been developed by the Center for HIV Information at the UCSF Medical Center (HIVInSite 2016).

In a seeming crescendo of enthusiasm, the workshop concluded with the voices of the newly trained birth attendants singing, praying, and giving speeches of gratefulness for the group of volunteers who had traveled from America to help them meet their need to prevent HIV infection. As the birth attendants began to depart, I was concerned about how they would manage to take their Doc in a Box with them as they returned to their villages; some had traveled more than twenty hours to get their training. I need not have worried—the women hoisted the boxes into the air, placed them on their heads, and joyfully danced as they began their journey home. It was a memory that would not be forgotten by any of the volunteers or by me.

As part of the training, Chris was intent on motivating the birth attendants to develop specific action plans and an associated timeline to be implemented on returning to their communities. During the workshop, Chris was carefully observing and listening to the birth attendants and selecting those who appeared to have leadership abilities. He was realistic about the training, realizing that it was only a beginning but one that could result in traditional birth attendants carrying out implementation of single-dose NVP for perinatal HIV transmission in their villages. Not all of them would be successful, but those whom he selected would be asked to return to Faith Alive to receive additional intensive training by a Faith Alive-appointed coordinator responsible for providing follow-up, record keeping, quality assurance, and ongoing education.

From a Small Beginning to Major Prevention and Care Programs

17

SENDING PRECIOUS DRUGS INTO UNSTABLE REGIONS AND WAR ZONES

The immediate outcome of the Faith Alive workshop in Nigeria was encouraging, but it was even more encouraging to observe what happened over the next several years. The model Global Strategies had employed to identify indigenous leaders was confirmed, and providing training and the tools to begin HIV prevention and care could be multiplied with additional resources beyond what Global Strategies had initially established.

In the first year following the workshop, ten of the traditional birth attendants received extended training and went on to perform voluntary counseling and HIV testing for more than two thousand patients in their communities. Also, within a year of the Global Strategies workshop, Dr. Isichei was able to use the data that had been accumulated from the trained health-care workers' endeavors to successfully apply for and receive funds from the US President's Emergency Plan for AIDS Relief (PEPFAR) (Nigeria was a designated PEPFAR country). Three months after receiving PEPFAR funds and ARVs, more than fifteen hundred HIV-infected men and women were recruited for treatment. Six years after the workshop, Isichei and his staff at Faith Alive were seeing more than nine thousand HIV-infected patients each month, providing them with HAART in a new hospital and clinic facility that had been designed, funded, and completed in 2006 by volunteers from the Bayside Church in Sacramento, California.

Rather than allowing HIV-infected individuals to languish until complex interventions could be implemented, beginning HIV prevention and care, even in the most adverse circumstances, was an essential step to Faith Alive's eventual success. The first step required the courage and trust that was part of Global Strategies' mission. The workshop in Jos, Nigeria, had been a concrete demonstration that infrastructure-poor regions, too often neglected in the "big picture" of the HIV/AIDS epidemic by much larger organizations, could successfully take modest beginnings and simple but highly effective interventions and use them to jumpstart and transform HIV-prevention programs into much larger and sustainable efforts.

There were also important lessons learned by each of the volunteers. During their time in Jos, each of them lived with families who were deeply involved in the

HIV/AIDS epidemic. They visited schools for orphans, spoke with widows who were infected with HIV, met with sexually abused young girls, and mingled with families that had experienced the premature death of mothers, fathers, and children. Initially strangers, the volunteers were allowed to enter into the lives of those affected by the HIV/AIDS epidemic to learn about their pain and suffering. They found that those they met had no choice in becoming infected—it was an epidemic that had descended on them and engulfed their daily lives.

With time, the workshop training extended beyond Nigeria's borders. Isichei and four of his coworkers even traveled to Buduburam, a Liberian refugee camp in Ghana, to assist in a training workshop for fifty health-care workers residing there. I will never forget Isichei's comment to his co-workers: "We must find a way to help these people; we have so much more than they do."

SENDING SCARCE DRUGS TO LIBERIA

When Dr. Chudy Nduaka from the United States contacted Global Strategies in 2003 to ask if it could provide ARVs for a program in Liberia, it was clear that granting the request would be difficult. Charles Taylor, the dictator president of Liberia, had lost almost all legitimacy, driven the countryside into rebellion, and precipitated the complete collapse of the country's social services. Faced with this situation, some humanitarian organizations decided not to send funds or medicines to the country. Yet, Global Strategies felt that the HIV-infected pregnant women in Liberia deserved as much help as those in any other country and therefore decided to respond, even while questioning what could be accomplished with the political uncertainties and confusion. To ensure the safe arrival of the NVP and rapid HIV-test kits, supplies were sent through contacts in neighboring Ivory Coast, who then moved the supplies to a clinic in Liberia. Thus began the first program in Liberia to prevent the transmission of HIV from mothers to their children.

A small West African country of three million people, Liberia was much in the news at the time, for unfortunate reasons. Originally founded as a refuge for freed African slaves, Liberia was now seeking refuge for its current residents from the country's interminable civil war and political chaos. Exhausted by war and in desperate need of humanitarian aid to meet basic needs, they pleaded for help from the outside world. The person seeking help to prevent HIV transmission—another consequence of the Liberian war—was Dr. Lily Sanvee, a surgeon at St. Joseph's Hospital in Monrovia.

A month after the supplies from Global Strategies arrived in Liberia, the fighting escalated. The news media contacted me to ask if supplying NVP for pregnant women to prevent HIV infection should have the same priority as supplying other drugs. Would Global Strategies continue to support an HIV-prevention program in the middle of a war zone? (The implication was that this was a luxury).[1] I responded with an explanation in the September 2003 *Global Strategies* newsletter:

> It is easier for individuals to understand things that are immediately seen—the terrible wounds of war. What are less visible are the long-term consequences. In many wars in developing countries, more people, especially women, will ultimately die from HIV infection than the immediate impact of war. It is still

vital that a balance be maintained in caring for both short-term and long-term victims. As troops invade, women and young girls are often raped. Those who flee to refugee camps often suffer similar injustices. Many women who are raped become pregnant and contract HIV from their attackers. Without medical intervention, many of their children will become HIV-infected as well. HIV is a kind of viral land mine left behind by invading troops. Its impact smolders for years. There are no second chances with HIV. Once the virus is transmitted from an HIV-infected mother to her infant, the infant is infected for life, and no amount of treatment can eradicate the infection.

My point was that something could be done to prevent the devastation of HIV. In addition to caring for the wounded, sheltering the displaced, and feeding the hungry, it was vital to save a future generation of Liberians from unnecessary suffering and early death.

Dr. Lily Sanvee was the defender of St. Joseph's Hospital in Monrovia, preventing its destruction by rebel forces through face-to-face confrontations. Sanvee was born into a family of twelve children, which explained, perhaps, why she was so tenacious in her goals. Following the successful completion of her basic education, Dr. Sanvee was accepted on a full scholarship to a medical school in Spain less than a week before classes began. She arrived in Spain with little money and unable to speak Spanish. Undeterred, she completed her medical studies and decided to return to Liberia. The brutal civil war under Charles Taylor drove Dr. Sanvee out of Liberia, but she eventually returned to care for her patients and to rebuild St. Joseph's Hospital and clinics. When she returned to Liberia, she discovered that she had lost her home, her land, and all of her personal possessions. That did not prevent her from completing her mission to provide health care for the poor of Monrovia.

As a survivor of the war years in Liberia, Dr. Sanvee lived with the hope and dreams of providing all HIV-infected women and children with lifesaving drugs. She spoke enthusiastically about this to Liberia's President Ellen Johnson-Sirleaf, Africa's first woman president. In the many years of conducting HIV prevention and care workshops at St. Joseph's with Dr. Sanvee, I realized that I had the great privilege of working with one of the distinguished and powerful women who led that country into freedom and advocated for justice and equity. One need only read the story presented by Leymah Gbowee, winner of the 2011 Nobel Peace Prize, in her book *Mighty Be Our Powers: How Sisterhood, Prayer, and Sex Changed a Nation at War*, to realize the political power of the women of Liberia (Gbowee 2011).

BRINGING HIV EDUCATION AND TRAINING TO A REFUGEE CAMP

Cori Stern was on the move again. She alerted Global Strategies of an opportunity to provide training on HIV prevention and care in a very different location than that of previous workshops. During the reign of Charles Taylor, there was a mass exodus of many Liberians across the borders to adjacent countries. Under the guidance of the UN High Commission on Refugees (UNHCR), certain countries agreed to host the refugees in camps on a temporary basis. One of the refugee camps, called Buduburam, was located not far from Accra, the capital of Ghana. Cori had been travelling through different parts of Africa and came upon the Buduburam refugee camp with some six thousand Liberian refugees in a semi-permanent state. It was quickly apparent that HIV and other STIs were a definite problem. Buduburam resident Reuben Gboweh, a bright and energetic Liberian with a history degree, was interested in what could be done on HIV prevention and care. After I spoke with Reuben, Global Strategies decided that a workshop would be an appropriate means to train health-care and community workers in the refugee camp along with the local hospital staff.

Because Dr. Chris Isichei from Faith Alive in Jos, Nigeria, had gained so much experience in education and training for HIV prevention and care following the 2004 workshop, I invited Isichei and his staff to take the lead in the 2005 Buduburam refugee camp workshop. Isichei brought with him Daniel Ossom, Sunday Obri, Ruth Garba, and Rita Wakili, all highly experienced individuals who were implementing HIV-prevention programs at Faith Alive. When the Buduburam workshop started, they were still painting the building where the workshop was held, an indication of the pride the refugees felt in conducting the workshop within the camp. The enthusiasm of the refugee community was encouraging, and it was exciting to see the leadership of individuals who had only several years before gone through the same process of learning about how to perform HIV counseling and testing and implementing methods to prevent HIV transmission from infected mothers to their infants. It was precisely the model that many working in HIV envision, often referred to as "train the trainer," but in this instance, training and education were provided in highly disadvantaged settings typically ignored by many organizations.

Isichei loved teaching and did so in a highly animated style. He had incredible eye contact and the ability to wander in and around the workshop participants eliciting questions as well as answers. He told the participants about the myths that surround HIV and sometimes result in denying its existence or fostering stigma and discrimination. Africans are fond of play-acting and are especially appreciative when individuals from other countries participate. The Liberians were delighted when I agreed to play the role of the infant tested for HIV, especially when, following the "finger stick," I imitated a crying infant.

Before we began planning the workshop in Buduburam, several logistical obstacles occurred that almost derailed the entire project. I had travelled to Accra several days before only to find that all of the printed materials were held up in customs. I found the customs officers sitting on boxes of the "Facts and Myths" booklet, which included cartoons about HIV and was very popular among the African participants as well as a good instruction tool for workshop participants to learn about HIV counseling, testing, and HIV transmission. Although Ghana had accepted the Liberian refugees, there was much ill will between the Ghanaian residents and the refugees based on the belief that the refugees were getting special treatment. One way to make the refugees' lives more difficult was to hold up anything in customs that was for their benefit, especially educational material. After several hours of negotiation, the booklets were released for use in the workshop. I hoped that during the delay everyone at the customs offices had taken the opportunity to read the booklet on HIV/AIDS.

The second obstacle came as a complete surprise but should have been anticipated. The UNHCR country director of the refugee camp had heard about the workshop and was concerned about what would be taught. She was about to call a halt to the workshop. An urgent meeting was held, and after an explanation was given, including the credentials of those teaching and attending, she realized the importance of the workshop, especially with increased rates of HIV and other STIs being observed. The turnaround was somewhat remarkable—on the workshop's opening day, the UNHCR refugee camp director provided words of welcome, stayed throughout most of the workshop, and expressed her appreciation for bringing a team of teachers and community health-care workers to Buduburam to address some of their urgent health-care issues. The workshop was a go. Each morning ten adults responsible for teaching at the workshop crowded into one van for the two- to three-hour drive to Buduburam.

As with many of the workshops conducted by Global Strategies, there was a special earnestness and eagerness to learn. Individuals in the community stood at the doorway and open windows, spilling into the meeting room to listen to the presentations. The eagerness was infectious, and additional individuals from within the refugee camp began attending. But, it was one thing to talk about what was needed and how to implement perinatal HIV transmission and quite a different thing for the Liberians in the refugee camp to gain access to ARVs and HIV testing, even though they were only a few miles from Accra, where HIV prevention and ART were available.

A final obstacle emerged at the conclusion of the workshop. Although the community health-care workers, nurses, and physicians at the refugee camp had been fully trained and were capable of performing HIV testing and administration of ART, when the Ghanaian Ministry of Health heard that individuals in the refugee camp were going to administer HIV treatment, even though they were trained nurses and doctors, it resisted, saying that it could not be done by individuals in a refugee camp but only by Ghanaians in Accra's hospitals. This was an unrealistic and vindictive attempt to exclude the refugees from HIV prevention and treatment. The refugee camp was miles from the hospital and at almost any time during the day the road was cluttered with cars and construction, sometimes resulting in four-hour delays before reaching the hospital. That would make it virtually impossible for a woman in labor to travel to the hospital to receive treatment and care.

Although the roadblock introduced by the Ghanaian government could be neither understood nor justified, in many ways it represented the same paternalistic attitude toward African countries that had been introduced to the implementation of perinatal HIV transmission by developed countries, especially the United States. This attitude implied that only an HIV expert could do HIV testing and administer treatment for HIV. And since there were a finite number of HIV experts in the entire world, this meant that the majority of HIV-infected individuals would have to forgo receiving life-saving treatment. The obvious paradox was that, worldwide, mothers were entrusted to give even more complex antibiotics to their infants for other infections, including otitis media, bronchitis, pneumonia, malaria, and TB.

I was particularly troubled about what appeared to be the demeaning attitude not just to Liberians but to African women in general. As a pediatrician who had for decades entrusted mothers to successfully administer antibiotics at home for the treatment of severe and chronic diseases in their infants and children, I felt that African women had been stereotyped as being less capable of caring for their infants—perhaps reminiscent of the US Agency for International Development (USAID) Administrator Andrew Natsios' comment that ART would not be practical in Africa because, "Africans don't know what Western time is . . . and many people in Africa have never seen a clock or a watch their entire lives."

During the Buduburam workshop, as well as in other workshops, it was often easy to identify those who would emerge as leaders moving forward HIV prevention and care programs in their own communities and even in their own countries. One such person was Rueben Gboweh, who continued his efforts to make a difference among his displaced people long after the workshop ended. On his own initiative, he summarized the material that was presented at the workshop, asked for a small amount of funding to have the workshop results printed, and then distributed it to key individuals on his return to Liberia. He realized the importance of documenting what was and was not available to combat the HIV/AIDS epidemic in Liberia and, again on his own, traveled throughout Liberia visiting hospitals and clinics in remote areas, generating a report detailing what resources were left after the devastation of Charles Taylor's reign. In the years that followed, Reuben continued working with the Liberian government, including the National AIDS Control Council, providing direction and the energy that was needed to keep the HIV prevention and treatment agenda moving.

A tangible piece of evidence that the Buduburam workshop had been successful occurred when I visited St. Joseph's Hospital in Monrovia in 2011. Dr. Sanvee was taking my coworkers and me through the hospital, and I was asked to see a baby who had just been born and was about to receive NVP to prevent the infant from becoming infected. As I looked at the nurse, I recognized her as one of the community health-care workers from the Buduburam refugee camp who had returned to Liberia and was now employed by St. Joseph's to perform prevention of perinatal HIV transmission.

Liberia's countrywide HIV prevention and treatment program had progressed significantly from its initial stages and the shipment of NVP from Global Strategies to Dr. Sanvee during Charles Taylor's reign. Once peace had been introduced following Taylor's ouster, attention could be directed to reconstructing health-care delivery, establishing a National AIDS Control Program, and developing national HIV prevention and treatment guidelines by partnering with large international organizations that, along with the Liberian government, could provide sustaining funds. Leaders within the government, such as Minister of Health Dr. Walter Gwenigale, who always welcomed me and my coworkers and had also endured Charles Taylor's reign of terror, were committed to seeing HIV come under control and Liberia having the ability to provide HIV prevention and care for all of its citizens.

INTO THE HEART OF DARKNESS

In 2003, Ted Ruel, a pediatric resident from the UCSF Medical Center (now a professor of pediatrics at UCSF), was looking for a clinical project in Africa. He had a close friend working in Rwanda who helped set up a project for health assessment of imprisoned adolescents. While there, he received a call from Lyn Lusi who, along with her husband Dr. Joe Lusi, an orthopedic surgeon, was the primary force behind getting medical assistance to Goma, in the eastern Democratic Republic of Congo (DRC), which had been ravaged by decades of fighting by rebel forces and devastated by the 2002 volcanic eruption of Mt. Nyiragongo. Their needs were desperate, and they asked Dr. Ruel to come and teach for one week before he returned to the United States. Ruel was impressed by Goma's dire situation after the volcanic eruption—the physical devastation, poverty, and lack of governmental infrastructure. But he was also impressed with the people—doctors, nurses, and health-care and community workers who continued to go to work every day even when they weren't getting paid, and the Lusis, who were clearly devoted to caring for people in the best way and by whatever means possible, using volunteers, NGOs, churches, faith-based organizations, and any other avenue available.[2]

Ruel had heard about the work that Global Strategies was doing in remote areas of Africa, and shortly after his return to the United States he called me to set up a meeting to discuss the situation at HEAL Africa in Goma. I was sitting in an office at the Center for HIV Information (CHI) at UCSF, listening to Ted Ruel relay his experiences on his travels to the eastern DRC. Ted conveyed how impressed he was with the way people were working together to rebuild the city in spite of the destruction. He was also impressed with how different religious groups were working together to care for those with HIV infection. However, they had virtually nothing to provide in the way of prevention or treatment. Ruel suggested that, in the glaring absence of any NGO or international organization, Global Strategies should visit to determine whether we would want to conduct a training and education workshop and assist in providing HIV testing, prevention, and treatment.

The DRC had a long history of death and destruction, not only from natural disasters, but also from bands of unopposed rebel armies that roamed the forests and countryside, destroying villages and killing innocent people (BBC 2014; Hochschild 1998). It is estimated that between four and six million people lost their lives from war-related deaths, diseases, and starvation in the DRC between 1998 and 2004. The Rwandan genocide directly affected eastern DRC as perpetrators of the massacre fled into the DRC to escape arrest and imprisonment. Goma, the city that Ruel had visited, was located in the province of North Kivu, one of the areas that suffered more than any other as rebels indiscriminately killed the Congolese people. Along with the killings, there were deliberate acts of physical and sexual violence against women. Often, these attacks included knowingly transmitting HIV infection in an attempt to destabilize communities. DRC politics with Rwanda, Uganda, and Burundi were complex, with some of the instability attributed to Rwanda's goal of accessing more land and other countries' desire to mine the vast mineral-rich regions of eastern DRC. The instability and lack of any formal government in eastern DRC meant that most international organizations had written it off as an area where not much could be accomplished in most areas of need, including HIV prevention and treatment. Neglecting the HIV/AIDS epidemic in the DRC was striking given that HIV was believed to have originated there and in the adjacent countries of Cameroon, Equatorial Guinea, Gabon, Congo-Brazzaville, and the Central African Republic. If HIV started in the DRC region, how could the epidemic ever be controlled without addressing its continued presence there?

THE VIOLENT HISTORY OF THE DEMOCRATIC REPUBLIC OF CONGO

The DRC's violent history goes back to colonial times, beginning in the 1800s with Belgian King Leopold II's exploitation of natural resources and enslavement of the Congolese.[3] The violence continued even after the country's independence from Belgium in 1960, with leaders such as Patrice Lumumba contributing to the ongoing instability. Over the last sixty-six years, the UN has been intermittently involved in unsuccessful peace-keeping operations. A seemingly endless parade of rebel leaders has contributed to destabilization, as they have not distinguished themselves as purveyors of peace but rather as disruptors of peace. Kasavubu, Tshombe, Mobutu, Bemba and, more recently, Kony, Bosco, and Nkunda have all contributed to the chronic instability, with surrounding African countries often facilitating rebel activity.

Following the 1994 Rwandan massacre, one million refugees that included Hutu extremists, Interhamwe militia, and deserting Rwandan military entered eastern DRC. In 1999, the UN Security Council established the largest contingency of UN troops in eastern DRC, but fighting continued between rebel and government forces. Between 1999 and 2004, various rebel groups and countries signed peace agreements with the DRC, and in 2005, a new constitution was adopted. Joseph Kabila, elected as president of the DRC in 2001, remains in power. In recent years, much of the rebel activity has ceased, but tensions remain high between Rwandan President Kagame and Kabila. Elections for president of the DRC are to be held in November, 2016, but many in the international community are concerned that Kabila will not step down.[4]

In September 2004, following Dr. Ruel's urging to establish HIV prevention and treatment programs in eastern DRC, and in spite of the region's dark history, I traveled to two locations in the DRC that looked promising as sites for working with indigenous leaders on HIV prevention and treatment—Good Samaritans Hospital in Kananga and HEAL Africa in Goma. Paul Tshihamba, originally from the DRC and now a missions pastor at Christ Presbyterian Church in Edina, Minnesota, was a critical partner in the journey. He knew the Congolese culture and spoke several of the local languages. It was he and Ruel who advocated that Global Strategies travel to the DRC. A four-hour flight was required from Goma to Kananga. The pilot of the single-engine plane was an ex-Navy pilot who was now flying individuals and groups to destinations in Africa for Missionary Aviation Fellowship. It was not a short flight, and although I didn't think to ask if a restroom were available on board, I should've known judging by its size. Three hours into the flight, I wished that I had not consumed my usual cups of extra-strong coffee before embarking. The plane carried seven passengers including the pilot. As it flew over the mountains, rivers, and forest, I was struck by the absence of roads below. Instead, I saw only small villages separated by huge areas of forest fondly referred to as "broccoli" by those flying over the terrain. Seeing the vast open spaces with the lack of transportation between cities, I began to understand why, although originating in the DRC, HIV had failed to explode there in the same manner as it had in other countries: HIV traveled with individuals going from one highly populated city to another. While more contagious viruses such as Ebola, which was first documented near the Ebola River in the DRC in 1976, were transmitted through direct individual contact and traveled from the DRC to other parts of western Africa, HIV was sexually transmitted and therefore more contained.

The first destination in Kananga was Good Samaritans Hospital, located in a remote section outside the main city. Kananga is in the Kasaï-Occidental Province in the south-central portion of the DRC. As the plane gradually descended, I couldn't help asking the pilot where the airfield was. Only when the wheels touched the ground with the propellers cutting shrubs as the plane landed did I realize that the "airfield" was merely a strip of dirt. As the Global Strategies team approached the medical facility, we could see a large amount of smoke alongside the hospital. Our immediate thought was that the smoke was related to some sort of rebel attack, but we were told that the smoke was coming from the monthly burning of outdated and unusable drugs that had been shipped to them from various organizations in wealthy countries. This reminded me of information I had read about pharmaceutical companies donating outdated drugs to low-income countries to gain corporate tax breaks. Within the hospital, the team was also shown a large room stacked to the ceiling with donated broken equipment that could not be repaired because of lack of parts or skilled technicians. After a day of assessment and an overnight stay, the Global Strategies team returned to Goma to visit with the staff of HEAL Africa, the medical facility that Ruel had originally mentioned. The logistical problems of reaching Good Samaritan Hospital, coupled with the expense involved in transporting both people and supplies to Kananga, meant that HEAL Africa in Goma would be the more logical first location for a Global Strategies program.

HEAL Africa was positioned on top of a lava flow from the Nyiragongo volcano eruption in Goma in 2002. On the hospital grounds and from the windows of the buildings it was easy to see the devastation. Rusted vehicles that had not been covered by the lava appeared as sculptures emerging from the lava flow. In spite of the volcanic eruption and the scars left from rebel activity, Goma had swelled to a population of more than one million people over several years' time. To get to the hospital, we had to travel over the lava-bed roads, often passing buildings that we thought were intact only to discover that the entire first floor was submerged under lava, and what we were seeing was actually the second floor, where businesses now conducted their activities. In the midst of desperate poverty and devastation, Dr. and Mrs. Lusi had worked to rebuild their hospital and clinic to meet the health and spiritual needs of those suffering from HIV, sexual abuse inflicted by rebels, malnutrition, and the impact of poverty. There almost seemed to be too many desperate needs in Goma, but the Global Strategies team knew we had to listen to the health-care and community workers about what they deemed were the most important. Conversations ended not with promises but with a commitment for Global Strategies to help in HIV prevention and care where we could, to advocate for the HIV/AIDS epidemic in eastern DRC, and to identify resources from whomever and wherever possible.

In February 2004, Global Strategies returned to Goma to conduct an education and training workshop and to work alongside community and health-care workers to address their desperate needs. The Global Strategies team was accompanied by a group of individuals under the leadership of Pastor Paul Tshihamba, who would just several weeks later pledge $1 million over two years for the programs of HEAL Africa and Global Strategies in Goma, which was the beginning of strengthening HEAL Africa's infrastructure. They worked with indigenous leaders and gave tangible proof to their message and belief that one can indeed make progress in HIV prevention and care, even in the most unstable regions of the world.

Despite initially limited financial resources, Global Strategies provided for HIV programs in North and South Kivu. With time, additional resources came from the Clinton Foundation, which donated the much-needed ARVs to treat HIV-infected infants and children, as well as from the Mennonite Central Committee, which purchased HIV rapid tests and two thousand doses of ARVs for PEP to prevent HIV in young girls and women who had been raped. In a period of eight years, HEAL Africa managed the largest program to care for HIV-infected and -exposed infants and children in the eastern DRC. Associations and contacts developed by Global Strategies throughout the epidemic were used to amplify programs where Global Strategies could not provide them.

The HIV prevention and care programs established by Global Strategies in the DRC had an extraordinary impact in spite of their location in a volatile and politically unstable region. Their success did not go unnoticed. In 2010, I received an email from Jacquelline Fuller at Google, asking that we apply for Google funding for Global Strategies' programs. I asked what size proposal was needed, to which Fuller replied, "Just a few pages submitted by email." I complied. A little over two weeks later, my wife Marilyn was opening the mail and found a plain envelope. I asked Marilyn to open it quickly. Inside was a check for $4 million. The "official" award statement came by email on October 27, 2010, announcing, "Based on Global Strategies for HIV Prevention's proven track record in preventing and treating HIV/AIDS, and your personal legacy of leadership and wisdom in providing care in regions such as Congo and Liberia, it is Google's intention to fund your project with $4,000,000 USD in 2010." It was signed by the 2010 Google Holiday Sales employees and was the largest health-care grant that Google had ever awarded. It was a morale boost not just for Global Strategies, but more importantly, for the many indigenous leaders in the DRC who had labored so hard over so many years under some of the most adverse circumstances: their work was being recognized. Global Strategies budgeted the $4 million over four years to strengthen and improve HIV prevention and care and to incorporate strategies to reduce infant and maternal mortality.

THE REALITY OF SEXUAL VIOLENCE IN THE DRC

The welcome news from Google tempered some of the concerns that dominated working in regions of violence, especially violence against women. I remember well when I first began to encounter the unimaginable. I had seen documentaries and read books about burning villages and unprovoked rebel attacks, but when I saw firsthand the physical and sexual violence against women I was overwhelmed. It should have been expected.

HEAL Africa in Goma was known for caring for women who had been subjected to extreme physical and sexual violence, but I had never seen an entire ward of a hospital devoted to women who had not one but multiple surgeries to try to correct vaginal and rectal fistulas caused by physical and sexual trauma. The women were housed by themselves because the odors from the draining fistulas were not tolerable to other patients. Women with fistulas in various stages of repair and disrepair congregated outside the hospital with their children. They cooked, ate, and slept together with their children, isolated from everyone else.

The problem of extreme violence against women extended from North to South Kivu. On my first visit to Bukavu in South Kivu, I met Dr. Dennis Mukwege, nominated for a Nobel Peace Prize for his efforts to quell the violence against women. His hospital, too, was noted for fistula repair. It was hard to ascertain the extent of the rapes.

"Official" numbers varied from as low as forty thousand per year in just one province to as high as one hundred thousand each year (Bartels et al. 2011). No matter the precise number, even four hundred would have been alarming enough. There are many reasons given for the widespread rapes—revenge by rebel forces; deliberate HIV infection to demoralize women, men, and their communities; lack of laws; police corruption; failure to punish perpetrators; and, the most demeaning and disturbing of all, the pervasive attitude of "that's what men do when they are deprived of sex in the forests for months at a time." Whatever the reasons for the physical and sexual violence against women, it was itself an epidemic of global proportions that, together with the HIV/AIDS epidemic, resulted in the DRC being labeled by some as the worst place for women to live.[5] For me, there were times when the physical and sexual violence seemed overwhelming and the efforts to repair and rehabilitate the women a mere token (Bartels et al. 2011; Orbinski, Beyrer, and Singh 2007). Yet, once again, whether at HEAL Africa in Goma or Panzi Hospital in Bukavu, the dedication and courage of health-care workers overcame my discouragement and provided hope that one day violence would end and people could return to their families, communities, and a life of peace.

As Global Strategies worked with indigenous leaders, we observed a component of rape that was not being fully addressed in either North or South Kivu. Although there were theoretical programs to provide PEP to women following rape, it was difficult to identify clinics or hospitals that had PEP kits containing drugs to prevent HIV infection and other STIs such as syphilis and gonorrhea, as well as unwanted pregnancy (Flexner 1998; Gerberding and Katz 1999; Kim, Martin, and Denny 2003). Curious as to why an organization the size of Global Strategies was repeatedly being asked to provide PEP kits, I tried to track down the organizations that I knew had received funding to provide PEP. They were either nowhere to be found or they were not fulfilling their obligations to distribute PEP kits even though they had received substantial funding from USAID and UNICEF. The whereabouts of the PEP kits was not known either to us or to our partners.

Even when PEP kits were available, few women who had been raped completed the entire course of drug prophylaxis. On investigation, I found that the PEP kits that were supposed to be used, or were available, contained six different drugs. The ARV in the kit had to be taken twice each day for thirty days, and it was one of the weaker ARV combination drugs. One of the antibiotics had to be taken four times a day for one week. Few women could endure the side effects of the drugs, which resulted in decreased compliance in spite of the desperate need to prevent HIV, other STIs, and unwanted pregnancy. It appeared as if the PEP kits had been designed by a committee of individuals with no firsthand experience.

I felt that Global Strategies could do better. Plans were made to streamline the PEP kits to make them more acceptable, less costly, and more available. There were four key individuals who worked to put this plan into action: Joseph Ciza, Cindy McWhorter, Dr. Givano Kashemwa, and Dr. Josh Bress. Ciza is a nurse who, armed only with a cell phone, traveled into rebel-held territory to rescue women who had been kidnapped by rebel forces. Ciza knew the circumstances surrounding rape and was aware of the lack of PEP kits, especially when rape occurred in a rural region several days away by foot from a clinic or hospital. Kashemwa is a Congolese physician and an expert in HIV prevention and treatment. We were fortunate to be able to work with him. His skills as an educator, physician, and communicator are extraordinary. McWhorter, always indefatigable and filled with compassion for the plight of the Congolese, was Global Strategies' international program director. Dr. Bress is an amazing pediatrician (he became president of Global Strategies in 2014) who spent one year in the DRC working with the indigenous health-care leaders to save the lives of infants and children, whether from HIV, birth asphyxia, sepsis, malnutrition, or the many other diseases that, year after year, establish the DRC as one of the countries with the highest infant mortality rates. Both McWhorter and Bress were committed to assisting the Congolese in their efforts to overcome what often seemed to be insurmountable obstacles to delivering life-saving health care.

Working together, Ciza, McWhorter, Kashemwa, and Bress realized that the PEP kits needed to be streamlined by reducing the number of drugs taken, using drugs that required only once-per-day dosing, and replacing outmoded medications with more potent ones, including ARVs, to prevent HIV infection. They moved quickly to compile PEP kits and to obtain resources to conduct special training workshops to teach that the medicines in the PEP kits needed to be taken within seventy-two hours following the rape. This meant that additional community health-care workers needed to be trained in rural regions and a simple mobile-phone tracking system was needed to determine where the rapes were taking place, where the medicines were located, and what supply of medicine was available at the nearest location. Undaunted by the fact that there was no simple mobile-phone system then available, McWhorter and Bress implemented a tracking system using mobile phones that could provide real-time data simultaneously in the DRC and in the United States, reporting how many rapes had occurred in what region of the DRC, whether PEP had been taken within the seventy-two-hour time limit, and how many PEP kits were available and in what locations.

There was one additional obstacle. The cost of the streamlined kit was beyond Global Strategies' resources. The ARV would need to be donated in order to make the PEP kit affordable. McWhorter, Bress, and I approached Gilead, the pharmaceutical company that manufactured some of the most potent once-daily ARVs. They not only agreed to donate their drug for PEP but also agreed to assume the anticipated shipment and customs fees and to provide additional funding for the education and training of health-care workers and the evaluation of the new PEP kit. Unlike funds from governments that are too often transient and ethereal, Gilead's provision of drugs and funds insured a continuous supply of life-saving PEP drugs for women in the DRC who had been raped.

Fully anticipating that we could rapidly provide PEP to the thousands of women who were being raped in eastern DRC, Global Strategies moved ahead with the plan to ship the drug and make it available as quickly as possible. But some had other plans. The national Congolese government, located in Kinshasa in western DRC, often considered the eastern DRC population as somehow inferior and was unsympathetic to their needs. They were not even providing the drugs listed in the outdated WHO recommendations for PEP and were now resistant to implement a newer, more effective, and much less expensive means to protect raped women from STIs and unwanted pregnancy. In all likelihood, they were also fearful of repercussions from WHO if they went against their recommendations. Thankfully, Paul Volberding at the UCSF Medical Center and

Kenneth Mayer at the Harvard School of Public Health Beth Israel Deaconess Medical Center in Boston, both renowned international experts on HIV prevention and treatment, agreed to provide their expert opinions. Armed with the most up-to-date evidence provided by Volberding and Mayer on the use of ARVs to prevent HIV infection, Givano Kashemwa journeyed to Kinshasa to "gently" persuade government officials to approve the streamlined PEP kit. Kashemwa's success confirmed the benefits and necessity of working with indigenous leaders.

One additional obstacle emerged that resulted in a delay of almost one year before the life-saving PEP kits could be delivered. The drug donation from Gilead arrived on time at the customs offices. Rather than extracting a "normal" customs fee, Kashemwa was told that $150,000 was being charged. The customs officials clearly knew the value of the drug and were attempting to extract a bribe—Global Strategies refused to pay bribes. The customs office was fully aware that the ARVs were desperately needed to prevent HIV infection following rape. Global Strategies was confronted with a dreadful ethical dilemma reminiscent of *Sophie's Choice*: holding up the drugs would mean that thousands of women might become HIV-infected, acquire other STIs, and become pregnant. In addition, the clock began to tick on the drugs' expiration dates. But succumbing to a bribe would mean that there would be no end to the payments extracted on future shipments. There was no choice but to resist until fortunately, at last, the customs office relented.

During my visits to Goma and Bukavu, I wondered how our collaborators, and now friends, in the DRC could survive the tragedies that were a part of their daily lives. They rarely spoke in emotional terms, perhaps to protect themselves from succumbing to being immobilized by the extent of the problem. Why would they stay in the DRC under such difficult circumstances, risking their lives and the lives of their families? This was the lesson I would learn—that in some of the most dangerous and unstable regions of the world, there are those who remain to help. It was also a lesson on why so many international programs fail. I witnessed the flight of international aid organizations when rebel activity increased or when rebel troops invaded regions of the eastern DRC. Those who remained were committed to the Congolese people, whom they could not bear to abandon even under the most difficult of circumstances. I observed that those who stayed were most often individuals from faith-based groups who were committed to partnering with the Congolese, whose sufferings were immense.

DEEPER INTO THE HEART OF DARKNESS

The Congolese were protective of those who worked with Global Strategies, but there were times when individuals like Ciza, who experienced some of the worst consequences of rebel activity, did not understand the long-lasting impact that it might have on others. Ciza and Dr. William Bonane asked me to travel with them into a region north of Goma to visit potential new clinic sites. Bonane had identified them as clinics where perinatal HIV prevention could be introduced. His hard work would continue for many years, and later we sponsored him to obtain a degree in public health, launching him as a credible leader in eastern DRC heath care.

The journey with Ciza and Bonane would forever alter my feelings about violence against innocent people. We started our journey from Goma, eastern Congo, early in the morning. Ciza, who had traveled to our planned destination many times to assist victims of rebel activity, said that that the region had been declared safe by UN security forces the evening before our departure. As an added measure of security, we were to travel in an ambulance with a conspicuous red cross on the side. We were also strongly advised that we should return before dark. Our goal was to reach a hospital and four clinics located in several small villages in the province of Rutshuru, a region situated between the volcanic mountains that border Rwanda and Virunga National Park in Congo. Years before, the area was host to the escaping Interahamwe, the militia formed by the Hutu ethnic majority of Rwanda. Together with the smaller Impuzamugambi and state army and police forces, they were responsible for more than 800,000 deaths in the Rwandan genocide of 1994 (Mandelbaum-Schmid 2004).

Ciza told us many stories about this region. Now he said that the people and health-care workers who lived there had asked that he return with training and medicines to begin HIV testing and treatment and care for HIV-infected pregnant women to protect their babies from becoming infected. We knew in advance that HIV was not their only concern. There were other pressing needs—shelter, food, and safety. But even in the midst of all these needs, HIV was seen as disrupting entire communities and taking away their future generation.

Our four-wheel-drive ambulance, initially traveling at thirty miles per hour, often stalled as we bumped and sometimes slid our way over half-gravel, half-mud roads climbing up into the recesses of the mountains. Our first stop was to see where a village had been two years before. Swept away by a lava flow, it was a symbol reminding us that we were entering an unstable area. Indeed, as we continued we witnessed the suffering of the people living in one of the most beautiful and seemingly peaceful mountain areas of the Congo. At our next stop, we knocked on the steel gates of the UN compound to let them know we were in the region. (The fact that no one answered was a bit unsettling.) We drove on and soon reached the first of four clinics that we were to visit during the next twenty-four hours. Thus began a drama that repeated itself at each stop, but with a changing cast and diminishing props.

The first clinic had been ravaged by the rebels. A male nurse and regional physician were there waiting for us (thanks to cell phones). On the rough table before us were a calculator and neatly arranged records containing data on the number of patients seen, how many were pregnant women, how many babies had been delivered, and an estimation of how many individuals might be HIV infected. We walked to where the counseling room would be (chairs would be needed), then to a dimly lit room where the HIV tests would be performed (better lighting would be required), and then to the room where the ARVs and antibiotics would be secured (the empty shelves would need to be filled with medicines). We returned to talk about how many nurses would need to be trained. Somewhat shyly, the nurse asked if we could provide financial support for four nurses. I asked how much that might be and braced myself for the reply. Thirty US dollars per month for each nurse—a total of less than $1,500 for the entire year. Simultaneously, I felt relieved at the small amount and embarrassed that I had even asked.

As we left the clinic, I was jolted by one of many paradoxes that unfolded. We were told that the Interahamwe had been at the clinic just one hour before we arrived. They had heard that we were coming (cell phone again) and wanted to be certain that their wives would also be tested and receive treatment if HIV infected. It was then, early in the journey, when I realized that we were not there to judge but to bring hope and healing to everyone.

As we proceeded along the road, I saw a pile of ashes in front of us. The driver drove over the smoldering remnants as I wondered why a fire would be built in the middle of the road. I glanced at the back of the ambulance and saw Ciza elbowing Bonane. Looking at me, he asked, "Do you know what that was?" When I answered, "No," they told me that it was the remains of two thieves that the rebels had caught, immediately sentencing them to being burned to death. Farther up the road we drove over several more smoldering piles of ashes, some still glowing from the night before. As we proceeded, we noticed an increasing number of rebels standing in the bushes, all heavily armed and watching us as we moved further north.

We drove farther into the mountains, visiting another clinic sparser than the first. Just before the Ugandan border, we turned "left" and entered the Virunga National Park. At first I thought Ciza had forgotten the purpose of our journey and wanted me to see the park's beauty, but I soon realized that we were on our way to the farthest clinic, bordering Lake Edward across from Uganda. As the warm breeze from the savanna blew through the open window, I thought how strange it was to be driving through this vast national park in an ambulance searching for those who needed care and compassion.

We reached our destination at dusk. The clinic appeared as suddenly from behind the trees as did the wild animals from behind the tall grasses. Nyakakoma was a fishing village to which HIV had been carried by Ugandan fisherman who derived a single night of pleasure from young women trading sex for food. The fishermen left more than food—they left behind a disease that would forever change those young women's lives. A disease that, without treatment, would cause their death. The nurse who greeted us smiled out of politeness, but I knew from the numbers on the chalkboard behind her that the epidemic was in full force.

On our way back, the sun was disappearing behind the mountains that border the Rift Valley and the park. We now traveled in the dark, never knowing what animal might decide to cross the road. It became obvious that, despite the warnings to leave before nightfall, we would need to stay overnight. We visited one more clinic, meeting the health-care workers and reviewing the records by the flicker of kerosene lamps.

I was now hungry and thirsty. Five of us had shared one loaf of bread and a bottle of water each the entire day. When at last we turned off the road, we entered the gates of the monastery where we would spend the night. I wondered how it had survived the rebel years. The monks, whom I never saw, had prepared a meal for us that we devoured by flashlight. I welcomed the bed and the mosquito net that covered it, even though I had no change of clothes or overnight supplies (I would have said overnight necessities, but since I survived without them, I can't really say they were necessities). As the sun rose, the proverbial rooster crowed, and I began to hear the deep and vibrating voices of Congolese monks chanting their morning prayers. Yet another paradox in this rebel-torn region: the chants enveloped my mind with an overwhelming sense that the new day would bring peace.

Leaving without breakfast, we stumbled into the ambulance and made one more stop at a hospital that had been built by Italians but abandoned during the rebel fighting.

It was now managed by Congolese health-care workers. The first sign I saw was printed with the name of the hospital, "Nyamilima," beside a symbol indicating that automatic rifles were not allowed inside. Despite the early hour, we were once again greeted by health-care workers pleading for assistance. I watched as we walked through the hospital wards, crowded with patients getting dressed and preparing their own food. They smiled at us in spite of it all.

Our return to Goma was emotional. Like the hard drive of a computer that has reached its capacity and groans before shutting down, I occasionally closed my eyes, no longer able to watch the constant stream of people struggling alongside the road. Their march was repeated every morning of every day—children the age of my grandchildren, seemingly hidden under the stacks of wood on their backs; women of who-knows-what age, wrinkled and bent like arbors from sacks of flour; men pushing stacks of sugar cane that stretched across the road as they struggled up the mountain on homemade wooden bikes; the lone man with one leg withered from polio who pushed an equally heavy load; a village of perhaps one thousand, set on top of a mud field where people lived in what resembled play houses made of torn canvas and sticks—they had become instantaneous refugees after their entire village was burned to the ground. When the road narrowed, we drove slowly past barely moving columns of women and children, so close that I could reach out and touch their faces, and, somewhere within me, I wished I could. How many of these were HIV infected, and when would the infection sap away their remaining strength and end their ability to care for their families?

As we entered Goma, I was relieved that we had made the journey safely. Strangely, after those twenty-four hours I felt no despair. I actually felt hopeful. I understood how people could live day-to-day with suffering and at the same time maintain hope. I, too, understood justice coupled with forgiveness. The children of the Interahamwe were as in need of protection from HIV as the children of the oppressed. Ciza knew that and so did the health-care workers and the doctors. Compassion, they realized, should have no political boundaries. Therefore, I felt sure that the first program for prevention of HIV transmission from mothers to infants in a rebel-dominated area of the eastern DRC would bring hope to tens of thousands of pregnant women each year, many of whom were already HIV-infected. It was a courageous step for those who would be doing the training, performing the HIV testing, and providing the medicines. Their belief in these people's value would be an encouragement for others to bring additional resources. Subsequently, as I reflected on my journey to the DRC, I did not feel hopeless. Instead, I remembered the perinatal HIV prevention programs in which I saw Dr. Bonane functioning in the midst of heavily armed rebels; the health-care worker who waited patiently in the clinic by the edge of Lake Edward; the faces of those refugees who daily marched along the road; the orphaned children—all these images are a reminder that we must never forget the suffering of those we cannot immediately see.

Looking back at the DRC programs during our decade of engagement, the words "conflict, hope, progress" sum up what transpired. In spite of increasing political instability, programs were successfully initiated that brought HIV prevention and care to tens of thousands of women and infants in eastern DRC, one of the most neglected regions of the world. It happened by investing in indigenous leaders who understood the obstacles and overcame them through dedication and hard work. During the most difficult years, much larger organizations such as UNICEF and USAID abandoned their programs due to unsafe conditions. Global Strategies continued to invest in indigenous leadership and even expanded the reach of its programs into rural regions, incorporating low-cost, high-impact, easy-to-use technology for monitoring patients, tracking drug supplies, and obtaining data to substantiate that the programs were working. Collaborations were formed with the Clinton Foundation to obtain the much-needed ARVs. The presence of Global Strategies brought increased numbers of volunteers—nurses, doctors, educators, engineers, architects, teachers, pastors, and palliative care workers—who, in turn, brought hope and skills to health-care workers and the embattled patients. Importantly, as people in the United States heard the success stories, they were willing to invest. Donations came from compassionate individuals, churches, and sympathetic foundations such as the Schmidt Family Foundation, the Caerus Family Foundation, Google, the Robert James Frascino Foundation, the Clinton Foundation, and the foundations of sympathetic pharmaceutical companies such as Gilead Sciences.

Why Wait? Start Now

18

ADVOCACY: THE LIFE-BLOOD OF PROGRESS AND OVERCOMING INDIFFERENCE

One of Global Strategies' many strengths was its ability to identify issues that slowed progress in expanding HIV prevention and treatment in neglected geographic regions and populations. Unencumbered by conflicts of interest or control by institutions or governments and armed with an ability to make rapid adjustments and changes to meet urgent needs, Global Strategies could move quickly to implement pilot programs, test them for effectiveness, and then advocate for strengthening and expanding successful approaches.

One example was the "Save a Life Program" initiated by Global Strategies in 2002.[1] Despite the exciting results of the HIVNET 052 NVP clinical research study in Uganda that demonstrated a 50 percent reduction in HIV transmission with an inexpensive and easy-to-use ARV intervention, the bureaucracies of ministries of health, WHO, and UNAIDS, along with increasing intrusions by academic researchers, took a simple intervention that could have been rapidly employed and made it sufficiently complex so that its implementation was delayed (Carr and Cooper 1996; Check 2005; IMPAACT 2015; Lallemant et al. 2000; Petra Study Team 2002). Global Strategies intervened by making donations of NVP and rapid HIV tests with simplified applications available on the Internet. The applications were reviewed quickly, and drug and HIV test donations were provided within months. Lack of funds was not an excuse for delaying implementation. The cost of NVP for both the mother and the infant was less than one dollar, and the cost of rapid HIV testing was less than two dollars.

The Save a Life donation program was not meant to be a sustaining program but rather one that could get a clinical program started and provide the basic tools for perinatal HIV prevention. It was intended to save lives but also to provoke ministries of health and larger organizations into action and remove excuses for delays. Within two years, seventy hospitals and clinics in eighteen countries had received sufficient NVP and HIV rapid tests for more than fifty thousand HIV-infected pregnant women and their infants. During that time, many hospitals and clinics were still waiting for resources from their health ministries or from some of the large international organizations such as WHO and UNAIDS.

The program was not without controversy. Dr. Costa Gazi, working in one of the poorest regions of South Africa, provided health care to women and children with HIV infection. Because of the complex political nature of the South African government, it was difficult for Dr. Gazi to openly provide ARVs. For Gazi, it became an ethical issue as to how long lifesaving drugs could be withheld. South Africa's new post-apartheid president, Thabo Mbeki, did not help the situation, because he had adopted the HIV denialists' stance. Gazi's own personal journey had included imprisonment by the apartheid regime for three years, and now he was being threatened by the current government for his use of ARVs to prevent perinatal HIV transmission.[2] In spite of the risk, Global Strategies provided Gazi with enough NVP and HIV rapid tests to treat 750 HIV-infected pregnant women and their infants.

DON'T NEGLECT LOW SEROPREVALENCE COUNTRIES WITH LARGE POPULATIONS

China was a country where advocacy was needed to get the national government to officially recognize that they were facing an impending HIV/AIDS epidemic (Ammann 2000a). My first visit to China was in 1998 at the invitation of Dr. Yunzhen Cao and the Chinese Academy of Sciences in Beijing. Cao and I knew one another from when we worked together on the Ariel Project, studying factors that determined perinatal HIV transmission. Cao lived through the repression of Communist leader Mao Zedong's Cultural Revolution, during which time she was prevented from obtaining an advanced education or going to medical school. The government sent her to a rural region of China with limited to no access to education. Eventually she succeeded in her aspirations, graduating from medical school in China and immigrating to the United States in 1986.

Cao's work in HIV began when she was invited to New York University. While working in the laboratory of Dr. Friedman-Kien, a well-known AIDS investigator, she first described the detection of antibody to HIV in the urine of infected patients. Four years later, she began working with David Ho at the Aaron Diamond AIDS Research Center in New York City. But she never forgot her homeland and was intent on working with public-health officials in China to address the emerging HIV/AIDS epidemic there.

China's population, the largest of any nation, stood at 1.4 billion; the country is home to more than 22 percent of the world's people. Yet it was not getting the attention that it deserved in the global HIV/AIDS epidemic for a number of reasons—the political tension between China and the US Congress was great, the HIV seroprevalence was considered low, the actual number of individuals infected with HIV was uncertain, and the Chinese government itself was resistant to acknowledging that the number of HIV infections was increasing.

The first individual with AIDS in China was reported in 1985 (Settle 2003). For the following three years, HIV infection was sporadically reported in small numbers—individuals who were either "foreigners," according to Chinese officials, or overseas Chinese. The government used the occurrence of HIV in foreigners to emphasize the "decadence" of other cultures, especially the United States. Rapid spread of HIV began in 1995 and continued with an estimated cumulative number of 300,000 HIV infections by 2000. The largest number of cases was in Yunan Province (southern China), followed by Xinjiang (northern China). The seroprevalence of HIV was particularly high in Xinjiang, which bordered Russia, Mongolia, Kazakhstan, Kyrgyzstan, Tajikistan, Afghanistan, Pakistan, and India. The dominant ethnic group in Xinjiang is the Uyghurs, who also had a high rate of intravenous drug use and needle sharing. In 2000, intravenous drug users accounted for 67 percent of HIV cases, but individuals came from all occupations, including laborers, private businessmen, commercial blood donors, and farmers. The latter were often referred to as "floating farmers" because they moved from rural to urban areas and back again and accounted for some of the spread of HIV across China (Solinger 1999).

A sobering account of the spread of HIV by blood donation and transfusion was reported in 2001 from Henan Province, where blood donation stations had been located for the manufacture of blood derived products (Settle 2003). (I had reported the documentation of HIV transmission by blood transfusion in 1982.) Unfortunately, it was a common practice to reuse needles and re-inject red blood cells into donors following plasma separation so that donors could keep giving blood. This was unheard of in almost all countries throughout the world, as such practices spread hepatitis and HIV (Yin et al. 2003). The practice almost assured that any infectious agent, including HIV, would be transmitted to the plasma donors. Tens of thousands of donor farmers and peasants were infected with HIV. Although the blood donation stations were closed down in 1995, a government cover-up ensued. On August 23, 2001, the Chinese government finally admitted that perhaps as many as thirty thousand to fifty thousand Chinese people who had participated in the donation program were likely infected with HIV (Settle 2003; Yin et al. 2003).

Compared with other high infection areas of the world, the total HIV-infection rate in China was relatively low. Nonetheless, because of China's vast territory and large population, the potential for spread of HIV had to be taken seriously. On my first visit to the Chinese Academy of Sciences in Beijing in 1998, I felt it was my responsibility, based on my having observed firsthand the expansion of the AIDS epidemic from a small number of individuals in 1981 to millions across the world within a short period of time, to warn them that HIV had taken hold in China and had the potential to spread quickly throughout the country (Ammann 2000a; Watanabe 1999).

Meeting in a fairly ordinary conference room, public-health leaders from the Chinese Academy of Sciences listened attentively as I pointed out that the major risk factors for spreading HIV were present—a recent increase in STIs that previously had been under control for decades, an increase in intravenous drug use, the occurrence of HIV in blood-transfusion recipients, and the population's increased mobility. I suggested that the recent increase in TB might also be related to HIV as a consequence of the HIV-induced immunodeficiency that made individuals more susceptible to TB (Gray and Cohn 2013). Interestingly, senior Chinese physicians denied that HIV was present in the new cases of TB or that patients with HIV had an increased incidence of TB, but later that day, several of the younger physicians, unwilling to contradict their seniors during the meeting, told me that they had indeed seen a dramatic increase in the number of patients co-infected with HIV and TB.

To illustrate where the HIV/AIDS epidemic might be headed in China, I showed several graphs I had constructed that demonstrated where the HIV/AIDS epidemic had been in the mid-1980s in the United States and in Africa, and the subsequent exponential increase in infections over the period of several decades. I then overlaid a second graph on the first, showing where HIV in China stood in 1998 and where it might be ten years later if measures were not taken to introduce strong HIV-prevention and treatment programs. I ended by saying, "With a strong investment in resources and a well-defined strategy, China could become the first developing country to avert an escalation of the HIV/AIDS epidemic to the proportions currently observed in Africa and India." I wasn't certain how my presentation would be received, but my Chinese hosts were cordial and appreciative, and at the end of my first visit they presented me with an honorary degree from the Chinese Academy of Science.

By 1999, it was obvious that HIV was expanding to almost every country in the world, whether it was being reported officially or unofficially. There was a special concern for countries with large populations, such as India and China. American relationships with China were not good in 1999, and while there were reports of an expanding epidemic, there was no simple way of finding out the details of what was happening without inviting Chinese officials to the United States. It was clear that there were pockets of rapidly expanding infection, and in a country with a population of over one billion individuals and extreme poverty, there was concern that China could become the new "Africa." A US congressional hearing seemed in order, but I soon found that setting it up and inviting guests from China were not easy tasks. I spoke to several organizations as well as the NIH, asking if they would share responsibility in sponsoring a delegation from the Chinese Academy of Sciences and if they would assist in getting clearance from the US government. No one was willing to take on the task, citing all kinds of governmental obstacles.

Finally, completely frustrated from rules, red tape, and bureaucracy, I (perhaps naïvely) decided to plan a congressional hearing on my own. Fortunately, my good friend Congressman James McDermott was sympathetic to the issues and, indeed, felt it was important to address the growing HIV epidemic in China. Congressman McDermott had personally witnessed the rapid expansion of HIV from a handful of patients in South Africa to a massive epidemic and had reported his observations to a somewhat indifferent US Congress. Global Strategies went forward with plans for the presentations, sent invitations to key leaders from the Chinese Academy of Sciences, made arrangements for payment of travel expenses and accommodations, and, on March 24, 1999, a congressional briefing on HIV in China was held.[3] Once it was announced, individuals and organizations that previously had refused to help came out of the woodwork asking to attend. Many even had the effrontery to request time to speak about their organization's interest in HIV in China. Both NIAID Director Anthony Fauci and Congressman McDermott recognized the importance of addressing the emerging HIV/AIDS epidemic in China and did as much as they could to draw attention to the issues that confronted the populous country. Following comments by Congressman McDermott, I provided the following introductory statement:

> It would be the height of public-health foolishness not to assist China with what we know is inevitable. We watched as Africa was overwhelmed by HIV. The epidemiological evidence is clear. Unopposed, additional tens of millions

of individuals could be added to this international HIV/AIDS epidemic. I would argue that if we have responded to natural calamities and circumstances that threaten far fewer individuals, then morally, we must respond to the HIV/AIDS epidemic in China at this time. There are two objectives for this briefing. 1) To present the status of the HIV/AIDS epidemic in China; 2) To convince you that, with adequate resources, China, with a population of 1.4 billion, could be the first developing nation to avert a new HIV/AIDS epidemic.

I then introduced the four visiting scientists from the Chinese National Academy. When it came his turn to speak, Ke-an Wang, president of the Chinese Academy of Preventive Medicine, a soft-spoken professional of youthful appearance, stated that in spite of the Chinese Ministry of Health being downsized, the Academy of Preventive Medicine "was approved to be set up, so it's a very rare situation, and it's a symbol of the central government paying attention to HIV and AIDS prevention in China," which was welcome news.

During the next several days, I escorted the visiting Chinese scientists from the moderately priced Capitol Suites Hotel conveniently located within walking distance of the House of Representatives Longworth Office Building to various places, including the Washington Metro and the NIH. On the second day, one of the scientists, somewhat shyly, said to me that usually when they visited other countries they were provided with limousine service from one location to another. I surprised even myself when I quickly stated, "I wanted all of you to experience what the real America is like and to mingle with ordinary people on the Metro going to and from work." It seemed to satisfy them and, in fact, they seemed to enjoy it.

During the months that followed the briefing, significant progress was observed between Chinese and US scientists as well as the beginning of increased availability of research funding (Watanabe 1999). On my last official visit to China, I could see that progress had been made in addressing the emerging issues of the HIV/AIDS epidemic. It was reassuring to see that the Chinese government had accepted the fact that HIV did indeed exist, even in Chinese nationals, and that there were measures that could be taken to prevent and treat HIV. I wondered how aggressive the Chinese would be in prevention of perinatal HIV transmission taking into account the one child policy—the loss of a single child in the family would mean the loss of the only child for the parents and for both sets of grandparents.

ADVOCACY BY GLOBAL STRATEGIES: A VOICE IN THE WILDERNESS

From the very beginning, in 1981 when the AIDS epidemic was first recognized and when I found the first infants with AIDS, I had known that advocacy for infants and children would be needed. Without advocacy, the plight of infants and children and their HIV-infected mothers would be lost in the much larger world of the adult AIDS epidemic. In the early years of HIV, advocacy was successfully led by highly visible individuals and foundations such as Elizabeth Glaser, the Pediatric AIDS Foundation, Mathilde Krim, amfAR, and the scientists and clinical researchers associated with these foundations. The marked influence of the Think Tank participants, coupled with my access to key scientists, congressional leaders, and government committees, extended advocacy into almost every area of public view.

As a result of advocacy, much of what had been sought after by the pediatric AIDS community had become a reality—increased funding for clinical research, increased drug approval for infants with HIV infection, recognition by the media and national and international political entities that HIV infection in infants and children was an integral part of the overall epidemic and could not be neglected, and increased calls from the activist community to bring a halt to pediatric HIV/AIDS infection.

However, by 1996 things began to change. In what seemed to be an incongruous shift in emphasis, implementation of known solutions to bring an end to the HIV/AIDS epidemic in infants and children was replaced by a greater emphasis on clinical research—almost to the exclusion of implementation. Treatment with HAART had changed the face of HIV-AIDS in wealthy countries, but the tragic delays in initiating treatment and prevention in poor countries allowed the epidemic to continue among the most disadvantaged. In this atmosphere of seeming abandonment, I realized that Global Strategies could play an essential role in advocating for the elimination of pediatric HIV/AIDS and in protecting HIV-infected women and children in low-income countries from exploitation.

The advocacy issues that Global Strategies and I identified had less to do with the need for more scientific discovery, which had by 1998 been extraordinarily successful, and more to do with justice and equity for the women and children who were part of the pediatric AIDS epidemic. Influential international organizations such as WHO and UNAIDS were creating obstacles that thwarted implementation of known HIV treatment and prevention measures. Pediatric researchers were denying that research advances applied equally to HIV-infected pregnant women and infants, unethical research studies were escaping the oversight of institutional review boards (IRBs), many of which lacked the expertise to protect vulnerable subjects from research exploitation, and clinical research participants in low-income countries were failing to obtain promised benefits from their participation. Most importantly, women and infants were not being protected from HIV infection and, when they were infected, were denied adequate treatment to prevent them from progressing to and dying from AIDS. Interventions and resources were focusing on downstream issues in women and infants, important in the short-term for those already infected with HIV, while upstream issues such as the lack of contact tracing to prevent HIV infection were ignored. There also was the need to accept the link between sexual violence against women and HIV—they both represented violent acts against women, and they needed to be addressed together to find legal, social, behavioral, and public-health solutions for how to protect women (Dunkle and Decker 2013; Jewkes et al. 2010).

One advocacy issue that Global Strategies addressed directly was the necessity of treating all HIV-infected individuals with HAART. As if living in two different worlds, I saw the HIV epidemic in the United States decrease dramatically as a result of the widespread use of HAART and HIV infection in infants virtually disappear to the point where the United States was hinting that perinatal HIV transmission had been eliminated in this country. Meanwhile, elsewhere in the world of vulnerable women and children, the HIV/AIDS epidemic continued, adding millions of infected individuals and deaths each year.

When Michel Sidibé, executive director of UNAIDS, visited San Francisco on June 20, 2012, he met briefly with a number of us who had been involved in the HIV epidemic since the discovery of AIDS in 1981. Seated at a table at San Francisco General Hospital, he asked each individual what needed to be done to end the epidemic. When my turn came, I said that I had only two words: "treat all." One month later, Global Strategies followed up with the "Treat All" campaign at the July, 2012, Nineteenth International AIDS Meeting in Washington, DC (Ammann 2012), for which we used both high- and low-tech advertising tools, including a website sign-on similar to the Durban Declaration and buttons prominently labeled "Treat All" that we distributed at the meeting. The campaign was primarily directed at the recalcitrant leadership at WHO, which in spite of recommendations from the USPHS and the sixteen thousand members of the IAS to treat all HIV-infected individuals, persisted in its refusal to change WHO guidelines to become consistent with the world's experts in HIV prevention and treatment.[4] In effect, WHO's flawed guidelines resulted in perpetuation of the HIV epidemic and condemned millions of HIV infected individuals to progression to AIDS and death.

Other advocacy issues were addressed using a combination of meetings with individuals, written commentaries and opinion pieces, communication with advocacy organizations, presentations, group meetings, conferences, and Internet publications on the website *ethicsinhealth.org*.

THE GLOBAL STRATEGIES IMPACT

There are many ways to determine an organization's impact. One is to list the accomplishments by numeric equivalents, and the other is to create a descriptive narrative of specific achievements. By both measures, I felt that Global Strategies was successful in its mission to empower communities in the most neglected areas of the world by improving the lives of women and children through health care.

In the eighteen years since Global Strategies was formed, it has raised more than $30 million to support collaborative programs, provided 125,000 women and children with ART, and, in recent years, implemented some of the first programs in low-income countries to utilize a "Treat All" with HAART approach for HIV-infected pregnant women in order to prevent HIV transmission to their infants. It has provided hundreds of thousands of HIV rapid tests in rural areas as well as over 1.2 million doses of CTX to prevent opportunistic infection in HIV-infected individuals. Through the Hope Walks program, more than two thousand children in nine orphan programs have received assistance, including ARVs for those who were HIV-infected. More than thirty HIV prevention and treatment workshops have been conducted in fourteen countries to provide education and training to more than 5,500 health-care workers. These numbers reflect interventions in neglected regions of the world and serve as proof that one need not be immobilized by seemingly overwhelming obstacles or inadequate infrastructure; there are interventions that are simple, inexpensive, and, when implemented, can begin a process of addressing much broader HIV prevention and treatment needs.

When I am asked to discusses the strengths of Global Strategies, I talk about the ability of a small organization, unencumbered by rules, regulations, politics, and bureaucracy, to move quickly into neglected and unstable regions of the world, declaring that everyone is deserving of advances in HIV prevention and care, no matter the circumstances under which they live (Bemelmans et al. 2014). Global Strategies has identified factors that are important to ensure that programs address local needs and provide universal access to HIV prevention and treatment, including the following:

1. Identifying strong indigenous leaders who are endowed with the ability to overcome local obstacles and develop strong relationships with community organizations that have the best knowledge of the health needs facing their community.
2. Investing in the professional development of indigenous leaders to increase their visibility and credibility.
3. Transferring building capacity to local health-care providers.
4. Allowing community and health-care workers to identify priorities for their local needs without imposing predefined programs.
5. Developing best practices, care models, data documentation, and resources to deliver health care.
6. Working with indigenous leaders to encourage collaboration between programs, to strengthen existing programs, and to identify future resources for self-sustainability.
7. Introducing low-cost, simple-to-use, high-impact, and sustainable technology to facilitate patient care and data documentation.

Going the Last Mile

The Obscure, the Neglected, and the Desperately Needy

19

WHAT GLOBAL STRATEGIES DISCOVERED

It was one the most remote sites to get to. Reaching Kaziba, which lay about forty miles outside the city of Bukavu in the province of South Kivu, DRC, required leaving the paved streets of Bukavu and winding up the mountains on potholed dirt roads in two four-wheel-drive vehicles of dubious reliability. Dr. Givano Kashemwa had visited more than twenty different potential sites for Global Strategies in search of partners for HIV prevention and care programs. Leslee Budge, Cindy McWhorter, and I were there to visit with the health-care workers Kashemwa had identified as potential leaders.

As we traveled up the mountains, we remarked on the beauty, the flowing rivers, the deep green forests, and the pleasant temperature. We told Kashemwa that this would be the kind of place, if it were in the United States, where people would build mountain cabins to retreat from the problems of the world. Only after we returned to Bukavu did Kashemwa tell us that the place of beauty we drove through was occupied by the much-feared Mai-Mai, formed to defend their local territory against armed groups such as Rwanda-affiliated Congolese rebels.[1] However, claiming that they were defending their own community did not prevent them from looting, robbing, or stealing cattle.

Almost at our destination, the dirt road changed from a loose, potholed gravel surface to one that was smooth and firmly packed, allowing the two vehicles to pick up speed, at least for a short period of time. Rounding a bend in the road, the lead car suddenly stopped. There before us was a monstrous haul truck, weighing at least forty tons, prominently labeled with the name of a Canadian mining company. Carefully driving around the haul truck with barely enough room to pass, we saw an elevation in the hills where there were two helicopters. Our host explained that this was a gold-mining region, and the Canadian mining company was likely under contract to the DRC government in Kinshasa. Kashemwa went on to explain that before the DRC government had "arranged" for a foreign company to mine the gold, people living the hills would walk along the streams after a rainstorm and pick up gold nuggets that provided them with an income. Now, that was illegal, in spite of rampant poverty, and anyone who violated the rules would end up in prison.

Just as abruptly as the new road began, it ended. We continued down the dirt road, and as we entered the village of Kaziba, we caught our first glimpse of brick buildings—a hospital and a school. The hospital had been established in 1922 by the Norwegian Pentecostal Church, and its work had continued until World War II, when financial help from Norway ceased. In the years that followed, widespread violence threatened the medical work, leading to a decision in 1960 to form a council of missionaries and indigenous leaders to assume responsibility for all primary schools and health care. The new organization was named CELPA, the Federation of Free Pentecostal Churches in Africa. Today the only networks operating in the region are the Protestant churches, the Catholic Church, and CELPA. Although they have trouble maintaining the hospitals and schools, they manage to keep them open and functioning, even as government structures collapse.

When Leslee, Cindy, and I met with the health-care workers at Kaziba, we quickly learned that the medical facility was devoid of almost all resources for confronting the HIV/AIDS epidemic. Pregnant women often traveled miles down the mountains to a clinic where they could be tested for HIV, but no treatment was available. An adjacent orphan program provided barely enough assistance to keep the children alive. It was obvious from looking at the orphans that they suffered from severe malnutrition and skin infections. Dr. Barhwamire LeBon from CELPA wasn't certain how many HIV-infected people relied on its hospital and clinic for care, but there were many more than it could test or treat with ARVs to improve their health and prevent the HIV-infected women's infants from becoming infected.

On the way down from the mountains and back to Bukavu, there was much discussion in both English and French about the paradoxes that we had seen. The gold-mining company was building roads and helicopter landing pads to increase the efficiency of extracting gold. They were using the human resources who were able to work for them. But neither the government of the DRC nor the Canadian gold-mining company seemed to care about those who lived around the gold mine, and the DRC government apparently did not require the Canadian gold-mining company to improve the local infrastructure of roads and schools or the health care of the people living by the gold mines. The experience confirmed my resolution to not accept a government's claim that there are insufficient funds to support health care. In most instances, the decision is based on what is deemed to be a higher priority, which usually means the government officials themselves and not the people they represent.

HIV, EBOLA VIRUS, AND VIRAL RESERVOIRS

On the way back from Kaziba, I wondered if, somewhere in the surrounding mountains we had just visited, HIV might have originated fifty or more years before.

Historians of infectious disease and epidemiologists know that microbes travel from animals to people and thereafter spread from one person to another. The origin of many epidemics can be traced back to remote areas of the world where an infectious agent "jumped" from animals to humans and then spread from human to human. There are no better examples than the HIV and Ebola virus epidemics and, more recently, the Zika virus. All three viruses are believed to have originated in Africa, and HIV and Ebola are likely to have originated in remote areas of the DRC, jumping from animal species to humans and then spreading by human-to-human contact. In the case of HIV, it was primarily through sexual contact; in the case of Ebola, it was through direct contact with secretions from infected individuals. The lessons that should be learned are that, in the world of global public health, remote and rural areas cannot be neglected without running the risk of some infectious agent getting a foothold in a mobile population and spreading, sometimes throughout the world, and all it takes to prevent the spread of a contagious disease is developing moderate infrastructure and training mid-level health-care workers to recognize the infection and learn how to prevent its spread. The consequences of ignoring "pockets" of infection in remote areas is a lesson that should not be forgotten for HIV or for the recent Ebola epidemic. Global Strategies wants to be certain that these consequences are not forgotten as it develops models to reach out, even to the "last mile." It is always easier and less costly to prevent an infection than to contain it once the infection has spread.

AN OPPORTUNITY SEIZED

After first visiting the eastern DRC in 2004, Dr. Theodore Ruel and I, both pediatricians from nonprofit organizations—International Pediatric Outreach Program (IPOP) and Global Strategies for HIV Prevention, respectively—saw war-torn eastern DRC as an opportunity to bring desperately needed health care to a neglected population. Motivated by the highly dedicated indigenous leaders who lacked even basic resources, we identified individuals within the DRC who could bring high-impact, inexpensive, and easy-to-use interventions to prevent HIV infection of infants and to reduce infant and maternal mortality. Within the decade that followed, Ruel and I worked together to support locally led programs in maternal/child health and HIV and saw a visible impact on the health of women and children in two of the most unstable provinces in eastern DRC—North Kivu and South Kivu. We learned that one need not stand back immobilized by political instability and uncertainty. Rather, we witnessed the benefits of investing in the indigenous leaders who were best equipped to develop a sustainable health-care program. In the process, we also learned a lot about refusing to abandon those in greatest need in some of the most impoverished regions of the world.

While many international organizations focus on easier-to-reach urban areas for HIV prevention and care, Global Strategies chooses to reach out to the "last mile." Our intent is to prove that these regions need not be neglected and to challenge the global public-health community by reminding them that HIV probably originated in rural regions of the DRC and surrounding countries, from whence it spread through travel and migration across Africa and worldwide. Failing to realize that these remote regions can act as ongoing "repositories of infection" almost certainly guaranteed a continuous source of HIV to replenish the HIV/AIDS epidemic (and the recurrence of the Ebola virus epidemic).

Global Strategies' philosophy is that of partnership and collaboration, rather than domination, brought about through strong indigenous leadership that can survive the most adverse circumstances. We continue to develop low-cost and highly effective models of intervention, and our mission is direct and clear: "Empower communities in the most neglected areas of the world to improve the lives of women and children through health care." Global Strategies' new chair, Anne Marie Duliege, expresses it well in the Global Strategies 2015 annual report, stating, "Our passion remains engaging with the most neglected communities in the world. Working hand-in-hand with local leaders, learning from their experience and then partnering with them to deliver innovative solutions, we continue to break new ground." The foundation's leadership and vision are in the hands of President Josh Bress and Chairwoman Anne Marie Duliege, working collectively with the board of directors, Program Coordinator Jean Armas, and Operations Manager Sloane Drake (*www.GlobalStrategies.org*). Their compassion is felt by those whom they serve in some of the poorest and most remote regions of the world, perhaps invisible to many, but very real to Global Strategies.

PART 3 Unexpected Obstacles: Institutions, Therapeutic Denialism, and Treatment Guidelines

All I maintain is that on this earth there are pestilences and there are victims, and it's up to us, so far as possible, not to join forces with the pestilences. That may sound simple to the point of childishness; I can't judge if it's simple, but I know it's true. You see, I've heard such quantities of arguments, which very nearly turned my head, and turned other people's heads enough to make them approve of murder; and they come to realize that all of our troubles spring from our failure to use plain, clear-cut language. So I resolved always to speak—and to act—quite clearly, as this was the only way setting myself on the right track. That's why I say there are pestilences and there are victims—no more than that. [Tarrou speaking to Rieux]

Albert Camus, *The Plague*

20

Pediatric AIDS and Drug Development

UNSAFE AT ANY DOSE: HIV-INFECTED CHILDREN IN NEED OF FDA-APPROVED DRUGS

The impact of AIDS activism on drug development and approval was revolutionary. For decades the FDA enforced a complex drug regulatory process that had evolved for over one hundred years to protect individuals from unsafe and ineffective drugs. But some felt that it had gone too far. As AIDS activists, many of them HIV-infected, learned about the drug approval process, they were appalled at the delays. They began attending FDA advisory meetings and asking pointed questions of FDA staff and medical consultants. Why did it take so long to get drugs approved? Why couldn't patients with potentially fatal diseases gain access to drugs before final approval? Why were the pharmaceutical companies and academic institutions not more aggressive in developing drugs for HIV infection, and why did they succumb so easily to FDA regulations? Within a short period of time, FDA regulations began to change, and new ARVs were approved in record time (HHS 1995; FDA 2014; White-Junod 2008). The story of drug approval for children was tragically different. Approval for ARVs for children was rapidly falling behind, just as it had for other drugs over the past five decades (Cohen 2003).[1]

Every drug approved by the FDA is required to go through a rigorous process of testing for dosing (pharmacokinetics), safety, and efficacy (does the drug do what it's supposed to do for a specific disease). Drug prescribing information is derived from the drug manufacturer's drug insert that accompanies the prescription or from various credible resources on the Internet or information on drug dosing in medical publications. After more than half a century of tragedies and advocacy related to the approval and use of drugs in infants and children, only about 20 percent of drugs approved by the FDA were labeled for pediatric use, forcing health-care professionals to resort to the age-old, unsafe and uncertain solution of estimating the drug dose based on studies in adults and administering the drug in "good tasting" liquids such as honey and fruit juices (White-Junod 2008; Pawar and Kumar 2002; Phelps and Rakhmanina 2011).

The history of the pediatric HIV/AIDS epidemic illustrates the problems of getting drugs approved for use in infants and children. While potent ARVs were developed and rapidly approved to treat HIV infection in adults, information to allow the same drugs to be used in infants and children was unavailable. Attempting to change the mindset of the pharmaceutical companies, the FDA, and pediatric clinical researchers in order to overcome well-identified obstacles for approval of children's ARVs seemed overwhelming. As the pediatric HIV/AIDS epidemic continued to escalate, the need for simultaneous approval of ARVs in adults and children was increasingly urgent. Paradoxically, institutions, organizations, and even pediatric AIDS investigators themselves often lost sight of their legal and moral obligations to insure rapid approval of ARVs. Anyone with the opportunity to review the multiple pieces of legislation put in place since 1994, allegedly designed and redesigned to make life-saving drugs quickly available to infants and children, would likely find themselves confused by their complexity and would perhaps conclude, as I did, that "Twenty years of legislation had failed to improve on the original FDA 1994 Pediatric Rule designed to provide infants and children with equal access to life-saving drugs" (Ammann 2016; Thaul 2012). The 1994 FDA Pediatric Rule clearly stated that separate studies of efficacy (long, complex studies which would take years to complete) where not needed in children if they had the same disease as adults. But it seemed that few in the pharmaceutical industry wanted to adhere to the rule. They worried about the liability of making drugs available for infants and children. And incredibly, few in the pediatric HIV/AIDS research community wanted to adhere to it either. To do so would mean that they would have to give up millions of dollars in research funds for studies that were not considered necessary.

The process of drug approval for children with fatal diseases came under increased scrutiny following the approval in 1987 of ZDV for use in HIV-infected adults but not for HIV-infected children. Two years later, ZDV was approved for use in HIV-infected infants and children (Kolata 1989; FDA 2011). The FDA's defense was that it had not received the required data from clinical research investigators or from Burroughs Wellcome, the manufacturer of ZDV, who had argued, without any scientific substantiation, that the disease was different in children and thus required a separate efficacy study. Unfortunately, this argument was promulgated by both the CDC in defining pediatric AIDS and by some pediatric researchers who were engaged (and funded) to conduct clinical research on HIV in children. They too, without scientific substantiation, claimed that HIV infection in children was different than in adults. It was not only a flawed decision but also one that would be lethal for tens of thousands. In contrast, those who were HIV clinical experts agreed that since HIV infection, whether in children or adults, was caused by the same virus, had the same clinical features, and, without treatment, had the same clinical outcome, there was no need to conduct additional complex clinical research studies of efficacy that would only delay access to lifesaving ARVs. The only scientifically substantiated difference between HIV infection in adults and children was that children died faster (Blanche et al. 1994; Becquet and Mofenson 2008; Violari et al. 2008; Kline and Shearer 1992). If anything, this observation should have caused everyone, including the FDA, pediatric HIV/AIDS researchers, and advocates for children and drug development, to demand more rapid approval of ARVs for children.

EXCUSES: QUESTIONABLE PROGRESS

High-level government officials and political appointees everywhere seemed to acknowledge the crisis of drug development for children. Admiral James Watkins, chairman of President Reagan's Commission on the Human Immunodeficiency Virus Epidemic, released a written report in 1988 stating, "One of the most pressing clinical trial needs is trials for pediatric patients" (Presidential Commission 1988). Why, then, if the FDA enacted special regulations for drugs to treat life-threatening illnesses, was pediatric AIDS not being included in new drug evaluation?

If HIV caused the same disease in children, and if children died even faster from HIV than adults, why not make ARVs available for infants and children at the same time as for adults? Why should lengthy clinical research trials for efficacy be conducted in children, which only served to delay the availability of ARVs? Why not just test new ARVs for safety and dosing, a process that would take only months instead of years? In media interviews, Dr. Sam Broder, director of the NCI and developer of ZDV for adults, and Dr. Phil Pizzo, director of the Pediatric Branch of the NCI who first extensively tested ZDV in children, had answers to these questions. They both argued that extensive testing of ZDV in children, other than for safety and dosing, was unnecessary (Culliton 1989; Kolata 1989; Stolberg 1997).

Broder stated, "I think the system is breaking down. We still don't have a recognized system by which ZDV can be given to sick children. I don't think that the normal pediatric clinical trial mechanisms have adequately kept pace with information emerging from adults." It was a statement severely criticizing the pediatric AIDS research community's failure to aggressively pursue the advances occurring in adult therapy. It was also a statement that remained true in the decades that followed. Referring to ZDV, Pizzo was even more blunt: "I think it's disgusting. There is enough data that this drug should be approved."[2] In fact, Pizzo's study of ZDV in children provided the data needed for eventual approval of the drug. He was able to complete the necessary studies with fewer resources and in a shorter period of time than many others in the national pediatric AIDS network's effort because he saw the suffering of children and felt the urgency to do something about it. While others offered reasons for delay, he produced the needed results.

Other prominent voices spoke out as well. Early in ZDV clinical trials in adults, Dr. Catherine Wilfert at Duke University argued that the drug approval process for children needed to be changed. Drs. Gwen Scott from Miami, Ed Connors and Jim Oleske from Newark, and Arye Rubinstein from the Bronx all repeatedly argued for rapid access to experimental and adult-approved drugs for children. Paradoxically, as funding for pediatric clinical research increased dramatically, calls for immediate approval of ARVs from pediatric clinical research investigators based solely on dosing and safety studies faded. Was it possible that a conflict of interest had arisen, even among those who had previously defended the need for infant's and children's early access to ARVs? Studies of dosing and safety in infants and children would require small studies of fewer than fifty to one hundred, while studies of efficacy would require the enrollment of thousands of children—ensuring that large sums of funding would accrue to both investigators and their academic institutions.

Also absent from the calls for immediate evaluation of new drugs for infants and children were groups that traditionally represented neglected children and advocated for child rights. The American Academy of Pediatrics, which had historically taken strong stands on issues such as physically and sexually abused children, nutrition, and immunization, was strangely silent. In addition, the Pharmaceutical Research and Manufacturers of America (PhRMA), the association that represented and lobbied for the majority of major pharmaceutical companies, voiced some of its strongest objections to requiring dosing and safety studies in children when the FDA began to indicate that it might start to require pediatric studies in order to approve drugs (Pear 1997b). PhRMA quickly distributed literature to Congress and the public claiming that pediatric studies were too costly to perform, even more costly than adult studies. I considered this argument disingenuous, as pharmaceutical companies were never prohibited from adding the cost of drug development to the ultimate price of the drug once it was approved for marketing. It is only when there is a significant public outcry about a drug price that any significant attention is paid to overpriced drugs. Even then, it is highly unusual for pharmaceutical companies to slash prices.

Another reason given by PhRMA for not performing pediatric studies was based on a deceptive ethical pretense. PhRMA claimed that it was unethical to perform studies on children, as children cannot give informed consent to participate in research studies. If taken at face value, the argument would mean that children with serious diseases would either have to be denied all drugs or that life-saving drugs would have to be administered without performing a single pediatric study for dosing or safety. This in itself would be unethical, as giving a drug to a child without adequate safety and dosing information would be the equivalent of performing an experiment on a child. Moreover, many tragic deaths had occurred when drugs of unknown safety and dosing had been administered to children (Mulhall, Louvois, and Hurley 1983; Pear 1997b).

WHERE WERE THE ACTIVISTS?

Perhaps more than any other event in the history of the FDA, the AIDS epidemic served to focus the need for urgency in reviewing and implementing specific regulations that governed the FDA drug-review process. Following the approval of ZDV in 1987, AIDS activists, always impatient with the pace of scientific progress, began to ask hard-hitting questions about HIV drug development, availability, and costs. Activists fought for compassionate-use protocols and accelerated drug development and approval, insisting that HIV-infected patients should be allowed to participate in experimental clinical trials and that drugs showing significant promise should be made available to patients even before receiving final FDA approval. The activists were initially viewed as arrogant, troublesome, and demanding, but over time this perception changed as various parties involved in the issue, including pharmaceutical companies, physicians, and the FDA, realized that they could collectively benefit from meeting the activists' demands. Whereas it had historically taken six to eight years to obtain full approval for a new drug, they were now being approved in as few as three years.[3] For each additional year that a drug was approved, the drug manufacturer stood to gain hundreds of millions of dollars in additional profits. The benefit to physicians and HIV-infected patients was that they had a greater choice of drugs available to treat HIV.

The FDA also benefited. They realized that the need to accelerate drug approvals could serve as a means to obtain increased staffing funds from Congress, and in 1992, Congress enacted the Prescription Drug User Fee Act (PDUFA), which allowed the FDA to assess a fee from pharmaceutical companies to fund the new drug-approval process

(FDA 2015). The PDUFA prompted the evolution of an accelerated drug-approval system that resulted in the largest number of new drugs approved in the shortest length of time on record.

The collective change in attitude toward drug development unquestionably brought about dramatic health benefits to tens of thousands. However, most of those individuals were adults, and the only group that continued to lose in the equation was the one that had been neglected throughout the history of new drug development—infants and children. All of the mechanisms for acceleration were focused on adult use, and it was clear that the approval process for pediatric drugs was falling farther behind. In the mid-1990s, clinical studies revealed that HIV progressed four to five times more rapidly in untreated infants than in adults, but even this revelation did not compel the FDA, the pharmaceutical companies, or the pediatric AIDS research community to focus on the urgency of approving ARVs for children.

Unfortunately, as the HIV epidemic continued, far fewer activists spoke out for rapidly approving ARVs for infants and children. But there were some who did. Bill Thorne, in a position paper written by ACT-UP San Francisco, strongly argued that children should not be excluded from access to experimental drugs. Martin Delaney from Project Inform accompanied me to Abbott Pharmaceuticals to argue for children's treatment; Greg Gonsalves, from the Treatment Action Group (TAG), and I made the case for enforcing the Pediatric Rule to the Presidential National AIDS Task Force on Drug and Vaccine Development; Mark Harrington, also from TAG, spoke up for more rapid drug approval in children at an Institute of Medicine meeting on surrogate markers (Weis and Mazade 1989).

THE FDA 1994 PEDIATRIC RULE SHOULD HAVE SOLVED THE PROBLEM

In December 1994, the FDA published its final Pediatric Rule regarding when pediatric studies were required for approval in the treatment of infants and children (FDA, Final Rule 1994). The Pediatric Rule clearly declared that separate clinical trials in children were not deemed necessary for proving efficacy, particularly for an infection like HIV that behaved identically in children and adults. There was no historical or scientific precedent to consider a virus responding to treatment differently in children versus adults. All this should have been an incentive for moving full speed ahead with the much shorter, less complicated, and less expensive pharmacokinetic and safety studies in infants and children without the need for considerably larger and more expensive efficacy studies that would delay the availability of lifesaving drugs for countless HIV-infected infants and children.

Ultimately, both the pediatric AIDS research community and the major pharmaceutical companies rejected the requirements of the Pediatric Rule, as it was not in their own interests to comply. I was deeply troubled by the pediatric AIDS research community's attitude. It clearly was in the children's best interest to make drugs available rapidly. Early in the epidemic, the pediatric AIDS research community was a strong advocate for making ARVs available to infants and children at the same time as to adults. Previously, they had demanded that infants and children have rapid and equal access to ARVs. Why the change? By 1994, the NIH had significantly increased the funding provided for efficacy studies in children. Although deemed unnecessary by the FDA and various HIV experts, they were perhaps too profitable for clinical researchers and their academic universities to admit that they were not required.

POTENT NEW TREATMENTS FOR ADULTS BUT NOT FOR CHILDREN

Two years after the 1994 ACTG 076 study that used ZDV as the sole ARV to prevent perinatal HIV transmission, potent new ARVs known as protease inhibitors were discovered. In preliminary studies in adults, these drugs appeared to be both safe and effective, producing the most dramatic declines in HIV blood levels that had ever been observed ("Protease Inhibitor" 1995).[4] These results prompted universal optimism that a new class of drugs had finally been discovered that could control the relentless progression of HIV to death. Understandably, many in the pediatric AIDS community were greatly concerned by the fact that no pediatric studies were planned, meaning that these drugs would not be available for children in the foreseeable future.

In 1995, while in Washington, DC, I was invited to a dinner meeting with a scientific director from Abbott Laboratories, a major pharmaceutical company that had sponsored adult clinical trials for RTV, their PI drug. As I listened to the results of preliminary studies on RTV, I was enthusiastic—the potential for this drug to treat HIV infection in children was great. Several other factors accelerated my enthusiasm; the first was that the clinical studies had been conducted by Dr. David Ho and his coworkers, in whom I had a high degree of confidence. If Ho was enthusiastic, it spoke volumes for the drug's potential to control HIV disease progression in both adults and children. Second, the drug was already available in a liquid formation, which could accelerate its evaluation in infants by months or even years. I interpreted my invitation to the Abbott Laboratories meeting to mean that RTV would soon be available to treat HIV infection in infants and children, which temporarily renewed my hope.

I was further encouraged that accelerated drug approval for infants and children was possible after I was contacted by Mark Rubin, a senior investigator at Glaxo Wellcome, which had initially introduced its new drug combination of Epivir (3TC) plus ZDV in a liquid formulation, having already performed safety and dosing studies in children. Rubin told me that they were soon going to present their data to the FDA Advisory Committee and asked me to preview the presentation. I hoped that the drug combination would be the first simultaneously approved ARVs for children and adults, proving that through the mutual commitment of pharmaceutical companies, clinical researchers, and the FDA, unnecessary delays in drug development for children could be avoided.

An FDA Advisory Committee meeting to review 3TC met on November 17, 1995. The meeting lasted all day and consisted of careful presentations and a review of complex data on safety, dosing, and efficacy. At the end of the day, I was invited to testify. I used my time to emphasize what could be done if a pharmaceutical company had the will, compassion, and ethical persuasion to recognize the needs of desperately ill children. To my great excitement, within days of the Advisory Committee meeting, the FDA approved the use of the combination drug for treatment of HIV in both adults and children (James 1995). What escaped many among the pediatric AIDS research community and NIH leaders was that the combination treatment was approved without separate efficacy studies in infants and children, vindicating the intent of the 1994 FDA Pediatric Rule (Schachter and Ramoni 2007).

The excitement sparked by the dual approval of ZDV plus 3TC was short-lived. Several months later, I learned that Abbott Laboratories would soon be appearing before the FDA Advisory Committee to seek approval for RTV, but they would not be presenting any pediatric data or seeking pediatric approval. I was shocked. Just a few months earlier, I had been led to believe that they were committed to moving forward with pediatric studies. When I inquired at Abbott as to the reason for their new stance, I was told simply that the liquid formulation of RTV did not taste good and therefore was not marketable to the pediatric population. Of course, I raised the obvious question— what infant enjoys the taste of any medicine? There simply had to be other reasons, most likely financial. Outraged, I decided to attend the upcoming FDA meeting and protest the lack of pediatric studies for RTV.

Before the meeting, I received a call from Dr. David Pizzuti, divisional vice president of medical affairs at Abbott Laboratories, who assured me that they were planning a meeting with pediatric investigators to design safety and dosing studies in children. However, this meeting was scheduled to take place after the FDA Advisory Committee meeting, meaning that the drug still would not be approved simultaneously for adults and children. It was an obvious attempt to prevent any adverse testimony at the FDA hearing.

The FDA Advisory Committee meeting took place on March 1, 1996, and was well attended, as expected. RTV was the first truly potent ARV up for approval, and all involved parties, from HIV/AIDS patients to activists to the FDA to Abbott Laboratories, hoped it would become one of the most rapidly approved drugs in the history of the FDA.[5] I knew that representatives from the major AIDS activist groups would be in attendance but also that none of those groups represented children. The best I could do was to find a patient advocate—preferably a mother and her HIV-infected infant. I called all of the major advocacy groups representing HIV-infected women and at last found a perfect witness—Ashami and her infected daughter, Celeste. Ashami was a young woman from southern California who had been HIV infected for many years and had transmitted the virus during pregnancy to her daughter, Celeste, who was now three years old. Ashami was doing well thanks to treatment with combination ARVs, but Celeste had been treated with ZDV alone, and she was getting sicker.

At the FDA meeting, Ashami and I were scheduled to speak during the public testimony segment, which would take place after Abbott presented its data on safety, dosing, and efficacy in adults. Abbott's presentation proved to be one of the most masterful examples of high-tech presentations by a modern pharmaceutical company. All of the data was fully digitalized, with Abbott employees positioned throughout the room, periodically muttering into their two-way headsets. Every question was answered with data that was instantaneously projected onto the screen, almost as if each question was known in advance.

With such a vast amount of data to address, and such intense scientific interest, the public testimony segment was postponed until after lunchtime. During the lunch break, Ashami and I walked across the street to an FAO Schwartz toy store to buy a gift for Celeste and perhaps to break some of the nervous tension. As I walked down the aisles, surrounded by towering stacks of toys, I couldn't help but reflect on the incredible paradox: all these toys were produced by hundreds of manufacturers who were putting all their efforts into convincing parents to purchase things that their children didn't really need, while just across the street, a wealthy pharmaceutical company was intent on not performing any studies on a drug that could save the lives of thousands of infants and children.

When the floor was finally opened to public testimony in the afternoon, the meeting had been so delayed that Ashami and I each had only five minutes to speak. The most arresting moment of Ashami's testimony came when she looked directly at David Kessler, head of the FDA, and asked, "What should I tell my daughter when she sees me take a medicine for exactly the same condition from which she suffers and asks, 'Why can't I take the medicine you're taking, Mommy?'" Nobody answered. In reality, Ashami's question had been answered two years previously by the FDA 1994 Pediatric Rule that Kessler himself had promulgated—separate pediatric drug studies were not needed before her HIV-infected child could get ARVs.

When I stood up before the packed room of FDA advisers, pharmaceutical representatives, and activists, I realized that I would only have time to present about half of the statement I had prepared. What follows is the abbreviated transcript of my statement:

> You are here to review the data for a drug to treat HIV. You are responsible for determining whether a drug which is to be used in all populations (and I quote from the Food and Drug and Cosmetic Act statutory and regulatory document) "contains data on a reasonable sample of patients likely to receive the drug once it is marketed." In the FDA's own words, this applies equally to the pediatric populations. You have no option but to recommend enforcement of these rules. HIV-infected children and women cannot be the only population denied lifesaving drugs, denied compassionate use, denied entry into the circle of lifesaving drugs. We, the pediatric HIV/AIDS community, are trying to do everything that we can. We are talking to pharmaceutical companies, we present recommendations to the right people and institutions, we participate in advisory meetings such as this, we make the needs known before the right people at President Clinton's National Task Force on AIDS Drug Development, we support incentives for pharmaceutical companies, we supported the Better Pharmaceuticals Act for Children, we have made the needs known to you. Today we have five specific recommendations for you. First: Approve this drug for use in adults. Second: As a condition of approval for use in adults, require pediatric safety and pharmacologic data. Third: If the company does not perform required pediatric studies, go to court to seek an injunction requiring them to do so. Fourth: Review all ongoing drug research for which you have been given permission for human clinical trials. When you find a drug that has potential pediatric use for a chronic or serious condition, review the research plan to see if the company is making adequate progress toward having pediatric safety and pharmacologic data at the time it seeks approval. If it does not, notify the company that you will not be able to grant approval for adults only. Fifth: Require that all compassionate-use protocols for drugs that have a pediatric use also include infants and children.[6]

I also reminded everyone of the scoreboard when it came to pediatric drug approvals: In the nine years following approval of ZDV, ten ARVs were approved for adults but only three for children. In the year preceding the hearing, the FDA Committee had approved five of the most potent ARVs in the history of the HIV/AIDS epidemic, but none of them were approved for children, a population that died faster than adults if left untreated. As I finished my testimony, I heard the encouraging sound of members of the AIDS activist groups chanting, "Give them the drug! Give them the drug! Give them the drug!"

Soon after my return to California, I received a phone call from Pizzuti at Abbott, informing me that an Abbott internal committee meeting had determined that I must retract my testimony. Pizzuti stated that unless I submitted a written retraction and allowed Abbott to respond on a yet-to-be defined television program, I would be prohibited from attending the upcoming meeting with pediatric investigators to discuss plans for conducting pediatric studies on RTV. First, I asked, "What television program?" Apparently some television reporters at the FDA Advisory Committee meeting had filmed my testimony, and this had triggered Abbott's apprehension about its public image. I replied that I wouldn't retract my testimony, and if they didn't invite me to the meeting, it was their choice, but I hoped the decision would be interpreted by others as evidence of Abbott's lack of concern for children.

One month later, I was invited to speak in California at a small community meeting of mothers of children with HIV to update them on pharmaceutical companies' progress in studying drugs in children. As I began to explain that RTV had been approved for adults but not for children at a recent FDA Advisory Committee meeting, one mother asked what she could do for her son, who was getting sicker every day. Although RTV was in a liquid formulation, her pediatrician could not prescribe it without knowing the proper infant dose. Moreover, because it was not yet FDA approved, she could not receive reimbursement from her insurance company and therefore could not afford it. She began sobbing uncontrollably, saying, "I see all the HIV-infected adults I know getting better on these new drugs and going back to work, and my son keeps getting sicker and sicker . . . I know he's going to die." I felt helpless and only wished that I could force executives at each of the major pharmaceutical companies producing ARVs to listen to the pleas of these women for their children.

A LOTTERY THAT CHILDREN COULD NOT WIN

As if anticipating that there would be a high demand for their new protease inhibitor ritonavir once it was approved, in December 1995, months in advance of the actual FDA approval of the drug, Abbott announced that they would have a lottery for the limited supply that would be available. This was yet another setback for HIV-infected infants and children, who would be asked to compete with a vast population of HIV-infected adults. At that time, the three most potent PI drugs that had been developed were on track to be approved for adults within the next year, but none of them had any of the pediatric safety and dosing data that would be necessary to make them available to infants and children. In spite of clinical research data demonstrating the potency of the PIs, the pharmaceutical companies did not anticipate the intensity of the demand, and when the drugs were approved for adults, they found themselves with insufficient supplies. To address the deficiency, Abbott Laboratories created a lottery system as a solution, announcing that it would make RTV available by lottery to two thousand AIDS patients, whose physicians were required to complete an application enrolling them in the lottery. The application clearly stated that the lottery would be limited to patients over the age of twelve. The limitation, and the failure to even mention children, incensed the pediatric AIDS community. It was a deliberate exclusion and particularly abhorrent considering that much of Abbott's profit was derived from pediatric products. When RTV was approved for adults in March 1996, it was estimated that within a year Abbott would reap profits of over $16 million, which would be more than adequate for funding the necessary pediatric studies to get the drug approved for children.

TOO EXPENSIVE FOR POOR PEOPLE

Beginning in 1996, clinical research studies performed in developed countries were proving the efficacy of cART. In 1996, HAART was being promoted as standard of care, and within four years the death rate for people with HIV infection plummeted by 84 percent ("HIV/AIDS Mortality" 1998). However, the cost of treatment was excessive for low-income countries. In the United States, HAART cost between $10,000 and $15,000 per person, per year—far too expensive for the ministries of health and local clinics in poor countries to consider as an approach for saving the lives of those with HIV infection. Interventions were needed, but activism of the kind that had successfully resulted in rapid drug approval and realistic pricing in the United States was absent in all but a few poor countries such as Brazil and South Africa. Further intellectual property laws that dominated income-rich countries also controlled what could be done in low-income countries to reduce drug prices, especially those who were members of the World Trade Organization (WTO).

Pressure on pharmaceutical companies to lower drug prices intensified when the issue of equity—rich versus poor, life versus death—began troubling an increasing number of individuals in the United States who were providing HIV prevention and care in income-poor settings. The discrepancy between the life expectancy of an HIV-infected individual living in a wealthy country compared to a poor country was jolting. Traveling between North America and countries in Africa, clinicians with patients on both continents would be shaken by just a twenty-four-hour journey, from a country where over thirty drugs were available to a country where only one was available.

The solution to high drug prices in low-income countries was to allow the use of low-cost generic drugs. A generic drug is a copy of a brand-name patented drug which is identical to the patented drug except that it is produced in a poor country and therefore at a much lower cost. The price difference was remarkable. For example, instead of the $10,000 to $15,000 per year for the patented drugs, CIPLA, an Indian generic-drug manufacturer, offered the same drugs for as little as $295 per person, per year. Some versions of triple-combination drugs were available at an even lower cost, as low as $64 per person annually.

In 2006, UNITAID, an international drug purchase organization, was established to ensure a stable source of funds for obtaining drugs to treat malaria, TB, and HIV. They partnered with the Clinton Foundation, and specifically with the Clinton Health Access Initiative (CHAI), negotiating with manufacturers of patented and generic drugs to continue to lower drug prices and to provide a stable source of the drugs. The cost saving was significant. As a result of these negotiations, over $600 million was saved over several years, allowing more HIV-infected individuals to be placed on treatment.

The dramatic decrease in drug prices should have resulted in WHO immediately revising their poorly conceived and economically driven HIV treatment guidelines, which recommended withholding ARV treatment until HIV-infected individuals reached advanced and sometimes irreversible stages of infection. The amount of money that it cost to treat a patient in 2002 could, in 2006, treat 150 more HIV-infected individuals than previously. However, it was not until September 2015 that WHO at last recommended treating all HIV-infected individuals with HAART.

Acronyms and Legislative Redundancy

21

REINVENTING THE FDA 1994 PEDIATRIC RULE

The year 1997 would prove to be one of intense activity and focus on the legislative process of speeding up drug development for life-threatening diseases for children, or at least it was meant to be. When proposed changes to existing rules were published by the FDA in the *Federal Register*, they seemed encouraging. On closer examination, they were worrisome.

In February 1997, I received a surprising phone call from Paula Botstein at the FDA. I had worked with Botstein on Clinton's National Presidential Task Force for HIV/AIDS Drug Development in 1994 and 1995. At that time, I was president of amfAR and carefully followed all FDA and congressional activity surrounding pediatric drug approval. Botstein informed me that an upcoming publication in the *Federal Register* was publishing new rules on pediatric drug development proposed by the government, and an important announcement would be made. She cryptically stated, "I can't tell you what it is, but be on the lookout for it. You will be interested." Over the next two months, I continuously scoured the *Federal Register*, but when I saw nothing of interest by April, I assumed that the announcement had been tabled. I had to wait until August 1997 to learn what it was all about, when I received a phone call from the White House staff inviting me to participate in a press conference where President Bill Clinton would announce his new requirement that the FDA require pediatric drug studies. I was optimistic.

The press conference took place on August 13, 1997, with President Bill Clinton, First Lady Hillary Clinton, Vice President Al Gore, and Secretary of HHS Donna Shalala in attendance. Also present were representatives from the FDA, congressional members, pharmaceutical-industry executives, physicians, lawyers, and journalists.[1] The speeches began with Shalala and ended with President Clinton—all addressing the issue's importance and outlining how the administration had always been interested in health-care issues involving children, not just drug development, but also children's vaccines and health insurance. Shalala stated, "Children are not simply small adults. Under the new rule, manufacturers of drugs likely to be used by children will be required to complete studies and place information on drug labels to help physicians make scientifically based decisions when prescribing drugs for children." President Clinton stated, "When a child gets sick, parents should never have to worry about whether a drug is safe for their child." He also declared, "Too many pediatricians are playing a high-risk game when they prescribe untested drugs" (Pear 1997a).

The press conference was designed to highlight the actions Clinton was taking to fulfill some of the election promises from his 1996 presidential campaign. Clinton's approach to pediatric health-care issues, ranging from drug development to daycare to vaccines to health insurance, was commonly referred to by the media as the "cult of the child." On the issue of drug development, Clinton stated that only 50 percent of drugs that are approved for adults but are known to have potential health benefits for children are in fact approved for the pediatric community. He then made the bold statement, "The rule I propose will put an end to unsafe drugs for children." Clinton announced proposed legislation requiring new drugs that were likely to be used on children to provide sufficient pediatric data for accurate pediatric labeling in order to be approved.

To me, the proposed rule was déjà vu. The1997 proposed Clinton Rule not only reiterated what had already been contained in the FDA 1994 Pediatric Rule, but it also added numerous provisions for deferrals and other loopholes for pharmaceutical companies if they refused to perform required pharmacologic studies in infants and children. The issues for equitable drug approval for infants and children could have been solved once and for all, but they weren't. Children remained vulnerable because the rule only addressed a small segment of untested drugs for children. Many drugs would still be unsafe at any dose, and the needs of the sickest children would continue to be at the mercy of guesswork and chance. For infants and children with HIV infection, drug approval would continue to languish, placing them at risk for adverse drug reactions and delays in drug availability. One of the most important questions remained unanswered: Who was going to enforce the FDA's 1994 Pediatric Rule?

Initially it appeared as if the supporters of Clinton's 1997 proposal had won; the proposed rule was signed into law on November 21, 1997, as part of the FDA Modernization and Accountability Act, championed by Congressman James Jeffords, chairman of the Senate Committee on Labor and Human Resources. It included a number of positive health reforms, such as a continuation of surcharges on drug development so as to provide increased revenue to the FDA to support the expedited approval of new drugs, as well as a measure requiring that more women be included in clinical research trials. In its final form, Clinton's measure required the FDA to develop and publish a list of already approved drugs for which more pediatric information was required in order to benefit the health of the pediatric population. The list was to be updated annually. Few in the audience knew that the proposed revision was merely a reiteration of the 1994 FDA version but with some troubling qualifications that would not benefit children.

After the *Federal Register* was published, I painstakingly went through the proposed revisions. In a seven-page public comment on the proposed Clinton Rule, I expressed my concerns, stating, "Since the initial authority given to the FDA was to ensure the safety and efficacy of the drug for all populations likely to use the drug, the FDA has both the regulatory and legal authority to require pediatric dosing and safety studies. The proposed new rule has a porosity which is unacceptable, will worsen the inequities which already exist regarding the availability of safe and effective drugs for children, and continue to segregate children into a category for which drugs for serious and life-threatening conditions are not evaluated for safety and dosing in a timely manner, if at all."

MORE LEGISLATIVE ACRONYMS BUT LITTLE PROGRESS

By 1996, the issue of pediatric drug approvals had come to a crisis point. Of the ten drugs that had been approved to treat HIV by that time, only three had been approved for use in infants and children. I began writing to every high-level individual I could think of who might be able to put pressure on the FDA and Congress to develop measures to accelerate drug approval for children. One of my requests was that Congress give full bipartisan support to Senator Nancy Kassebaum's Best Pharmaceuticals for Children Act (BPCA, H.R. 4277, 104th Cong.). Kassebaum first introduced this bill to the Senate in 1992, then again in 1997 with the co-sponsorship of Senators Kennedy, Dodd, DeWine, Mikulski, and Simon. The bill acknowledged that pharmaceutical companies would always drag their feet on performing pediatric studies if they were simply required to do so by FDA regulations, which, in some inexplicable way, the FDA was not able to enforce. The BPCA presented an alternative, which was to offer financial incentives to pharmaceutical companies to combat the frequent excuse that pediatric studies were simply too costly. The bill stated that for drugs that were still on patent, a six-month patent extension would be granted if pediatric studies were performed that resulted in the drugs being labeled for a pediatric indication.

A number of potential problems immediately stood out. First, how could there be any incentive for companies to do pediatric studies on the hundreds of drugs that were already off-patent and on the market? No one had the authority to request this. Second, would a six-month patent extension prove to be a sufficient incentive? PhRMA responded to the bill with demands that the extension be raised to three to five years, which would mean billions of dollars of additional income for pharmaceutical companies but would result in ongoing high costs to consumers while generic drugs remained unavailable. Third, would pharmaceutical companies cherry-pick drugs that could be easily and inexpensively studied rather than drugs that were of utmost priority for life-threatening diseases? Fourth, what age groups would drugs have to be tested on? There are marked differences in dosing and safety among infants, children, and adolescents, but nothing in the bill would stop a pharmaceutical company from simply doing studies on adolescents and claiming that they therefore deserved patent-extension approval—and that's precisely what happened.

Unfortunately, more than just theoretical concerns came to light. The BPCA included an initial list of 450 drugs that required pediatric labeling changes, yet from 1996 to 2001, only fourteen drugs received labeling changes that reflected new data. Meanwhile, pediatric drug sales were rising approximately 28 percent each year—faster than drug sales for any other age group. The pharmaceutical companies were simply prioritizing pediatric studies on their income-producing drugs so as to obtain patent extensions that would bring in the most revenue. For example, both Schering-Plough and Eli Lilly gained an additional $1 billion in additional revenue from patent extensions on Claritin and Prozac. In fact, Eli Lilly won that extension by submitting pediatric studies that had been performed on Prozac in 1995, two years before BPCA was passed.[2]

A detailed 2011 GAO report to the Committee on Health, Education, Labor, and Pensions explained why the BPCA was not effective in solving the problem of drug availability for infants and children. The BPCA was overseen by a number of organizations. To begin the process, the FDA worked with HHS, in consultation with the NIH, to submit a written request to a drug manufacturer to include pediatric data. If the drug manufacturer refused, the FDA could make a written request to the NIH, which would either fund and perform the study itself, or award up to $200 million to other organizations to perform the studies instead. The Institute of Medicine was also under contract to conduct a study on best practices relating to pediatric research and, along with the Eunice Kennedy Shriver National Institute of Child Health and Development (NICHD), had oversight of the BPCA's effectiveness. Not surprisingly, the involvement of multiple government organizations resulted in a diffusion of responsibility, lack of coordination, poor communication, and an inability to define who had final decision-making authority.

THE PEDIATRIC RULE REINVENTED AGAIN

In 1998, the FDA put forward its own revision of the 1997 Clinton Pediatric Rule. That meant that there were now three separate Pediatric Rules without addressing the most fundamental question—of what value is a rule if it is not enforced? The means for getting drugs approved for infants and children with HIV and other life-threatening diseases was not more rules or legislation but enforcement of existing rules. Dr. Janet Woodcock, director of the Center for Drug Evaluation and Research, first outlined the new FDA Pediatric Rule. In my interactions with Woodcock, I found her to be thoughtful, courteous, and motivated to offer guidance on FDA rules and regulations. She seemed especially interested in drug approval for infants and children and agreed with former FDA Commissioner Kessler that drugs should be approved for pediatric use if the disease was sufficiently similar in adults and children and if pediatric safety and pharmacokinetic studies were completed along with efficacy studies in adults.

It was not surprising that the revision once again caused discontent among pharmaceutical companies, but it was surprising that the Association of American Physicians and Surgeons (AAPS) opposed the change and, in 2000, sued to block implementation (Arshagouni 2002). AAPS represented adult patients, not children, and it made some extraordinary claims in the lawsuit, including that the new FDA Pediatric Rule would delay approvals for adult drugs, which was clearly spurious, as the rule stated that pediatric studies must be initiated early in the drug-development process but only after efficacy had been shown in adults. It also claimed that the rule would expose children enrolled in clinical trials to unnecessary danger, which obviously failed to acknowledge the fact that children were already being put in danger through the unapproved use of drugs that had never been tested for safety, or by simply not having drugs available at all. Interestingly, the arguments made in the lawsuit by AAPS and PhRMA were similar.

In a move that surprised everyone, including Woodcock at the FDA, in October 2002 Federal District Court Judge Henry J. Kennedy Jr. ruled in favor of the AAPS and struck down the FDA's revision of the Pediatric Rule, stating that the FDA had overstepped its authority (Arshagouni 2002). Judge Kennedy's decision was largely based on an incorrect interpretation of the BPCA. Kennedy claimed that the FDA did not have the legal authority to require pediatric studies for drug indications that weren't explicitly claimed by the manufacturer—even if it was known that a drug was being used on children, and even if that drug was desperately needed to save lives. Kennedy further argued that an incentive approach approved by Congress would be more appropriate than a mandatory requirement, a surprising conclusion for someone practicing law. There were a number of inconsistencies in Kennedy's ruling, not least of which was the fact that the FDA had been given authority by Congress in past rulings to ensure the safety of drugs for all populations in which a drug was to be used. It seemed that Judge Kennedy had failed to do his homework on the FDA and congressional legislation in reaching his decision.

In 2003, President George W. Bush signed into law the Pediatric Research Equity Act (PREA), which was intended to restore the protections that the FDA had been granted under the 1998 Pediatric Rule and strengthen the FDA's ability to require pediatric drug studies. The act was met with intense optimism from pediatric advocates and organizations. EGPAF stated, "The PREA of 2003 will give the FDA the authority to require manufacturers to test the safety and dosing of all new medicines and some already marketed medicines for children. It will also ensure that drugs are available in forms that young children can readily use, such as liquids and chewable tablets."[3]

Sadly, the initial optimistic interpretations would not hold true; ultimately, multiple government entities and pediatric clinical research organizations funded by the US government proved to be the greatest violators of the Pediatric Rule. Today, it is clear that much of the complex legislation passed between 1996 and 2000, as well-intentioned as it may have been, served only to undermine what should have been a simple process of enforcing the FDA's authority to protect infants and children from unsafe drugs and make compulsory the rules that were already in place in 1994. Involving multiple government agencies only served to further confuse the issue. There was little accountability or ability to track progress, there was no central plan that would cover all of the multiple agencies involved, and the responsibility for performing the critically needed pharmacokinetic and safety studies on severely ill infants had been placed in the hands of inexperienced pediatric investigators who would ultimately fail.

As pharmaceutical companies had the option to decline requests to perform studies under the BPCA, much of the responsibility shifted to the NIH, which sponsored studies by the Pediatric AIDS Clinical Trial Group, NICHD, NIAID, and multiple academic institutions. This division of responsibility diffused the accountability for who would be ultimately responsible for closing the gap between approved and unapproved drugs in children. In the end, the complex legislative measures failed to accomplish their stated purpose. Countless hours and dollars were spent in trying to correct what only needed to be enforced from the very beginning—the 1994 Pediatric Rule. HIV-infected infants and children were the losers.

Facts Speak Louder Than Words

22

Examining Efforts That Failed

AN IDEAL EFFORT THAT FIZZLED

In 1996, *Science* writer Jon Cohen, referring to Clinton's Presidential AIDS Drug Task Force, concluded, "AIDS Task Force Fizzles Out" (Cohen 1996). When the task force first convened in 1994, it seemed that it would work. The invitation to join came directly from President Clinton and was extended to major decision-makers from the US government, NIH, the pharmaceutical industry, and advocacy organizations, who would all be in the same room at the same time. The formation of the fifteen-member task force was announced at a November 30, 1993, news conference by HHS Secretary Donna Shalala and Assistant Secretary of Health Philip Lee, who was named as head. I received the official invitation on February 8, 1994, from Donna Shalala on behalf of President Clinton. I felt honored to be personally invited to the task force and to experience the early optimism over our potential impact on drug development. It seemed possible that at last something could be accomplished to truly accelerate the development of new drugs, rapidly introduce promising treatments to HIV-infected patients, and, importantly, simultaneously make them available to infants and children.

After reviewing the high profiles of those participating in the task force, I was encouraged that it would be successful—Harold Varmus, NIH director; David Kessler, head of FDA; Phil Lee, assistant secretary of HHS; Anthony Fauci, director of NIAID; Roy Vagelos, chairman and chief executive officer of Merck and Co., Inc.; Edward Skolnick, president of Merck Research Laboratories; Moises Agosto, of the National Minority AIDS Council; and White House AIDS policy coordinator Kristine Gebbie.[1]

Almost as if speaking with one voice, academic and pharmaceutical scientists as well as government officials stated that they hoped the task force would have a strong and positive impact on the research and development of drugs to treat HIV infection. The announcement, however, was not met with uniform optimism. Some in the activist community were more cautious than others. Derek Hodel with the AIDS Action Council in Washington, DC, stated, "Those of us who are optimistic hope that the task force will be effective at its charter in identifying barriers to research and to drug development, of which there are many. If it's well-appointed and well-staffed, it's quite likely that it could have a major impact" (Cohen 1996).

The first meeting of the AIDS Drug Task Force was held on April 14, 1994, in Arlington, Virginia, concentrating on identifying the problems that were hampering the development of promising new drugs for HIV treatment. During the meeting, almost everyone emphasized the fact that "risk" of evaluating new drugs needed to be increased—financial risk on the part of the pharmaceutical companies, regulatory risk on the part of FDA, and risk on the part of HIV-infected patients by allowing them to determine whether they wanted to participate in new drug clinical research trials.

At the meeting, I asked, "How do you balance life-threatening disease and possible drug toxicity? Perhaps we need to take these risks." FDA commissioner David Kessler was more cautious, stating, "We have to know that the drugs work first, and then that the people have access to them." During the first days of the meeting, there was much discussion about the balance between accelerating drug approval and the risk that patients would have to take with drugs that were not fully evaluated. Sitting back in his chair, Peter Staley, an activist and advocate for new drug treatment, pointed out that the real problem was that there were not enough drugs in the pipeline to even debate the issue thoroughly.

Three committees were formed. The first dealt with specific recommendations to identify potential new drugs and to move them quickly into the development pipeline. The second committee was given the task of identifying ways to move drugs more quickly from the bench to the clinic. The third committee, which Staley and I chaired, was to suggest ways to facilitate collaboration between government and private research. Having worked both at the Genentech biotechnology company and at UCSF in academic research, I felt that communication between organizations was poor, and there were too many egos wanting to reach success for new ARVs, which caused both pharmaceutical companies and academic researchers to want to go it alone.

On April 15, 1994, I was asked to present the "pediatric view" of drug development, or rather the lack thereof. I had decided to divide the presentation into two parts—those issues that could be resolved quickly and those issues which would require more discussion and interaction. Included in the former was action by the FDA to enforce the 1994 FDA Pediatric Rule, which did not require separate efficacy studies of lifesaving drugs if the disease were the same in adults and children. I also emphasize that if those in academia were to be engaged in pediatric HIV drug development, they needed to conduct the studies as quickly and as efficiently as the pharmaceutical industry did.

I wanted to end my presentation with optimism, so I used two examples of highly successful experimental treatments that had been first evaluated in infants and children and had resulted in great widespread life-saving treatment for adults as well as children. Both studies had carried significant research risks for the infants and children involved. For the first example, I used bone-marrow transplantation, first evaluated in infants with congenital immunodeficiency disorders and now used in children and adults for the treatment of malignancies (Gatti et al. 1968). For the second example, I used the illustration of the ACTG 076 ZDV study that had shown that ZDV, a minimally effective ARV, prevented HIV transmission from mothers to infants—a result that had enormous potential for ending the HIV epidemic by preventing sexual transmission of HIV, preventing transmission of HIV following accidental inoculation in health-care workers and following rape of girls and women, and ending perinatal HIV transmission (Folkers and Fauci 2001; Fauci and Folkers 2012).

Initially, the meetings and the subgroups' reports were encouraging. Certainly the HIV experts, representatives of NIH, academics, FDA, pharmaceutical companies, and government officials were all present at the same time and were exchanging ideas in a non-confrontational manner. But soon other issues began to creep into the agenda, including special legislation to extend patents on drugs that had little to do with HIV. Some high-level HHS representatives were not even aware that Medicaid did not cover all treatment of the ARVs or limited the monthly allotments to amounts that were utterly inadequate. A representative of the National Institutes of Child Health and Development presented a long list of ARV drug studies for infants and children and implied that the studies were in progress, but when I questioned her, she backtracked and said they were studies that they were planning to do, not studies that were already in progress.

At one point during one of the many meetings, I became frustrated with issues that seemed to be unnecessarily holding up approval of potent new drugs to treat HIV infection in infants and children. Raising my hand to be recognized during a particularly contentious and drawn-out session, I explained, "I like that rule. It's a good rule. But this is bigger than rules. This is life and death." Heads began to nod in acknowledgment, but little did those in the room know that the quote was from the movie *Babe*, which I had recently seen with my grandchildren, spoken by the duck as he convinces the pig to break the rules and enter the farmer's house.

Perhaps I should not have been so optimistic about the potential impact of the Presidential Task Force on AIDS Drug Development, but it seemed to me that all of the critical factors had been identified, and the essential individuals from the various interest groups had the opportunity to express their concerns as well as their solutions. Nevertheless, as individuals dispersed it became obvious that, as critical as the task force could have been, in the long run, personal, corporate, and academic self-interests would prevent accelerated approval of life-saving drugs for infants and children. The task force had a lifespan of just two years and could have ended with objective accomplishments. *Science* reporter Cohen was correct: it began with a "bang" but ended with a "fizzle" (1996).

WHEN ACADEMICS WOULD BE A PHARMACEUTICAL COMPANY

Sometimes efforts to fix a problem only make it worse. In 1997 a National AIDS Task Force Working Committee on Pediatric AIDS Drugs was established and given the mission of identifying drugs for life-threatening illnesses in infants where FDA-approved formulations did not exist or where relevant pharmacokinetic studies had not been performed. The committee was to address marketed drugs only. Drugs were divided into two categories: those used for acute life-threatening diseases and those used for chronic life-threatening diseases. The list was to be submitted to relevant federal government agencies and organizations engaged in studies on drug development for infants and children. After considerable deliberation, twenty-seven drugs were identified. Seventeen years later, in 2014, only six of those identified in 1997 had sufficient information for a full pediatric age use.

Another attempt to accelerate approval of drugs for infants and children was the costly network of Pediatric Pharmacology Research Units (PPRU), established by the NICHD. The total amount of funding provided to these units is difficult to obtain, but it must have been considerable, as there were seventeen units scattered across the United

States that were funded from 1994 until 2010. In addition to whatever funds they received from the NIH, in 1997 they received $500,000 from the American Medical Association specifically for pediatric pharmacology research. This funding was accompanied by a statement that "75 percent of all medications marketed today do not carry FDA-approved labeling for use in children, and only five of eighty drugs frequently used in newborns and infants are labeled for pediatric use."[2] Clearly, the priority for PPRU was to conduct clinical trials that would lead to pediatric labeling of drugs commonly used off-label to treat children. As time progressed, the PPRUs began to divert their efforts by including pediatric research into preclinical research models, biomarkers, and drug delivery systems. Examination of the publications listed by the PPRU indicate that there were only six during the six years that the seventeen PPRU units existed that were relevant to development of ARVs for infants and children. During the first five years, only seven drugs were evaluated that contributed to pediatric labeling. (The PPRU website still exists but contains only archived information.)

Another solution for accelerating drug approval for infants and children was the Pediatric Drug List and Research Fund. Legislation had authorized the FDA commissioner to consult with the director of NIH to study drugs that were not already being studied by pharmaceutical companies. The law authorized $200 million in 2000, as well as "Such sums as are necessary for each of the five succeeding fiscal years." Along with this authorization, the HHS secretary could refer a drug to the foundation if he or she determined that there was a need relating to the drug's use and the manufacturer had refused to conduct a study. A foundation was established by Congress in 1990 as a 501(c)(3) public charity to accept funding. Their 2012 annual report does not list any investigations that were done on pediatric drugs to gain FDA approval. Interestingly, of the twenty-nine board members on the NIH foundation, seven were from the pharmaceutical industry.

But perhaps the best means of determining the success or failure of the various attempts to accelerate drug approval in infants and children is to examine the data derived from a review of the drug inserts that the FDA requires for all drugs that it approves. The inserts give not only basic information on the drug structure and uses, but also drug doses. They also provide warnings about drug safety and, importantly, whether the drug has been approved for use in certain populations, such as infants, children, and pregnant women.

In 1996, there were ten ARVs approved for use in adults and only three for children. Today, the numbers are worse—there are over twenty-five ARVs approved for adult use. Only ten of these have been approved for use in infants and children, and many lack data that would allow a physician to treat an infant less than three months of age, a critical time for preventing disease progression and, based on recent studies, even the eradication of HIV infection itself (Persaud et al. 2013). Fifteen of some of the newest and most powerful ARVs include the following statement: "Safety and effectiveness have not been established for this drug in children younger than sixteen years of age." These results contrast with a recent analysis of drugs approved by the FDA primarily for adults: "A third of new drugs are currently approved on the basis of a single pivotal trial; the median size for all pivotal trials is just 760 patients. More than two thirds of new drugs are approved on the basis of studies lasting six months or less." The goal of accelerating approval of new drugs by the FDA is being achieved for adults but continues to languish in infants and children (FDA 2011).

It would be difficult for even the most ardent supporters of government regulations to claim that providing the necessary dosing and safety information for life-saving ARVs in infants and children has been successful. After decades of legislation and millions of dollars invested in academic approaches to solve the problem, evidence of success is lacking. Perhaps Marian Wright Edelman, founder and president of the Children's Defense Fund, was correct: "Children don't make campaign contributions, and many of their parents are too busy struggling to make ends meet to get involved in campaigns. If change is to come, it will happen because people like you respond in an aggressive, sustained, and even outraged way" ("Look at Me!" 2011).

FORMATION OF ADULT AND PEDIATRIC CLINICAL RESEARCH UNITS

By 1995, there was mounting criticism that in spite of increased funding for research in HIV/AIDS, progress was not adequate to stem the epidemic. William Paul, director of the Office of AIDS Research, had agreed to push forward an outside evaluation of the NIH-funded research programs by a review panel of 114 leading scientists and representatives of pharmaceutical companies, the community, AIDS advocates, and academia, headed by Arnold Levine of Princeton University. (See Chapter 27 for more on the Levine Panel Report.) Their conclusions were reported to the NIH directors and made available to the public (Altman 1996; Kolata 1989).

The consensus was that fifteen years of AIDS research had brought impressive discoveries, but greater scientific oversight and review by non-government scientists was required. Specific areas of criticism were identified with questions raised as to whether some NIH-funded clinical research studies could be carried out equally well and more rapidly by pharmaceutical companies. The Levine Panel Report was also instrumental in refining the research objectives of the adult and pediatric ACTGs. The National Institutes of Allergy and Infectious Diseases had formed the adult ACTG in 1987. Its accomplishments were many, and it was easy to point to the progress that it had made in pioneering clinical research for the diagnosis of HIV infection and the development of drugs to treat infection. In addition, although there was a question of whether the ACTG or the pharmaceutical companies had the primary responsibility, the NIH studies were pivotal in providing data for the approval of new ARVs as well as combinations of drugs, setting treatment initiation and follow-up criteria, and defining the pathogenesis and clinical features of HIV infection. Clinical studies that showed the impact of combination ARVs could only be assumed by a non-pharmaceutical company approach, since intellectual property hampered the evaluation of combinations of drugs if one drug were patented by one pharmaceutical company and the second or third drug were patented by a different company.

The Levine Panel Report certainly was an impetus for the ACTG to become a dominant player in the clinical research agenda with funds supported by the NIH. In 1995, the ACTG was restructured, and a self-governing structure was created with internal evaluation for establishing priorities and directing spending to specific focus areas. That same year, the PACTG, which split off from the adult ACTG in 1991, officially became its own entity. But questions began to arise about the ability of the PACTG to conduct studies efficiently and have accountability independent of the larger and more experienced group of clinical researchers that contributed to the adult ACTG research. The

Levine Report specifically recommended that funding for the PACTG be decreased, as its current level was not necessary, especially given the already apparent impact of the ACTG 076 ZDV study in reducing the number of HIV-infected children in the United States (Conner et al. 1994). The recommendation was ignored, and over the years that followed, funding for pediatric research increased dramatically, directly contributing to duplicative and unnecessary efficacy studies in children.[3]

In 1997, Dr. Stephen Spector from the University of California at San Diego became the group leader of the PACTG and director of the Coordinating and Operations Center, which was managed by a contract organization called Social and Scientific Systems, located in Bethesda, Maryland. At that time, there were twenty-one pediatric AIDS Clinical Trial Units (ACTUs) at major university medical centers under the ACTG umbrella. Each was the recipient of major funding from the NIH, and given this significant amount of support for research, one would have expected dramatic progress in the prevention and treatment of HIV in infants and children. This was not the case, however. Providing ZDV to HIV-infected pregnant women in the United States was beginning to significantly reduce the number of HIV-infected infants, and when HAART was used for preventative therapy, the number of perinatal HIV infections dropped even more ("Perinatal HIV Down" 1997). This meant that the number of HIV-infected children in the United States was inadequate for conducting any clinical trials of efficacy. Nevertheless, the PACTG moved forward with planning myriads of studies, even though it was obvious at the outset that it would be difficult to obtain the number of children required within a short enough time. The ensuing delay would significantly impede the evaluation of ARVs in children.

THE PEDIATRIC HIV/AIDS COMMUNITY DENIES HIV PREVENTION AND TREATMENT ADVANCES

The list of goals that could be accomplished within five years, first articulated at the 1995 Pediatric AIDS Foundation Think Tank on Early Treatment with Combination ARVs, included a reduction of perinatal HIV transmission to less than 2 percent in five years. In just three years, that goal was achieved in the United States, according to data compiled by the CDC. The achievement confirmed that the goal had not been theoretical but based on the implementation of advances in HIV prevention and treatment that were changing the course of the HIV/AIDS epidemic in the United States. The goal was reached without conducting additional large and expensive clinical research trials in HIV-infected women and their infants. It happened because physicians caring for HIV-infected patients had acted on existing evidence and had begun to treat all HIV-infected individuals with HAART—men, women, pregnant women, and children.

In spite of HAART's success in HIV prevention and treatment in the United States, pediatric HIV/AIDS researchers conducting international clinical trials chose to dismiss previous recommendations from an NIH-appointed panel of experts and from other experts such as Ho, Montaner, and Havlir at the 1996 Vancouver IAS Conference to treat all HIV-infected individuals with HAART, even though their pleas were based on multiple well-controlled research studies (Havlir and Lange 1998; Ho 1995; Montaner et al. 1999; Report of the NIH 1998). Also dismissed were decades of clinical experience and well-established, evidence-based principles that called for treating an infectious disease immediately following diagnosis—not waiting until the infection progressed to advanced disease. As Dr. Paolo Rossi from the Children's Hospital "Bambino Gesù" in Rome stated at a hearing on recommendations to delay ARV treatment: "This is prehistoric medicine." Delaying treatment and failing to use HAART in research and implementation were lethal decisions that had no precedent in the modern history of treating infectious diseases. The consequences would be grave. (Two research studies conducted in the 1940s, referred to as Tuskegee and Guatemala, withheld treatment for STIs and were subsequently deemed as unethical. They are discussed in Chapter 25.)

The gap between the adult and pediatric HIV/AIDS research community increased in 1995. The latter had argued that HIV infection of pregnant women and children was different from HIV infection in all other populations; therefore, the response to treatment would also be different. Although no evidence was presented to support this hypothesis, they argued that it warranted splitting the ACTG in two: one branch for adult and one for pediatric, allowing them to distance themselves from the vast body of scientific advances elsewhere. The move delayed the full implementation of HAART in women and children internationally and isolated the pediatric HIV/AIDS community from scientific and ethical oversight by the broader HIV research community. The risks of this isolation were highlighted in the 1996 Levine Committee review of NIH-sponsored research and the conclusions of the Whitley–Feinberg Panel on the research goals conducted by the PACTG ("Major Report" 1996; "Review and Reform" 1996; NIH 1996). Both reviews recommended an overhaul of pediatric research—a recommendation that was subsequently ignored, even though both the committee and the panel were commissioned by the NIH.

I participated in the Whitley–Feinberg Panel review, and I recall listening to presentations which suggested that the ARVs required separate evaluation in all pediatric populations—infants, children, and adolescents—not just for pharmacokinetics but also for efficacy ("Review and Reform" 1996; NIH 1996). I pointed out that the FDA did not require separate efficacy studies in all populations. Performing efficacy studies was not only unnecessary and therefore perhaps unethical, but also costly and time-consuming and would needlessly delay the availability of life-saving drugs for children. Listening to the discussion that followed, I wondered whether the increase in the number of research studies being proposed was related to the increase in funding available for research in pediatric HIV/AIDS.

Had early initiation of HAART been implemented by the pediatric AIDS research community, I sincerely believe that the goal of achieving less than 2 percent of perinatal HIV transmission could have been achieved internationally within five years as originally proposed in the 1995 Think Tank. In a perplexing turn of events, the pediatric HIV/AIDS research community took the unprecedented step of denying existing scientific data and delaying initiation of known highly effective treatment until HIV infection progressed to AIDS or infants became infected with HIV. It was not the lack of funding or the lack of convincing data that delayed the control of the pediatric AIDS epidemic—it was the result of a form of therapeutic denialism that crept into some corners of academic research and rejected the results of multiple studies demonstrating HAART's ability to reverse the course of HIV infection (CDC 2006).

The pediatric HIV/AIDS research community and WHO contributed equally to delaying implementation of HAART. The details of why and how their lethal decisions were made are discussed in Chapters 23 and 24, but it required both the pediatric

HIV/AIDS community and WHO to choose an Orwellian path of denying scientific evidence, declaring that HAART was not effective in vulnerable women and children, ignoring international ethical guidelines for standard of care, failing to protect human research subjects from exploitation, ignoring principles of informed consent, engaging in conflicts of interest, distributing benefits inequitably, and revealing an inexplicable indifference to the plight of hundreds of thousands of vulnerable women and children.

Over the decades that followed, the gap between the adult and pediatric clinical research community would widen even further. Separate committees were formed, and separate funding mechanisms were established. The pediatric clinical researchers funded through the NIH were thus able to develop their own research priorities, duplicate studies that had already been completed, claim that new studies were needed to answer questions that had already been answered, and avoid review by outside scientists and ethicists.

THE WHITLEY–FEINBERG PANEL: PEDIATRIC HIV/AIDS RESEARCH UNDER SCRUTINY

The Whitley–Feinberg Panel consisted of pediatric clinical researchers from both the pediatric and adult communities, along with activists and advocates. I had been asked to attend and comment on research completed by the PACTG and also on its proposed future direction. This was a more detailed review of NIH-sponsored pediatric research than that conducted by the Levine Panel, as Whitley–Feinberg focused solely on pediatric research. Lurking in the background was the fact that the PACTG was up for renewal that year, and the Whitley–Feinberg Panel members were fully aware that the Levine Panel Report had recommended significant reductions in their funding allocations ("Review and Reform" 1996; NIH 1996).

The PACTG had a modest beginning—only three clinical research sites received funding from the ACTG in 1986. By 1991, there were a total of twenty-four clinical research sites. Clinical research in pediatrics was not limited to the PACTG but was also performed by other NIH institutes, primarily the NICHD. Many of the clinical research sites were initially reviewed only by a contract organization rather than through the NIH's traditional peer-review grant process. The lack of sufficient scientific expertise within the contract organization may have been why some research studies moved forward in spite of objections by scientists who argued that they were not scientifically sound and ethically questionable.

By 1996, the PACTG had developed seventy-three clinical trials but had completed enrollment for only thirty-two. The cumulative enrollment of patients from 1987 to 1995 for all of the studies was only 8,836 infants and children, a number far too small to conduct timely studies of ARV efficacy. Increasing the numbers by enrolling adolescents with HIV infection did little to increase the numbers—over the same time period only 528 adolescents had been evaluated, and many who had become pregnant were also participating in studies of perinatal HIV transmission.

Because the cost of pediatric HIV/AID research was a concerning issue, the Whitley–Feinberg Panel examined the PACTG studies' per-patient cost and concluded that they were extremely high compared to adult studies. One in particular, conducted by the National Institutes of Mental Health, was designed to assess the development of HIV-infected children, a theoretically relatively straightforward observational study. The study was initiated in 1992, but by 1996 it had enrolled only 50 percent of the patients needed—it was projected to run for three additional years at a cost of $2.5 million each year. The calculated cost for each child enrolled was in the hundreds of thousands of dollars ("Review and Reform" 1996; NIH 1996).

Given the number of clinical research units focusing on pediatrics, there should have been a large list of accomplishments following ten years of funding and expansion of resources. However, the only truly successful study (ACTG 076) for which the PACTG could take sole credit was the prevention of HIV transmission from pregnant women to their infants. The study had been conducted in three years and consisted of only 694 patients to achieve its results. In contrast to the clear success of the ACTG 076 study, one of the PACTG's stated accomplishments was the observation that intravenous immunoglobulin could prevent serious bacterial infections in children with HIV. However, it was already known that intravenous immunoglobulin was effective in preventing bacterial infection in immunodeficient children. Outside the PACTG, this research study raised questions about unnecessary research duplication and exploitation of children.

A third accomplishment that the PACTG listed was one that showed that didanosine (DDI) and DDI+ZDV were superior to ZDV monotherapy in children who were symptomatic with HIV infection. Once again, this research study was unnecessarily conducted in children and actually had come to the wrong conclusion. DDI was not a drug that would survive the rigors of safety evaluation in infants and children, and adult studies were already showing that combination drug therapy was more effective than monotherapy.

The final major accomplishment listed by the PACTG in 1996 was the development of guidelines for preventing PCP in HIV-infected children. Before the study was even started, however, guidelines had already been developed for children with inherited immunodeficiency disorders and had established the widespread use of treatment with a common antibacterial agent known as trimethoprim-sulphamethoxazole. Therefore, this PACTG study was again unnecessary.

The Whitley–Feinberg Panel discussions identified an urgent need for developing infant formulations for the new ARVs, although we recognized that there was little financial incentive for pharmaceutical companies to develop pediatric products, and they always touted liability as an obstacle, regardless of its dubious significance. The panel recommended encouraging the earliest possible development of formulations, employing a systematic collaboration between the NIH and industry, using industry to provide assistance with formulations, and urging the PACTG's simultaneous evaluation of drugs for infants and children.

Unfortunately, not long after these recommendations were made, congressional legislation confused the role of the FDA, pharmaceutical companies, and the US government in developing these formulas. The population that lost out in the confusion was the infants, who were more dependent on chance interest than integrated concern.

There seemed to be agreement between the PACTG and the Whitley–Feinberg Panel that there were inadequate numbers of children in the United States to conduct many of the proposed clinical research trials—the only option seemed to be to move ahead with research in low-income countries where there was an unlimited number of infected or at-risk infants and children available (NIH 1996). I felt uneasy at the idea of conducting research using women and children in low-income countries without a preliminary, detailed, scientific and ethical evaluation of conducting studies in poor countries. In all likelihood, these countries would not directly benefit from the research, which could be construed as exploitation. Given the significant differences in economics, politics, culture, and language, the potential for research subjects' abuse was too great for comfort. I worried that US researchers were targeting poor countries to "mine" vulnerable individuals for research purposes: On the one hand, bringing clinical research to poor countries might be good news if it also brought the long-term benefit of access to newly discovered prevention and treatment. On the other hand, the potential for conflict of interest and exploitation were significant if the benefits of research proved to be greater for US HIV-infected individuals, clinical researchers, and their academic institutions.

There had been previous discussions about using research subjects from poor countries to evaluate products that were beneficial to individuals in the United States but would have no benefit for those in poor countries because of cost and lack of infrastructure. Would studies designed in the United States that enrolled vulnerable infants and children in poor countries take into account the priorities of the local health-care community? What if studies of the most potent and expensive ARVs were shown to be effective in poor countries but not available because of cost—would that be exploitation? Many thought it would.

The Whitley–Feinberg Panel concluded by developing a list of opportunities for clinical research beyond 1996. Perhaps the most important was a recommendation to evaluate early treatment of infants and children with HIV infection—the greatly increased rate of disease progression and death in children made this a priority (Blanche et al. 1994). Unfortunately, the recommendation was dismissed as future clinical research using children in developing countries defaulted to comparing inferior treatment strategies that delayed the initiation of treatment.

Given the early observations that 75 percent of HIV-infected infants in Africa died before five years of age, it is hard to understand why a study of early treatment initiation was not started immediately (Blanche et al. 1994; Becquet and Mofenson 2008; Violari et al. 2008; Kline and Shearer 1992). Instead, a delay of ten years followed, during which time infants and children could have received accelerated treatment with ARVs. In 2005, almost one decade after the Whitley–Feinberg Panel recommendations, incongruously, an NIH-supported study was designed to delay treatment in HIV-infected infants and compare this to early initiation of treatment. The study was conducted in South Africa and funded by a new iteration of NIH-supported clinical trials termed the Comprehensive International Program of Research on AIDS (CIPRA). As anticipated by critics of the study's science and ethics (who were not, however, able to stop the research from being conducted), the study was halted prematurely by the DSMB because of excess HIV infection and death in the children receiving delayed treatment (Violari et al. 2008). It was an unnecessary loss of vulnerable African children's lives.

Guidelines Can Become Rules

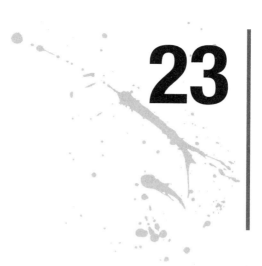

WHO IS WHO?

WHO is viewed as the major international organization dealing with global health and responsible for developing guidelines for the prevention and treatment of disease worldwide. The organizational structure is complex and its interaction with other UN organizations confusing. Their headquarters are based in Geneva, Switzerland, with six regional offices throughout the world and 147 individual country offices. The WHO headquarters in Geneva alone include a staff of eighteen hundred workers—there are eight thousand additional public-health experts, including doctors, epidemiologists, scientists, managers, and administrators scattered through hundreds of regional offices around the world. Its size, complexity, and insulation in decision-making have been a source of major criticism. Approximately 80 percent of WHO's current budget comes from wealthy countries, foundations, other multilateral bodies, non-governmental organizations, and private interests, such as pharmaceutical firms. Often the donated funds come with strings attached, requiring WHO to focus on specific diseases such as malaria and polio and leaving less room for flexibility or a rapid-response structure, which perhaps explains their delays in addressing the rapidly emerging Ebola virus epidemic in 2014 (WHO 2016).[1] But the slow response was not unique to Ebola; it was also evident in the emerging AIDS epidemic. An internal WHO memo in 1983, two years following the description of AIDS, stated that the organization did not need to be involved in AIDS because "[AIDS] is being well taken care of by some of the richest countries in the world where there is the manpower and the know-how and where most of the patients are to be found."[2]

DON'T TREAT THEM UNTIL THEY ARE REALLY SICK

In 1997, WHO published its first, much-delayed "Informal Consultation" on the treatment of HIV infection, which immediately sparked controversy—and with good reason. With an apparent paucity of expert scientific and economic opinion, WHO based its 1997 recommendations and its subsequently expanded 2002 guidelines on the short-term financial costs of treating millions of HIV-infected individuals. It was likely they were using what is now considered to be an outdated analysis of medical costs—cost-benefit, rather than the more realistic (and compassionate) cost-effectiveness analysis, whereby the long-range impact of investing in health care and stopping a rapidly expanding HIV epidemic is analyzed.

But the major difficulty with their guidelines was their unprecedented recommendation to treat only those individuals with advanced disease and to withhold treatment from millions of HIV-infected people. To put this into perspective, an international group of advisers headquartered in Geneva, Switzerland, with little to no responsibility for the care of patients with HIV/AIDS, no direct responsibility for their welfare or responsibility for the consequences of their decisions, assembled guidelines under which tens of millions of HIV-infected individuals worldwide should be treated, including when treatment should be started and what drugs should be used. The guidelines were meant to apply to countries affected by the HIV/AIDS epidemic regardless of the number of patients within those countries and regardless of whether the countries were economically advanced or extremely poor.

WHO treatment guidelines contrasted sharply with what was happening in practice in the United States. Once effective treatment became available for HIV/AIDS, healthcare professionals moved quickly to place all infected individuals on treatment, fearing that the disease would advance to irreversible complications and death, for which they might be personally responsible. One could only imagine the outcry and demonstrations from advocates and activists as well as patients themselves if, for example, physicians in the United States were to tell their patients, "I have drugs to treat your HIV infection, but you need to come back to me when you are sicker."

Few in the international community asked WHO to justify their authority to develop universal international guidelines that recommended withholding treatment until patients got sicker. WHO was entering new territory, usurping physicians' professional and ethical responsibility to make treatment decisions on their own patients and in their best interest. This trajectory was exactly the opposite of what individuals in low-income countries were asking for—they wanted to benefit from the same life-saving treatment that was available elsewhere, and they wanted their doctors to make a decision that was best for them.

EVIDENCE BASED, BUT WHOSE EVIDENCE?

WHO claimed that their treatment-guideline recommendations were evidence based. They were not. In fact, there is no evidence in the long history of treating infectious diseases that withholding treatment is of any benefit to the patient or to controlling an infectious-disease epidemic. In the past, formal attempts and studies of withholding treatment for an infectious disease were few, but in each instance they were ultimately deemed unethical. Now, WHO had embarked on a much more frightening path.

WHO's "evidence-based" conclusion came about by their simply stating that the evidence was not sufficient to recommend treating all HIV-infected individuals, which de facto ignored the recommendations of HIV experts, who since 1996 had been treating their patients with HAART. In fact, it is impossible to come up with an example of an infectious disease, or any other disease for that matter, where known effective treatment is deliberately withheld until patients advance to mostly irreversible phases of disease. Just think of withholding insulin for diabetes, cancer treatment for individuals with metastatic disease, or antibiotic treatment for pneumonia until the patient progresses to a more advanced level of the disease or even death.

One of WHO's other justifications for treating only the sickest of HIV-infected individuals was that, with limited funding, the sickest individuals should be treated first. Although on the surface this might seem a logical and compassionate decision, there was no clinical evidence that this approach would be the most effective in reducing mortality from HIV infection or in slowing the ever-increasing numbers of individuals who were becoming infected. At the time that WHO was promulgating its guidelines, evidence had accumulated that early treatment of HIV infection with cART could slow progression of HIV to AIDS, decrease medical visits, decrease the complications of infection, prevent the spread of TB, and prolong the lives of men, women, and children.

WHO's decision to promote these guidelines was destined from the outset for a tragic outcome. Spread of HIV by sexually active, untreated HIV-infected individuals continued, and the long-term cost of treating millions more HIV-infected individuals strained all national and international budgets. Lurking in the background was the inevitable development of HIV strains with multiple drug resistance, which would require more potent and expensive ARVs. In the long run, the human and economic toll of delaying treatment of HIV-infected individuals was costly and deadly.

WHO'S MISSTEPS AND DELAYS

The Economist news magazine was particularly harsh on WHO concerning the Ebola virus epidemic. In a commentary in the December 13, 2014, issue titled "Heal Thyself," they point out that in both the HIV and Ebola epidemics, WHO "dawdled" as the virus spread, leaving understaffed NGOs and faith-based organizations to pick up the slack.[3] A panel led by Dame Barbara Stocking, former chief educative of Oxfam, reviewed WHO's failed response to the Ebola epidemic. The panel's experts concluded that bureaucracy and politics coupled with a mismanaged response were responsible for WHO's failure. They recommended that a new division with new staff and a new director be established within WHO to coordinate emergency preparation, coordination, and responses to public health emergencies.[4]

WHO's response to the panel report was predictable. Having failed, they stated that they needed more money and promised that, in the future, they would be more accountable. It was a familiar pattern—repeated failures, repeated requests for more funding, and repeated promises of greater accountability. Just how greater accountability could be achieved was not made clear, but certainly it could not occur without removing many individuals with conflicts of interest in decision making and without enlisting detailed review by outside individuals who had nothing to gain personally. Perhaps, too, the funding formula for WHO needed to be changed to an industry standard—failure results in decreased funding; success results in increased funding.

In addition to recommending treating only those HIV-infected individuals with the most clinically advanced disease, WHO's recommendations for treatment included performing a CD4 cell count as a measure of impaired immunity, yet this is an advanced laboratory test that is unavailable to millions of HIV-infected individuals due to cost or lack of equipment.[5] Therefore, physicians practicing in rural regions of high-seroprevalence countries such as South Africa faced an ethical dilemma. In one study,

HIV infection rates were over 39 percent in pregnant women, but no CD4 counts were available for the majority of them. Investigators estimated that 70 percent of the women should have gotten HAART, but most did not solely because of unavailable CD4 counts (Hussain et al. 2011). Advanced technology was unnecessarily preventing health-care providers from giving HAART to needy individuals.

Following a workshop in 2007 on prevention and treatment of HIV that I conducted for mid-level health-care workers in Jinja, Uganda, I experienced a heartbreaking example of how WHO guidelines curtailed the willingness of health-care professionals to use their own clinical judgment. Early one morning, I accompanied two health-care workers who were making home-based care visits to HIV-infected individuals. One of their first visits was to a woman who was HIV infected and also had TB. Normally, this would have made her eligible for ART. She had lost a significant amount of weight since they had made their last home visit; however, I was told that she could not receive ARVs in spite of her known co-infection with TB and weight loss until a CD4 count was performed. The Ugandan Ministry of Health guidelines, modeled after the WHO guidelines, required a CD4 count before ARVs could be initiated, yet there was no immediate prospect of the woman's obtaining a CD4 count. A readily available and inexpensive total lymphocyte count would have solved the problem, or she could simply have been placed on ART without either a CD4 count or a total lymphocyte count, since she had two major criteria for AIDS diagnosis—advancing TB and weight loss. Had I been able to, as a physician responsible for the care of patients with HIV/AIDS, I would have placed her on treatment immediately, no matter what the guidelines said. After all, they were guidelines, not rules, and she would not survive much longer without ART. It was a striking example of how guidelines can replace sound medical judgment by becoming inflexible rules, to the detriment of the patient.

In contrast to Uganda's Ministry of Health (MOH), in 2012 Frank Chimbwandira, director of HIV/AIDS programs for Malawi's MOH, approached the situation in his country realistically and compassionately, stating: "We needed to do something. We found that we didn't test all the positive women for CD4 counts, and even those we did, there wasn't any systematic follow-up. We needed to protect the mother and the baby better, so we decided to put the HIV-positive women on treatment for life, which would save the mother and the baby" (UNICEF 2012).

Malawi did not have the economic or infrastructure capacity to provide universal access to CD4 cell-count testing, which would be needed to fulfill the WHO recommended requirements for implementing prevention and treatment. Chimbwandira used sound clinical judgment and saw the requirement for CD4 counts as an unnecessary obstacle to saving the lives of HIV-infected women and their infants in his country. He realized that each year there were tens of thousands of HIV-infected pregnant women who desperately needed ART but were not receiving it. Malawi's MOH therefore implemented a modified approach to prevention and treatment, in which all HIV-infected pregnant and breastfeeding women would be given lifelong ART regardless of CD4 count or clinical stage. This, of course, was precisely what pediatric activists had been demanding since 1996. Within the first year of implementation, Malawi realized a 748 percent increase in the number of pregnant and breastfeeding women who started ART, an increase from 1,257 to 10,663 women.

However, going against WHO guidelines, in spite of Malawi's success in saving lives, had international repercussions. The bureaucratic regulators did not look at the results showing numbers of lives saved in one of Africa's poorest countries. They saw only a country that dared to go against their guidelines. What was one of the poorest developing countries in the world doing setting their own standard for prevention and treatment of HIV infection? International funders of Malawi's HIV programs— including the United Kingdom Department for International Development, the World Bank, and the Global Fund to Fight AIDS, Tuberculosis, and Malaria—threatened to remove hundreds of millions of dollars of funding for Malawi's "violating" WHO guidelines and related issues. Ironically, years later, WHO, the Global Fund, PEPFAR, and the pediatric HIV/AIDS research community all adopted Malawi's approach to treating HIV-infected pregnant women and preventing perinatal HIV transmission as the universal standard of care.

GUIDELINES MAY NOT BENEFIT EVERYONE

Over the years, I repeatedly debated the validity of guidelines for the treatment of HIV-infected individuals. In 1985, in an article in the *Annals of Internal Medicine*, I argued that the CDC classification of AIDS was for epidemiologic purposes only, not to determine when treatment should be initiated (Ammann 1985). While the CDC had publicly stated that its classification of AIDS was only meant to help study the epidemiology of HIV and AIDS and was not meant as a guideline for treatment, just as with WHO years later, government regulators used the guidelines to deny treatment to HIV-infected individuals. The guidelines were in fact being used to classify HIV-infected children as well, resulting in underestimating the number of infants and children with AIDS in the United States. Because many of the HIV-infected infants did not have the classical symptoms of AIDS found in adults, they were denied medical, social, and psychological assistance. I publically stated that the approach to diagnosing and treating HIV-infected patients should be no different than any other infectious disease—treat as soon as a diagnosis is made. By 1985, an antibody test for HIV was available; it was a simple matter of performing a blood test to determine if an individual, no matter his or her age, was infected. If so, regardless of clinical features or other laboratory tests, treatment and care should be provided immediately.

The CDC guidelines also excluded women with HIV infection from obtaining access to care and treatment. In 1986, while working at Genentech, I meet with Dr. Jim Curran from the CDC. Curran knew almost everything that needed to be known about the HIV/AIDS epidemic—where new infections were occurring, risk factors for acquiring HIV infection, and how the virus was spreading throughout the United States and the world. On the evening of his visit, scientists from Genentech and I met Curran for an informal dinner at the Hong Kong Flower Lounge in Millbrae, California. Not surprisingly, most of the conversation revolved around HIV, what Curran knew about the epidemic, and the emerging science at Genentech related to HIV vaccine research. During the conversation, I brought up the issue of the misuse of CDC guidelines to exclude HIV-infected women and children from treatment and care, pointing out that a diagnosis of chronic and drug-resistant vaginal candidiasis was not considered an AIDS diagnosis in an HIV-infected woman; therefore, they were ineligible for treatment and care, even though their physicians knew that this represented an advanced stage of infection. Curran explained that when they proposed expanding the criteria for diagnosing AIDS, the US Office of Budget and Management had determined that expanding the AIDS diagnosis to include vaginal candidiasis would be too costly for Medicaid/Social Security disability. While Curran privately revealed the basis of the CDC's decision, it was never acknowledged publically.

Terry McGovern, a lawyer and senior fellow at the Ford Foundation, was well aware of the discrimination against women that resulted from the CDC guidelines. She was responsible for the program "Reducing HIV/AIDS Discrimination and Exclusion" and had firsthand experience with women who were being turned away from receiving benefits in the 1980s. "There were these women who were coming in because they couldn't get Medicaid, they couldn't get Social Security disability, they were losing their children because they couldn't work, and they clearly had AIDS," she said.

McGovern filed a class-action lawsuit in 1990 against the Social Security Administration, stating that they were violating race, gender, and disability laws. She highlighted a pattern across the United States in which women were excluded from HIV treatment and care. McGovern prevailed in the lawsuit, and the guidelines were changed. This was a clear victory, but one that was confined to the United States. The absence of comparable activism and legal representation for women and children in low-income countries was devastating. Governments were all too willing to forgo the demands of providing standard of care for citizens by deferring to the WHO guidelines that recommended less than the best of ART and to US-sponsored clinical research studies that employed inferior treatment standards.

UNDERMINING THE PHYSICIAN'S
RESPONSIBILITY FOR PATIENT CARE

An additional consequence of WHO treatment guidelines for income-poor countries was the power they had to remove the medical decision-making responsibility from practicing health-care professionals and place it in the hands of an often unsympathetic, uncaring, and unresponsive bureaucracy. During my travels to low-income countries, I often encountered health-care professionals fearfully reluctant to violate the WHO/ MOH guidelines. It was not just a matter of whether ARVs were available—government-controlled health ministries, indifferent to the needs of their people, even prohibited the use of donated ARVs because they were not listed on WHO's approved list of treatments. In some instances, government health-care officials prohibited the use of PEP drugs to prevent HIV infection and pregnancy in women who were raped because the treatment provided was not the package WHO recommended. Thousands of women who had been victims of sexual violence went without preventive therapy—many of them became pregnant and infected with HIV and other STIs.

How the guidelines became a means of prohibiting individual physicians from providing standard of care became clear to me while I was attending a workshop in Liberia in 2014 along with Dr. Susa Coffey, a San Francisco physician who was treating a large population of HIV-infected individuals with HAART. After listening to a long litany of requirements that the government had put in place before a health-care professional was permitted to start HAART, Dr. Coffey leaned over to me and whispered, "It looks to me like the WHO treatment guidelines are designed to keep as many patients as possible off of lifesaving treatment rather than putting them on treatment." Indeed, it seemed as if fewer patients were being put on treatment than kept off. Yet Coffey remained incredulous that a set of guidelines could usurp the authority of physicians to provide the best care for their patients.

In the days that followed, Coffey and I returned to San Francisco, where all HIV-infected patients could be placed on ART. It seemed the height of injustice that the same was not true in Liberia, the DRC, Zimbabwe, Tanzania, and a host of other countries where the cost of ARVs had plummeted to levels that could no longer justify withholding treatment based on economics. The stubborn refusal of WHO, the undue influence of US researchers who employed inferior treatment regimens, the insensitivity to the welfare of individual patients, and the indifference to an ethical standard of care were the major roadblocks.

WHOM DOES WHO REPRESENT?

By 2000 activism and advocacy in wealthy countries had subsided considerably as the most aggressive US activists were benefiting from the over thirty antiretroviral drugs and combinations of drugs available. Increasingly, oversight of the ethics and science of international prevention and treatment recommendations lay within the purview of highly selected individuals and organizations. Even the interpretation of the ethics of health-care delivery and research lay in the hands of a limited number of academics who were closely allied with those who made decisions on health-care delivery in poor countries. Many of these individuals acted as advisors for developing WHO guidelines and participated in scientific and ethical reviews of clinical research protocols. Too often these people consisted of friends and colleagues of investigators conducting research studies—or even the investigators themselves. They controlled the prevention and treatment decisions made in low-income countries and excluded outside criticism. Avoidance of self-criticism and adoption of unquestioned group thinking was a consequence. Also worrisome was the fact that many of them were supported by NIH funding that depended on continuing clinical research in low-income countries—an overt conflict of interest for many.

Absent from the decision making were the activists that had been present at almost every treatment decision-making event in the United States—individuals who fought for those who were most affected by HIV and were dying without ART, especially HIV-infected women and children. In the early days of the AIDS epidemic, HIV-infected individuals actually sat at the same table as representatives of the FDA, US government health agencies, the NIH, pharmaceutical companies, and clinical researchers, fully participating in the decision-making process that would directly affect their lives. In low-income countries, it was a very different situation. Poor women and children couldn't get to the meetings where the decisions determining their destiny were being made. If women were present, they were usually tokens used to avoid the criticism that they were being excluded. Today, examples can easily be found in which exclusion of outside opinion resulted in government or academic committees and organizations refusing to accept responsibility for the unethical conduct of a study or for failing to offer standard of care treatment.[6]

During this time an important question troubled me. Why did WHO fail to recommend the same standard of care treatment for individuals in low-income countries as was being recommended in the United States and Europe? Were they too isolated or too remotely involved in the suffering caused by HIV/AIDS? Was there some sort of conflict of interest within WHO, and if so, what could it be? Writing in *Foreign Affairs*, Christy Feig and Sonia Shah addressed a related issue: "Voluntary contributions from private interests and others now bankroll four out of every five dollars of the WHO's budget," and they raised the question of whether substantial sums of money from the United States, including large and influential foundations, can disguise hidden agendas and trade and commercial interests under the umbrella of public health.[7] Accusations can be made, but direct links are difficult to identify. Still, an increasing number of individuals are concerned that the large donations from highly influential foundations and the political influence of US government institutions may influence the direction and priorities of WHO's public-health decisions, especially since, increasingly, large donations are being made by a relatively small group of organizations with closely held beliefs on which public-health issues should be emphasized.

WHO's annual estimated budget of over $4.5 billion comes from a number of sources—$1.5 billion is derived from voluntary donations from member states, the UN, and other international institutions. It is hard to imagine that any of these sources could exert influence over WHO's treatment recommendations for HIV-infected individuals. However, this possibility was raised at a 2014 meeting of the International Alliance of Patients' Organizations in Ascot, England, where I was asked to speak. At the meeting, attended by numerous nonprofit groups from around the world representing patients with diseases ranging from diabetes to multiple sclerosis to chronic pain, a common theme emerged—patients felt that they were not getting standard of care and their needs were not being met. In other words, the regulators of health care were not listening. During a break in the meeting, I spoke to a former WHO employee about the complexity of some of these issues and used the illustration of the WHO guidelines on treatment of HIV infection as an example of the disconnect between international organizations, governmental organizations, and patient treatment needs. I further explained my frustration with trying to understand why WHO produced treatment guidelines that recommended inferior standard of care and delayed treatment until HIV had advanced. The former WHO employee explained that it was not difficult to understand at all—WHO might not want to risk making recommendations for treatment that would be costly to member states that were not interested in spending money for the health of their citizens and might, if threatened, choose to discontinue their donations. Member states might instead choose to spend their funds on military weapons or some other priority rather than on health care for their citizens. I was therefore provided with a possible explanation for WHO's recalcitrance in recommending a universal standard of care, but I still had no evidence that it was correct, even though the former WHO employee insisted that it was.

The next day, Marie-Paule Kieny, a WHO representative, addressed the International Alliance of Patients' Organizations conference attendees regarding the availability of health care in low-income countries. In the speech, she promised that WHO would listen to the voices of patients around the world and take into account their needs when making WHO recommendations for universal health care and treatment. As I continued to listen, the person sitting next to me realized that I was becoming agitated and urged me to "say something." I waited until the speech was completed and then, as politely as I could, considering my inner emotional turmoil, asked, "If what you just said was true, then why in eastern Democratic Republic of Congo are there hundreds of thousands of women who have been raped and are in need of PEP and hundreds of thousands of HIV-infected pregnant women and their infants who are pleading for ARVs for treatment and prevention but cannot get standard of care, even if drugs are donated, because their governments are adhering to WHO's inferior treatment and prevention guidelines?" My question went unanswered.

Treatment Guidelines

Not without Risks

Guidelines for the diagnosis and treatment of specific diseases are necessary to provide health-care professionals with information and direction on the best means of caring for their patients. All guidelines have, somewhere in their text, the statement that the guidelines are simply that—guides that are not meant to supplant individual decisions made by health-care professionals who are ethically and legally responsible for the welfare of their patients. Increasingly, however, guidelines become rules as they are used by large health-care providers and governmental agencies to control costs and determine what can or cannot be done based primarily on economic benefits to the health-care provider rather than the patient's best interest. Individual patients who object to how they are being treated by their physicians may find that decisions on their treatment are based on guidelines developed by the insurance company, health maintenance organization, or national government.

Concerns about the influence of health-care guidelines are not confined to low-income countries. Recently, physicians in the United States have been confronted with an avalanche of new guidelines for diagnosis and treatment, most of which have been highly controversial. For example, outside of the field of HIV, recommendations for the use of routine mammograms for the early detection of breast cancer and the treatment of hypertension are in constant flux, with much tension ensuing between health-care providers on the one hand and physicians and their patients on the other. In their recently published book *The Death of Cancer*, recounting the long and often frustrating history of treating the disease, Vincent DeVita and Elizabeth DeVita-Raeburn suggest that hundreds of thousands of individuals in the United States die needlessly from cancer each year, and rules and guidelines are partially to blame: "Guidelines are backward looking. With cancer, things change too rapidly for doctors to be able to rely on yesterday's guidelines for long. These guidelines need to be updated frequently, and they rarely are, because this takes time and money. . . . Reliance on such standards inhibits doctors from trying something new" (2015). The conclusion is that physicians and patients need to beware of rapid proliferation of government-generated guidelines for health care, especially under the umbrella of "health care reform." It is too tempting for health-maintenance organizations, health-insurance companies, and the US government to transform guidelines into rules in an effort to maximize saving money while neglecting to provide the best medical care to the patient. Rules, of course, hold greater weight than guidelines, and for that reason they are often used by national ministries of health to deny treatment to patients, especially under circumstances where treatment is provided by the national health-care system. "He who pays, decides what treatment is given" is a widespread interpretation of guidelines except, of course, in countries such as the United States, where there is a strong activist community challenging treatment decisions, and malpractice or legal repercussions for failing to give the best of care to an individual patient are a threat. But even in the United States, there are other ways to enforce guidelines to prevent health-care professionals from providing the best of treatment for their patients. One of them is to refuse to reimburse for the treatment.

The first widespread use of international guidelines to determine the health and welfare of HIV-infected individuals was the 2002 WHO guidelines for the prevention and treatment of HIV. Within years of their release, the guidelines became "rules."[1] Because WHO wields great international power, national ministries of health were reluctant to deviate from WHO guidelines and hid behind these guidelines by making them rules, especially when they were less costly to the national government. Individuals could therefore be denied the best standard of care simply because the current international standard of care was not included in the WHO guidelines followed by their country. Such was the case with WHO guidelines for the treatment of HIV, which from the onset recommended inferior treatment regimens and delayed treatment of HIV infection. Contesting the guidelines was virtually impossible. The activist community in low-income countries is less powerful and often unable to demand standard of care for any disease, let alone HIV infection. Legal remedies and malpractice are practically nonexistent and therefore offer little help.

What could have motivated WHO to take a shortsighted view of treatment and care for HIV-infected individuals? One reason perhaps was that they wanted to give the public impression that they were treating all of the HIV-infected individuals that needed treatment. Short of "smoke and mirrors," WHO calculated the percentage of individuals that were receiving recommended treatment under their guidelines by defining "treatment" as only for those with advanced disease. Of course, in reality, all HIV-infected individuals needed treatment, and there were tens of millions who did not have advanced disease but who equally required lifesaving treatment. They were excluded from WHO's calculations. Under their guidelines, WHO could claim 50 percent of those who needed treatment were receiving ARVs. However, if all HIV-infected individuals had been included in the calculations as requiring antiretroviral treatment, then only 12.5 percent were being treated.

There was certainly a need for an influential international organization such as WHO to develop health guidelines that helped low-income countries determine priorities, yet WHO used their own criteria rather than an international standard of care based on principles of treating infectious diseases. Failing to halt HIV transmission and infection with the universal use of HAART resulted not in controlling the HIV/AIDS epidemic but rather in perpetuating it. In the years that followed the publication of WHO's initial guidelines, the organization used its failures to argue for an increase in its role in treatment and prevention and, as also occurred in WHO's failed response to the Ebola virus epidemic, to call for even more financial support, even as it was failing its mission and the public's trust.

In some ways, it is not surprising, given the insulated way in which WHO operates, that the development of their treatment guidelines was so disconnected from the well-established principles and practices of infectious-disease medicine.[2] In their book *Tinderbox*, Craig Timberg and Daniel Halperin point out that the war against AIDS was directed by individuals who viewed the epidemic through "Western eyes," which resulted in recommendations that failed to recognize that HIV was finding new victims faster than it could be prevented and individuals treated (2012).

Only those who participated in the development of WHO's HIV treatment and prevention guidelines know how and why their recommendations were made and whether some of the decisions served the best interest of the consultants and ministries of health rather than the HIV- infected individuals from low-income countries who could not attend the meetings. What is known, however, is that WHO was consistently out of step and more than a decade behind the vast body of expert physicians, scientists, and health-care workers who were medically and ethically bound to provide their patients with the best standard of care. These experts knew best how to treat HIV infection and prevent new infections and, in the long run, how to slow the HIV/AIDS epidemic in all populations. They knew, too, how to transform those who were HIV infected into individuals with normal, healthy life expectancies, no matter where the patients lived. They looked at the WHO guidelines and asked, "What kind of standard of care is it if it only recommends what is affordable and not what is the best treatment available?"

THE RISE, FALL, AND RETURN OF STANDARD OF CARE TO HIV/AIDS TREATMENT GUIDELINES

The first informal US recommendation for the treatment of HIV infection was published three years following the approval of ZDV. A 1990 "state-of-the-art" conference sponsored by the NIH concluded that treatment should be initiated at a CD4 count of <500 cell/mm3 (the lower limit of normal) based on the results of a 1989 ACTG study that had shown that ZDV could delay HIV disease progression with minimal side effects in infected patients with CD4 counts <500 cell/mm3 (Fischl, Richman, Causey, et al. 1989; "State-of-the-Art Conference" 1990). Less than a year later, the FDA approved ZDV for HIV-infected individuals who were either asymptomatic or mildly symptomatic with <500 cell/mm3. The importance of this approval was that it acknowledged that even HIV-infected individuals with normal CD4 counts or who had minimal clinical symptoms should receive treatment.

An important aspect of the recommendations was emphasizing that CD4 counts are highly variable in individuals from week to week and even day to day. The purpose of the qualification was to point out that physician judgment was needed to determine when an individual should be started on ART. Given these precautions, as well as the complexity and cost of conducting CD4 counts in low-income countries, it is difficult to understand why WHO- and NIH-supported clinical researchers subsequently incorporated CD4 counts as a requirement for initiating treatment. With the passage of time, the WHO CD4-count guideline became as rigid as the WHO guidelines themselves. An individual could be denied treatment because his or her CD4 count was 500, but if it were repeated the very next day it might be 450, which would allow treatment.

The first formal ART treatment guideline was developed in the United States in 1993 by a group of HIV/AIDS experts during a time of intense scientific and clinical enthusiasm and AIDS activism (Sande et al. 1993). Not surprisingly, with few exceptions, treatment of all HIV-infected individuals was recommended.[3] By 1996, results of several clinical studies using combination ARVs in over six thousand HIV-infected individuals were available, indicating that the use of two or more drugs had greater benefit in controlling HIV disease progression than monotherapy. The IAS was the first organization to formally develop treatment guidelines incorporating some of these recent studies (Carpenter et al. 1996, 1997). They recommended that all symptomatic individuals be treated regardless of CD4 counts and once again recommended that asymptomatic individuals with CD4 counts of <500 cells/mm3 be placed on treatment. Additionally, for the first time they recommended that individuals with CD4 counts >500 cells/mm3 be placed on treatment if they had high viral loads (>5,000 HIV RNA copies/mL). The introduction of viral load to determine when treatment should be initiated was based on clinical studies indicating that the combination of a low CD4 count and high viral load predicted progression to AIDS. IAS also introduced the suggestion that treatment with three drugs would be better than two based on data that the new PIs had a dramatic effect on decreasing viral load and increasing CD4 counts. The treatment guidelines developed by the IAS reflected many clinical researchers' and physicians' optimism that at last HIV could be brought under control. It also reflected traditional infectious-disease principles that were shared by health-care professionals and activists—the earlier treatment was started, the more likely HIV could be brought under control and prevent HIV progression to AIDS.

In 1998 the OAR convened a panel of HIV experts to define eleven principles of treatment. The principles should have formed the scientific and ethical basis of all future treatment recommendations and clinical research study design—unfortunately they did not, and for HIV-infected pregnant women and children, ignoring the principles in formulating research studies and implementation strategies had dire consequences. The panel concluded its recommendations with this statement: "These topics and other data assessed by the Panel in formulating the scientific principles were derived from three primary sources: recent basic insights into the life cycle of HIV, studies of the extent and consequences of HIV replication in infected persons, and clinical trials of anti-HIV drugs. The principles and conclusions discussed in this report have been developed and made available now so that practitioners and patients can make treatment decisions based on the most current research results" ("Report of the NIH Panel" 1998).

The dichotomy of the strong recommendations coming from the NIH-sponsored panel of experts and the failure to act on them in subsequent WHO guidelines and NIH-sponsored research of perinatal HIV transmission suggested a lack of scientific and ethical integrity. Had the emphasis been placed on practitioners and patients jointly making treatment decisions as suggested, perhaps the outcome of the pediatric HIV/AIDS epidemic would have been different.

Erosion of the 1998 NIH panel of experts' recommendations came quickly and from within the NIH itself. Hidden within the 1998 meeting of the US Public Health

Service Task Force on ARV Treatment of HIV-Infected Pregnant Women was a statement that was predictive of the future direction of perinatal HIV prevention research on early initiation of HAART and which resulted in withholding treatment from HIV-infected pregnant women in low-income countries:

> Although more potent antiretroviral combination regimens that dramatically diminish viral load also may theoretically prevent perinatal transmission, no data are available to support this hypothesis. The efficacy of combination antiretroviral therapy to decrease the risk for perinatal HIV-1 transmission needs to be evaluated in ongoing perinatal clinical trials. Additionally, epidemiologic studies and clinical trials are needed to delineate the relative efficacy of the various components of the three-part ZDV chemoprophylactic regimen. Improved understanding of the factors associated with perinatal HIV transmission despite ZDV chemoprophylaxis is needed to develop alternative effective regimens. Because of the dramatic decline in perinatal HIV-1 transmission with widespread implementation of ZDV chemoprophylaxis, an international, collaborative effort is required in the conduct of such epidemiologic studies and clinical trials. (US Public Health Service Task Force 1998)

Unfortunately, this denial of scientific and clinical data went unchallenged. It did not bode well for ending the pediatric HIV/AIDS epidemic, and it was fatal for those who were destined to be denied effective ART. The statement falsely declared that there was no evidence that potent ART would reduce viral load and prevent HIV transmission from HIV-infected pregnant women, when in reality multiple studies had proven that the more potent the ART, the more the viral load was reduced and the greater the reduction in HIV transmission (Dickover et al. 1996; Sperling et al. 1996; Thea et al. 1997). Additional data that had been published reporting the results of US government-sponsored clinical research and epidemiologic data presented by the CDC had confirmed the association of viral load and HIV transmission. Further, the impact of implementing HAART had been documented by the CDC in 1997, demonstrating that the number of newly infected infants in the United States plummeted from two thousand per year to fewer than one hundred per year coinciding with early initiation of HAART in HIV-infected pregnant women ("Perinatal HIV Down as Treatment Increases" 1997).

The criteria for initiating ART recommended by the two major organizations engaged in developing treatment guidelines, the US Public Health Service and WHO, began to change in 2008. Gradually, the recommendations for starting ARVs based on CD4 counts crept upward from 250 to 350 and then in 2011 to 500—the level that was originally recommended in 1990 when only ZDV monotherapy was available. By 2012, IAS and the US Public Health Service finally released guidelines that recommended treating all HIV-infected individuals, regardless of CD4 counts or clinical symptoms (Thompson et al. 2012; DHHS Panel 2016). WHO and some pediatric academic researchers continued to resist changing their guidelines for more than three years until they were forced by scientific and public opinion to do so in 2015 (Beyrer et al. 2015).

In 2015, within three months of each other, two critically important announcements were made—one by the NIH and one by the International Maternal, Pediatric,

Adolescent AIDS Clinical Trials Network (IMPAACT) / Promoting Maternal and Infant Survival Everywhere (PROMISE) research team supported by NIH funding. They both declared that all HIV-infected individuals should receive lifelong treatment with HAART, including HIV-infected pregnant women. The announcements were based on the NIH-sponsored START study (Strategic Timing of AntiRetroviral Treatment) that had enrolled 4,685 HIV-infected men and women and had shown that approximately 50 percent of research subjects who started treatment at CD4 counts over five hundred had fewer episodes of AIDS, serious non-AIDS events, or death. The study was stopped prematurely by the DSMB based on the significance of the results. The official NIH announcement declared: "We now have clear cut proof that it is of significantly greater health benefits to an HIV-infected person to start antiretroviral therapy sooner rather than later . . . early therapy conveys a double benefit, not only improving the health of individuals but at the same time, by lowering the viral load, reducing the risk they will transmit HIV to others" (McNeil 2015; NIH 2015).

Also in 2015, at the IAS conference, almost twenty years after the first IAS Vancouver conference, during which treating all HIV-infected individuals had been first articulated, the 2015 "Vancouver Consensus" made it impossible for international organizations, researchers, or scientists to continue to deny treatment to any HIV-infected individual: "Medical evidence is unambiguous. At this point, further delays threaten not only millions of lives but also threaten a resurgence of this pandemic. But if we act rapidly, we can drive down HIV incidence, death, and long-term costs. Political will is needed to complete the work of what can be one of the most effective public health interventions in history" (Beyrer et al. 2015).

The announcements were a pyrrhic victory for advocates and activists who had demanded immediate treatment for vulnerable HIV-infected women and infants since 1996, but they were also too late for the millions of HIV-infected people who had been denied treatment between 1996 and 2015 and had succumbed to the virus. Readers must conclude for themselves what might have motivated WHO and certain clinical researchers to withhold potent treatment from HIV-infected individuals in spite of the pleas to "treat all" emanating from leaders in infectious disease and HIV such as Havlir, Richman, Ho, Markowitz, Montaner, Gulick, and over six thousand other scientists; health-care providers; political, community, and business leaders; journalists; governmental, non-governmental, and intergovernmental representatives; and people living with HIV/AIDS who attended the 1996 International AIDS Conference in Vancouver. Describing the dramatic results of early initiation of HAART, Julio Montaner, co-chair of the IAS conference, declared, "We have an obligation to decide whether the evidence is enough. We've waited too long to do what we know is right. Enough is enough. We need to move to implement."

Had these pleas been acted on in 1996, I wonder if we would be looking at a very different epidemic in 2016 and not one that still claims the lives of more than 1.5 million men, women, and children each year.

WHEN THERE IS A CHOICE BETWEEN SIMPLE AND COMPLEX, REGULATORS WILL CHOOSE COMPLEX EVERY TIME

What could be simpler than the following directive? "Test all sexually active individuals for HIV infection. If they are infected, start treatment immediately." Testing and screening for all sorts of diseases are done regularly in both high-income and low-income countries. An HIV test requires a simple finger stick, the test costs only two dollars, and it can be performed by mid-level health-care workers and even traditional birth attendants. Diagnosis leads to treatment, and treatment saves lives and prevents HIV transmission. Health-care professionals around the world know how to treat infectious diseases, many of which are as complicated as or even more complicated than HIV infection. But regulators from high-income countries seemed indifferent to the need for simple and concise HIV-treatment guidelines that could be used in low-income countries. Complexity reigned. Recalling the words of Dr. Susa Coffey at a workshop in Africa, "It looks to me like the WHO treatment guidelines are designed to keep as many patients as possible off of lifesaving treatment." The guidelines became a roadblock.

The first treatment guideline published by WHO in 2002 was over 160 pages long. The criteria for initiating ART read like a Chinese restaurant's menu.[4] There were multiple tables listing the various WHO staging criteria, which differed between adults and children. Other tables listed immunologic criteria for initiating treatment, and separate tables depended on what laboratory tests might be available in low-income countries. For the majority of HIV-infected individuals and the health-care professionals caring for them in some of the poorest regions of the world, rather than facilitating access to treatment, the guidelines became an almost insurmountable barrier to prevention and treatment.

The staging of HIV infection was a holdover from the early days of the epidemic when a test for diagnosing HIV infection was not available. The CDC had developed a list of laboratory and clinical features that defined AIDS. WHO followed the CDC's lead: Stage I was asymptomatic, Stage II consisted of early manifestations of HIV infection, Stage III had more advanced clinical manifestations, and Stage IV was the most advanced form of HIV infection. WHO decided to use Stage IV as the clinical criteria for initiating treatment, the stage that usually occurred some five to seven years after initial HIV infection and preceded death by mere months to several years. There was no evidence that this was where treatment should start in spite of WHO's insistence that its recommendations were always evidence based. In fact, what they were using was an "educated" guess. Within the different stages of HIV infection, there were specific diseases that were almost impossible for health-care providers in most areas of the developing world to diagnose or treat—central nervous system toxoplasmosis, cryptosporidiosis, cryptococcosis, etc. An individual who had lost 10 percent of his or her body weight would be classified as WHO Stage III and therefore ineligible for ART. But if the 10 percent weight loss was associated with diarrhea for over one month, that same person would be classified as WHO Stage IV and eligible for ART. What confusion!

A major obstacle to initiating treatment was the requirement for a CD4 count (see Chapter 23). The lack of a CD4 count often excluded individuals from receiving HAART. CD4 criteria for initiating treatment persisted until, in 2012, the IAS and USPHS guidelines stated that all HIV-infected individuals should receive lifelong treatment regardless of their CD4 count. But it was not until 2015 that all international public-health agencies and clinical researchers completely eliminated the requirement of a CD4 count before initiating HAART (Beyrer et al. 2015; McNeil 2015).

From the very beginning of developing treatment recommendations for HIV, a simple statement based on decades of treating all other infectious diseases would have sufficed—"Treat all HIV-infected individuals." It would have allowed the time, energy, and funding to focus on training health-care workers on how to correctly use the potent ARVs that had been discovered. And even more importantly, it would have saved the lives of millions of individuals from HIV infection and prevented the expansion of the HIV/AIDS epidemic.

The WHO treatment guidelines took a long time to develop, translate, print, and distribute. For over twenty years, costly workshops were conducted throughout the world to train health-care workers on the guidelines' intricacies. Ministries of health developed their own medical records or registries to track the patients that had been tested for HIV and required categorization before treatment could be initiated. For many, it seemed as if once training was completed and registries printed, a new set of guidelines inching closer to treating all those who are HIV-infected would appear, and training would begin all over again. In my travels through Africa, I observed health-care workers struggling to remember and define what stage of HIV infection individuals belonged to. I witnessed their discouragement when they were required to refuse treatment for an individual who fell into a non-treatment category.

In 2015 all of the previous staging categories and CD4 testing criteria were rendered moot as the recommendation to treat all HIV-infected individuals was declared universal. In 2105, after the new treatment criteria were published, I visited Zimbabwe, a country with a high seroprevalence of HIV but where much progress had been made in prevention and treatment. I still saw health-care workers in clinic after clinic filling out detailed registries and laboriously recording the WHO stage of disease and CD4 count. Contrary to the 2015 recommendations, health-care workers were still using CD4 counts to deny treatment, even as the pharmacy shelves were lined with enough ARVs to immediately treat all of their HIV-infected patients. At that point I wondered how long it would take to retrain all of the thousands of health-care workers and whose responsibility that would be—WHO, the NIH, the national ministry of health, or all of them? Arguably, WHO and NIH need to accept the major share of responsibility, having for decades incorrectly instructed health-care workers to deny HIV-infected individuals treatment based on CD4 counts, a laboratory test that should never have been used to begin with.

PART 4 Stalled
Losing Sight of the Mission

During the second phase of the plague their memory failed them, too. Not that they had forgotten the face itself, but—what came to the same thing—it had lost fleshy substance and they no longer saw it in memory's mirror.

He tried to recall what he had read about the disease. Figures floated across his memory, and he recalled that some thirty or so great plagues known to history had accounted for nearly one hundred million deaths. But what are a hundred million deaths? When one has served in a war one hardly knows what a dead man is, after a while, and since the dead man has no substance unless one has actually seen him dead, one hundred million corpses broadcast through history are no more than a puff of smoke in the imagination.

Albert Camus, *The Plague*

Damn the Ethics, Full Speed Ahead

THE STORY OF ESTHER AND HER BABY

Esther was a nineteen-year-old pregnant woman who lived in a rural village outside of a major city in sub-Saharan Africa. Her country ranks among the poorest in Africa. Esther became pregnant when she was coerced into having unprotected sex with an older man in exchange for food. After she told him she was pregnant, he disappeared.

Despite her unstable circumstances, having a baby of her own was very important to Esther, and she wanted to be certain that the pregnancy and delivery went well. However, in her village there are only traditional birth attendants. She had heard she could get better care at a medical center that received funds from America, and many of the doctors there had been trained by American physicians.

It took Esther over two hours by matatu minibus to reach the medical center. Once there, she had to wait an additional two hours before she was seen by a health-care worker. The prenatal-care clinic at the hospital saw between fifty and sixty pregnant women each day. It provided basic clinical care, education on self-care during pregnancy, and performed a handful of routine laboratory tests. At the end of her first visit, Esther was asked to attend a group session of about fifty to sixty women, where she was given additional information on pregnancy and infant care. During the group session, Esther was told that the clinic would test her for HIV unless she didn't want to have the test done. Clinic staff informed Esther how HIV is spread and explained the purpose of the test. All of the women in the group session were told that only the clinic workers would know the test results. Esther had heard about AIDS before; she knew that some young women had become very sick from an infection they got from men. She thought it was a good idea to get the test done, especially since she could receive the results before making the trip back to her village.

Esther waited in a large room with other women, many of whom had infants and children with them. After several hours, Esther was called into a private room to speak to a health-care worker. She noticed that the other women were watching her walk into the room. Esther observed that not every woman who had agreed to an HIV test was being called back, and she wondered if only the women who were infected were being asked to return. A health-care worker told Esther that her HIV test was positive, and that a second test was needed to confirm the result.

The second test confirmed that she was indeed infected. The health-care worker provided Esther with additional information and explained that Esther might need treatment for HIV. The worker also suggested that Esther might need additional treatment to keep her unborn child from also becoming infected. However, additional blood tests would be required to determine if Esther was eligible for such treatment.

It would be another four weeks before Esther was seen in the clinic again. As before, she took the long trip on the matatu minibus and waited to be seen, this time by a different health-care worker, who told Esther that she was not eligible for treatment of her own HIV infection, but that treatment could be given to her to prevent her baby from becoming infected with HIV. Esther did not understand why she was being offered treatment just for the baby. Why couldn't she receive treatment, too? She was reluctant to ask any questions, however, and wished that there were someone with her who could explain what she was being told.

The health-care worker then asked if Esther would like to participate in a clinical research study sponsored by the American NIH. The study would compare two different treatments to see which one worked best to prevent Esther's baby from becoming infected with HIV. One treatment would be given for a long time and one for a short time. She would not know which treatment she would receive. Esther was again confused—why wouldn't everyone get longer treatment? Wouldn't that be better? What was the NIH, and why were Americans interested in her? Once again, however, she was afraid to ask questions, but she wondered why no one seemed concerned about her HIV infection.

Later, more details were provided to her, including the benefits of breastfeeding and not breastfeeding. Esther was also told that she would need to attend regular clinic visits until her infant was nine months old, and if she did not want to be in the research study, she could still be seen in the government clinic. It was unlikely, however, that Esther would receive the same treatment at the government clinic that she would if she were to participate in the research study. Although the health-care worker was speaking Esther's tribal language, he used many words that she did not understand. Esther was illiterate and thus dependent on the health-care worker to translate the information from English to her tribal language.

The health-care worker had a printed document that described the benefits and risks of the research. It consisted of seventeen pages in English, which Esther could not read, and was called an "informed consent." As the health-care worker turned the pages, he referred to many things that Esther did not understand, such as randomization, research, experimental drug, antiretroviral drugs, allergy, and her right to receive compensation for injury. The health-care worker also talked about something that might affect her central nervous system or cause inflammation of the liver or severe muscle pain, but she didn't understand any of these words. Time was short, so the health-care worker spoke quickly as he explained that if there were better treatments available elsewhere, she would be told about them. When the interview was completed, the health-care worker asked Esther if she wanted to be in the research study and, if so, if she had any questions. She had none. All this happened in less than thirty minutes. Esther was then asked to sign the "informed" consent that had just been read to her. Her signature would indicate that Esther had agreed to be enrolled in the clinical research study and to abide by its rules, including regular visits to the clinic during pregnancy, delivery at the hospital, and nine months of post-delivery follow-up visits. (An example of an informed consent used in Africa is provided in the endnotes.[1])

Esther believed that what she being was told would help her and her baby. She wasn't being offered any special treatment at her village, and the health-care worker said that Esther would only get treatment to keep her baby from becoming infected with HIV if she enrolled in the research study. He also stated that she would receive a small amount of money to help defray the costs of traveling from her village to the hospital. Esther placed an X as her signature on the last page of the informed consent, indicating that she understood the risks and benefits of participating in the study. The health-care worker co-signed the informed consent, indicating that he had provided her with all the necessary information about the research study and that Esther understood what she was told. The research protocol required random assignation to one of the two available treatment programs, and when Esther returned to the clinic two weeks later, she began her randomly assigned program. She faithfully kept her scheduled return visits, using the small amount of money she'd been given to pay for transportation expenses.

The birth and delivery went well. Esther and her baby were given frequent blood tests, and on her last visit to the clinic, Esther was told that, unfortunately, recent tests indicated that her infant was HIV-positive. There was also evidence that Esther's own HIV infection had advanced, and the health-care worker told Esther that she might be eligible for treatment of her own HIV infection as well as treatment for her infant. However, she could not continue to receive care at the clinic she had attended for the last eighteen months because the research study had ended. Esther would instead need to go to the government clinic to ask if they had treatment available. Esther did not understand why she couldn't get treatment at the current clinic. The health-care worker explained that under the terms of the informed consent that Esther had signed, neither the clinical researchers nor the NIH had any obligation to continue her treatment. When Esther went to the government clinic, they told her that they did not have any of the medicines that she had taken in the research study and could not help her. Esther felt abandoned.

WEAKENING OF THE ETHICAL PROTECTION FOR CLINICAL RESEARCH

Although Esther's story is a hypothetical scenario, it is based on actual facts and observations that are far from unique. Thousands of vulnerable women and children in low-income countries have had similar experiences and indeed continue to experience a process of inadequate informed consent and randomization into one of two or three treatments. Esther's example illustrates some of the major ethical issues confronting clinical research today, such as which therapeutic products are selected for evaluation; who determines the priorities for selection; what benefits research subjects accrue from their participation; whether the research exploits vulnerable individuals (especially women and children); do informed consents truly inform; what is the definition of standard of care; and what obligation do clinical researchers have to continue care and treatment once a study has been completed. International ethical guidelines established to prevent exploitation determine the process by which research in humans is conducted and how informed consent is obtained. It is not an easy task, and it has been made more difficult by the complexity of research studies and the extraordinary proliferation of clinical research performed to prove the efficacy of a large number of new therapeutic products. A clinical research study sponsored by the US government or a nonprofit foundation must go through an ethical review in both the United States and in the countries where the research is being performed. If an experimental drug is involved that is also studied in the United States, the FDA also has oversight.

Much can go wrong, and it often does, especially when studies are performed in locations where careful monitoring is difficult and when there are differences in culture, language, legal protection, liability, and understanding of ethical guidelines. It is therefore not surprising that clinical researchers often attempt to simplify, reinterpret, and even bypass ethical guidelines, including the informed consent process. Past ethical guidelines are sometimes seen as irrelevant to current research seeking to address global health issues. Altering existing ethical standards is a risky practice which fails to consider that the guidelines deemed "irrelevant" were, in fact, established because of prior research abuses often caused by paternalistic attitudes that presumed research subjects, especially those in low-income countries, did not have the intellectual capacity to understand the risks and benefits of the research.

At this point in the discussion, it is essential to acknowledge the importance of clinical research. This book chronicles the remarkable medical discoveries that identified the virus that causes AIDS, the ability to diagnosis infection, and the means to identify all of the ways HIV is transmitted. Clinical research also resulted in the discovery of more drugs to treat HIV infection than any other viral disease. It would be unimaginable to think what the global HIV epidemic would be like if it were not for the successes of basic science and clinical research. Clinical research also sorted out what worked and what didn't work, providing benefit to millions and also protecting them from treatments that might be harmful. But undoing or weakening ethical guidelines to facilitate research cannot be justified or accepted. The rapid pace of new research discoveries necessitates an even greater call for ethical standards, justice, equity, and concerns for the safety and benefits of research participants who often place their own lives at risk for the benefit of others.

PLACEBO-CONTROLLED CLINICAL RESEARCH STUDIES

The primary goal of scientifically conducted clinical research studies is to test a hypothesis, prove that one treatment is more effective than no treatment, or that one treatment is superior to another. Some clinical research studies compare two or more treatments to determine whether or not the treatments are equivalent. The designation "treatment arm" is used to indicate that there are two or more comparisons. Ethical guidelines approve of the use of placebo comparisons only when no proven treatment is available. The first debate about the use of placebos in studies of HIV-infected individuals was the ACTG 076 study on prevention of perinatal HIV transmission. Following that study it was generally agreed that future use of placebos in studies of HIV-infected pregnant women and their infants was unethical.

Placebos are used to allow investigators to draw meaningful conclusions from shorter studies and smaller sample sizes. If successful, shorter studies allow life-saving treatment to be available sooner and to a larger number of individuals. But despite these benefits, when there are known effective drugs available, it is unethical to give patients a placebo, thereby depriving them of known effective treatment. Clinical research studies, especially those that use placebo comparisons, are conducted under well-controlled conditions with oversight by a DSMB, which can stop a study early if the data conclusively show either a marked benefit or marked detriment of the research drug.

At a 1997 congressional hearing on bioethics, the Public Citizen's Health Research Group—a national, non-profit consumer advocacy group—criticized the use of placebo in clinical trials. They expressed concern that studies comparing placebo versus known effective drugs would be done in low-income countries (Angell 1997; Lurie and Wolfe 1997). This concern arose from the use of a placebo in the ACTG 076 ZDV study, which had been approved by academic institutions and the NIH. Their criticism was quickly embraced as countries targeted for future studies—such as Uganda and Thailand—caught wind of these plans. Placebo trials were compared to the Tuskegee syphilis studies, in which treatment was withheld from infected African Americans in order to study the progression of untreated syphilis.

In 1997, the *NEJM* published two articles arguing that placebo trials were unethical and would deny vulnerable individuals a proven beneficial treatment (Angell 1997; Lurie and Wolfe 1997). Soon afterward, two prominent members of the editorial board of the journal resigned: Dr. David Ho, who was subsequently named *Time*'s Man of the Year, and Catherine Wilfert, who was an influential researcher, advocate, and professor of pediatrics at Duke University. Both were opposed to the strict, unyielding positions regarding placebos. They suggested that an outright dismissal of placebo use could significantly delay development of life-saving treatments by increasing the size of clinical research trials and lengthening the time between the initiation of the research study and obtaining results. Importantly, however, both Ho and Wilfert insisted that placebos could only be used in clinical research studies if there were no known effective treatments already available.

That same year, Dr. Joseph Saba, head of UNAIDS, and I co-authored an op-ed for the *New York Times* responding to the *NEJM* articles ("A Cultural Divide on AIDS Research," September 20, 1997). We outlined the stance shared by non-profit foundations, such as amfAR and UNAIDS, that placebo-controlled clinical research trials conformed to international ethical guidelines if there were no known effective treatments available. This opinion was shared by many physicians and leaders in low-income countries, such as Dr. Edward Mbidde, chair of Uganda's AIDS Research Committee. Mbidde declared that the arguments of the Public Citizen's Health Research Group were patronizing and a form of ethical imperialism. He believed that placebo trials were essential to determining whether shorter courses of antiretroviral therapies, which were more affordable than costly long-term treatment in low-income countries, could be equally effective in preventing perinatal HIV transmission.

Initially I was sympathetic to Mbidde's argument. Unfortunately, this opinion, unique to a specific time in the HIV/AIDS epidemic and clinical research, eventually led to conducting clinical research trials in poor countries and justifying clinical research based primarily on economic considerations. Rather than conducting studies that compared the standard of care to a potentially more potent and effective treatment, studies began to appear that compared treatment regimens that were less than standard of care to even more ineffective treatments based on theoretical economic advantages. The "new placebo" became inferior treatment regimens.

INADEQUATE INFORMED CONSENTS

Informed consents are essential for ensuring that research subjects understand both the risks and benefits of participating in a research study. Through the Freedom of Information Act, I was able to review several of the informed consents used in NIH-funded clinical research on perinatal HIV transmission. Many of the informed consents omitted critically important information and some misrepresented what was considered standard of care for HIV treatment and prevention of HIV transmission. In some instances, HIV-infected pregnant women were not told that the standard of care in income-rich countries was to provide lifelong HAART. Instead, the consent suggested that the answer was not yet known. Informed consents used in the NIH PROMISE clinical study for prevention of mother-to-child HIV transmission, which sought to enroll thousands of HIV-infected pregnant women and their infants in Africa, stated, "Stopping the anti-HIV medications after use for prevention of transmission to the baby in the women who would not be on the medications for their own health is often done in the United States and other countries."[2] The statement was in fact not true, suggesting that misinforming pregnant women about standard of care may have been used to encourage their participation in the research study. In addition, many of the informed consents had not been updated and approved annually as required by NIH ethical guidelines. In a recently announced NIH-sponsored study, VRC01, HIV-infected pregnant women will be asked to sign a complex fourteen-page informed consent while they are in labor to allow the experimental evaluation of a monoclonal antibody in their infants that was stated by the researchers themselves to be of no benefit to either the mothers or their infants. Additionally, if the mothers are illiterate, they can place an X at the end of the consent form to acknowledge that they understand the risks (NIAID 2016).

Other problems were apparent. While many of the informed consents also included risks such as the side effects of multiple drugs, the terminology they used, such as "lactic acidosis," "anxiety," and "immune reconstitution syndrome," were difficult to translate and understand. Many details important to individuals agreeing to participate in the research studies were omitted. For example, HIV-infected pregnant women were not informed that if they participated in the study and ART was stopped, they would run the risk of disease progression and might develop untreatable opportunist infections or that the ARVs might not work when restarted. Research participants were also not informed that the inferior treatment they were being offered was not recommended in income-rich countries or even in some neighboring countries of equal or even lesser economic status. None of the research participants were told that the studies they had volunteered for could not be performed in the United States, where offering inferior treatment without proper informed consent would be deemed unethical.

As I continued reviewing the content of other informed consents, I felt that the potential benefits of research were emphasized while potential risks were minimized or even omitted. The informed consents had evolved into an exercise of fulfilling a regulatory purpose rather than accurately informing research participants of risks versus benefits. As the motivation to conduct more research in HIV/AIDS as well as other diseases intensified, linked with dramatic increases in funding for research, the informed consent process began to be viewed by some researchers as an annoyance or even an obstacle to research.

Surprisingly, the February 2014 issue of the *NEJM* published an article written by highly respected ethicists suggesting a radical departure from requiring informed consent for all research studies, arguing that under certain circumstances an informed consent might not be needed to conduct ethical research. Ruth Faden, Tom Beauchamp, and Nancy Kass stated in their article: "One major question is whether informed consent should always be required for randomized comparative–effectiveness studies, particularly studies conducted in a learning health-care system." They were suggesting that academics know best when informed consent is required for certain types of studies and when it is not, and they should be trusted to make the decision. It was a plan that would eliminate the "annoying" ethical requirement of informed consent for certain studies and would allow research to be conducted without letting an individual know about it.

In an accompanying article, Scott Kim and Franklin Miller, two ethicists at NIH, considered Faden, Beuachamp, and Kass's proposal as "paternalistic," countering that individuals have the right to determine whether they participate in research regardless of the investigators' viewpoint. They added an additional concern—physicians would be engaging in deception, actively concealing the patient's inclusion in a research study, if informed consents were to be eliminated (Kim and Miller 2014).

TWO STANDARDS OF CARE: ONE FOR WEALTHY COUNTRIES AND ONE FOR POOR COUNTRIES

For decades, clinical research and economics were mostly distinct disciplines. However, as the cost of health care increased disproportionately to other costs, greater attention was given to the use of clinical research to evaluate the economics of health care and its affordability. Today it is not unusual to read some of the most prominent medical journals and find entire issues that focus on the economics of treatment and health-care delivery rather than the science of research and the practice of medicine. As the disciplines of clinical research and the economics of health care have merged, so too have the justifications for research become conflated. Economic factors are now used to justify research studies that compare an established standard of care to inferior treatment, with the purpose of determining if less costly but inferior treatment might be as effective as standard of care. To the economist, who is not directly responsible for the welfare of the patient, this type of study may seem logically required to define the cost of population-based health care. But for individual patients who participate in research studies and receive inferior treatment, the results can be disastrous. For physicians caring for their patients, making health-care decisions that give greater weight to economics degrades accepted principles of medical ethics. Historically, physicians have believed that their primary ethical duty is to provide the best standard of care to their patients. Costs are considered, but they are not the final arbitrator in determining treatment.

On the surface, it may seem that performing studies using less costly but inferior treatment comparisons might be ethical and an efficient means of defining economical ways to prevent and treat HIV in low-income countries. After all, if a country can't afford the best standard of care, what harm would there be in providing sub-standard care? At least "they" will get something. But this is an illusion, as it may inhibit working toward providing the best standard of care. The harm resulting from inadequate treatment and prevention may also be far greater than anyone wants to acknowledge—HIV infection is allowed to progress to full-blown AIDS and transmission of HIV in these countries, bringing with it a host of deadly and costly complications.

Standard of care definitions have long guided the ethics of clinical research and the practice of medicine. Many considerations regarding standard of care were derived from major ethical abuses of research-study participants in the past, such as in Nazi Germany and the infamous Tuskegee research studies in the United States.[3] But some have argued that it is unclear how standard of care is defined when considering clinical research that is performed at one extreme in income-rich countries and at the other extreme in low-income countries.

The definition of standard of care has been debated for many decades among organizations attempting to establish ethical principles of clinical research. The World Medical Association's revised *Declaration of Helsinki* put forward the view that all research trial participants in every country are entitled to the worldwide best standard of care. This is sometimes referred to as a universal standard of care defined as "the best current method of treatment available anywhere in the world for a particular disease or condition." (WMA 2013). Those who oppose this view argue that it is sometimes ethically permissible to provide less than the best worldwide standard of care to research participants and that, in some situations, research-study participants should be offered the best treatment available from their own national health system. Further, opponents of universal standard of care argue that there is a benefit in performing clinical research using individuals in low-income countries, as "something is better than nothing." The latter interpretation assumes that research subjects have little value beyond research and raises worrisome questions as to how far this argument could be carried. What if, for example, a poor country provides no treatment for a certain disease? Could clinical researchers preferentially select that country to justify the use of placebos or the evaluation of a treatment that would have absolutely no benefit? This would be considered exploitation of research subjects solely for the benefit of wealthier countries.

The use of economic factors to justify research studies of less costly but inferior treatment in a country that fails to offer standard of care must be viewed with suspicion. Will the research result in supporting misplaced political priorities? An example is South African President Mbeki's public position that there were inadequate funds to provide ARVs to prevent perinatal HIV transmission, while simultaneously spending $750 million, along with an unknown amount for kickbacks, for diesel-electric submarines. South African treatment delays continued even after they were receiving as much as $590 million per year by 2008 from the US PEPFAR program, more than enough to treat all of the HIV-infected pregnant women to prevent perinatal HIV transmission (Schneider and Fassin 2002). In another more recent example illustrating the fallacies of succumbing to an economic argument that all low-income countries lack sufficient funds for health care, the March 21, 2015, issue of *The Economist* reported that just a few Kenyan officials, ministers, and businessmen misappropriated an amount of funding that could have paid for ARVs for every HIV-infected patient in the country for a decade. Kenya is one of the many countries receiving funding from PEPFAR and the Global Fund to Combat AIDS.[4]

While economics is an important factor for determining how health care is delivered, it should not be a factor in defining standard of care. As understood by most practicing physicians, standard of care is the best level of care that can be delivered to the patient, not what can be done for the least amount of money. Regrettably, the introduction of an economic basis for determining standard of care resulted in a restructuring of ethical standards for HIV-related research in poor countries. Using the criteria of the most economical treatment to prevent perinatal HIV transmission, the number of clinical research studies for prevention of mother-to-child HIV transmission proliferated. The studies which were conducted in multiple low-income countries evaluated less expensive but inferior variations of drug combinations, varying treatment lengths, and whether ARVs were given to HIV-infected pregnant women, to their the infants, or to both. The studies could only be conducted by withholding known highly effective antiretroviral treatment (HAART) from HIV-infected women and children, raising scientific and ethical questions about the types of research studies that NIH should, or should not, be supporting.

There have been several widely reported clinical research studies of withholding lifesaving treatment from vulnerable research subjects. The two most infamous are the Tuskegee study conducted between 1932 and 1972 and the Guatemala study conducted between 1946 and 1948 (Katz et al 2008; Semeniuk and Reverby 2010; Reverby 2011; Mays 2012). Neither of the studies was declared unethical during the time it was conducted, and in the case of the Guatemala studies, the unethical nature was not discovered until 2010, more than sixty years after its completion, as Susan Reverby was conducting research on the Tuskegee experiments. There are disturbing similarities between the Tuskegee, Guatemala, and NIH-sponsored HIV/AIDS studies involving vulnerable women and infants—the studies were conducted by US-supported researchers, the research was approved by their academic intuitions, fundamental ethical research guidelines were violated, informed consents were nonexistent to inadequate, the populations enrolled were poor, disadvantaged, poorly educated, and vulnerable to exploitation, standard of care was not provided, the studies could not be conducted in income-rich populations, and the benefit to the researchers was greater than the benefit to the research subjects. Given similarities between the studies, it is likely that with time, medical historians will view the withholding of lifesaving antiretroviral treatment from HIV-infected women and children as comparable to the Tuskegee and Guatemala experiments except for the greater magnitude of the HIV studies. The combined number of research subjects in the Tuskegee and Guatemala studies is fewer than 2,500—the number of vulnerable women and children affected by the NIH research sponsored studies is difficult to calculate precisely, but it certainly exceeds 100,000.

The Tyranny of Research

26

RESEARCH SUBJECTS ARE REQUIRED
TO BENEFIT FROM RESEARCH

Ethical principles for clinical research were codified following major ethical abuses. The National Commission for the Protection of Human Subjects of Biomedical and Behavioral Research was formed in 1974 to address ethical abuses in research conducted in the United States. This commission issued the Belmont Report in 1979, which provided ethical guidelines for clinical research and outlined three major ethical principles to guide the conduct of research in humans. The first of these was justice, defined as the equitable enrollment of research-study participants and avoiding individuals that may be exploited because of vulnerable circumstances such as poverty, minority, or imprisonment status.

The second principle was autonomy, defined as the right of each individual participating in research to make an informed decision regarding participation. The principle of autonomy finds expression in the informed consent document, which should provide a detailed description of the research study, the risks, the benefits, and any treatment alternatives. After presenting the informed consent, patients should be given sufficient time to ask questions and clarify issues.

The third principle was beneficence, defined as the obligation to maximize benefits for the individual participant while minimizing their risk of harm. Certain clinical research studies emphasize beneficence as not just applying to the individual but also to society as a whole. Using the principles articulated in the Belmont Report as a guide, there is evidence to suggest that some current US-sponsored studies are deviating from ethical norms as well as from sound scientific principles that determine whether there is sufficient evidence to conduct the research in humans.

In the hypothetical story of Esther, all three of the above ethical principles are either violated or diluted. Concerning justice, Esther is enrolled in the study because as a poor, vulnerable woman she has little to no access to treatment. The clinical researchers and the study sponsors do not offer Esther extended care after the study is completed or any assurance that, if there is a future pregnancy, she will receive treatment that is proven successful. In regard to autonomy, the amount of time allotted to review the informed consent, the length of the informed consent, and the language obstacles raise questions as to whether Esther has truly given informed consent. Finally, there is a question as to what benefit Esther actually derives from enrolling in the study. At the time of the study, the clinical research investigators are aware of other, more effective treatments that their study will not provide.

The large US investment in research has resulted in the proliferation of new treatments, all of which must be tested for safety and efficacy before they can be approved by the FDA for use in humans. However, the US "pool" of individuals from which to draw research subjects is becoming insufficient, primarily as a result of successful HIV prevention and treatment. Evaluating a new antiretroviral treatment in US patients who are already taking three or more highly effective drugs is virtually impossible, as it would require patients to either stop taking their medications or to add an additional drug to an already successful regimen, making it difficult to prove the benefit of the new drug. As such, there is an increasing demand for research subjects who reside in poor countries and who do not have access to antiretroviral treatment. These individuals, referred to as "treatment naïve," make it easier for researchers to evaluate a new drug and also to reduce the number of research subjects required for a study. Further, conducting research studies in poor countries is much less expensive than comparable studies in the United States due to a number of factors, including lower salaries, less expensive and fewer laboratory studies, and little to no liability costs. For these reasons, it is tempting to move clinical research studies from the United States to low-income countries.

Complicating the approach to using research subjects in low-income countries is the fact that many of the drugs are exceptionally costly and, even if highly efficacious, are unlikely to be available in the poor countries where the studies are performed. Under these scenarios, the fallback reasoning and frequent justification for research is that it is "for the good of humankind," a rationale used increasingly to justify conducting research in poor subjects, including women and children, that is of no direct benefit to them.[1]

Several research studies have been conducted in poor countries because, ethically, they could not be conducted in the United States. One such study was sponsored by the NIH and performed in Uganda beginning in 2004. The study proposed using an antibody preparation called HIV hyperimmunoglobulin (HIVIG), which consisted of concentrated antibody obtained from HIV-infected individuals. The study's hypothesis was that infants became infected with HIV because the antibody transferred from their mothers was too weak to prevent infection (Onyango-Makumbi et al. 2011).

Even before the study was performed, it failed to meet the rigorous scientific scrutiny of several well-known scientists. Because there was a lack of convincing laboratory and human evidence that antibody could prevent HIV infection, scientists objected to this study, which they felt placed mothers and their unborn children at undue risk. In fact, a study conducted in the United States a full five years before the proposed Uganda study had not shown any clinical, immunologic, or preventative benefit of HIVIG in HIV-infected pregnant women and their infants (Stiehm et al. 2000). Since the study was halted in the United States by the DSMB, plans were made to conduct a similar study of HIVIG to prevent perinatal HIV transmission in Uganda.

When the results of the Uganda study were released in 2011, they not only failed to show any benefit, but they also demonstrated a statistically significant increase in HIV infection in the infants who received HIVIG, possibly related to the fact that antibody treatment may have facilitated HIV infection.[2] Art Caplan, a well-known bioethicist, referred to the study's numerous ethical violations and raised the issue of exploitation, arguing that "something ought not to be studied in a population which could not reasonably benefit from it" (Ammann, Gough, and Caplan 2012).

It is difficult to obtain an independent review of the ethics and science of a research study once it has been approved by academic institutions and their committees when the request emanates from an "outside" individual. When the request comes from a research study subject, it is even more unlikely to be honored. Frustrated by a seemingly failed ethical and scientific review of a study, I contacted various US government and academic institutions and requested a review of the study by an independent group who had no direct involvement or interest in the study. After more than a year of writing letters and emails requesting an investigation, I felt I was being stonewalled. No one seemed willing to accept investigatory responsibility for the study's questionable science and ethics. I even wrote to the director of the NIH, Francis Collins. In Collin's reply, he suggested contacting the Presidential Commission for the Study of Bioethical Issues, precisely where I had started one year before.[3] Reflecting on my frustration, I concluded that if a well-established researcher, academic, and leader in the field of HIV/AIDS could not get answers to his questions, there was no way a research subject in an income-poor country could obtain legal or ethical protection.[4]

WHAT IF THE RESEARCH HYPOTHESIS IS INCORRECT?

Howard Temin, who won the Nobel Prize in 1975 for his discovery of reverse transcriptase, taught me that all scientific investigation must be supported by a sound scientific hypothesis. He was not a believer in proceeding with research that was based on a false or weak hypothesis or wanting to conduct research for the sake of research. When I first learned of the hypothesis promoted by the PACTG that ARVs would not be as effective in HIV-infected pregnant women and infants in low-income countries as in adult males and non-pregnant women in wealthy countries, and therefore warranted independent research studies, I immediately recalled his words of wisdom. The hypothesis proposed by PACTG contradicted almost every well-established scientific principle and regulatory policy on drug evaluation and efficacy. Hundreds of studies conducted throughout decades of research in infectious disease, cancer, and HIV indicated that the major benefits of treatment occurred when treatment was started early before complications of the disease occurred—usually immediately following diagnosis. Additionally, the FDA had repeatedly declared that separate studies of drug efficacy were not deemed necessary in all populations for proving efficacy, particularly for an infection like HIV (FDA, Final Rule 1994). Delaying treatment with HAART in HIV-infected pregnant women and their infants until research studies were completed in low-income countries was unwarranted.

Previously published data which contradicted the PACTG hypothesis was dismissed, including studies that reported that without treatment, 50 percent of HIV-infected infants died by two years of age, five times more quickly than HIV-infected adults, an observation that should have called for immediate treatment of infected infants (Blanche et al. 1994). Also rejected was an Italian Registry study of the response of HIV-infected infants and children to HAART, documenting that they responded better to ART than adults (De Martino et al. 2000). Undeterred by the facts, the pediatric HIV/AIDS research community decided to conduct a study that compared early treatment of HIV-infected infants to delayed treatment. The study was called the Children with HIV Early Antiretroviral (CHER) Randomized Trial (Violari et al. 2008).

The CHER trial was designed to test the scientifically unsupported hypothesis that delaying antiretroviral treatment of infants might be of benefit to them. The study was conducted under the leadership of Avy Violari, a South African researcher, and involved more than eighty investigators from Africa, the United States, and Europe. HIV-infected infants were randomly assigned to a group receiving ARVs as soon as HIV was diagnosed, while the other group had treatment withheld until they reached certain clinical and immunologic end points of advanced disease. The study could never have been conducted in the United States at the time the study was initiated in South Africa. Many scientists outside the pediatric community objected to the study as unethical from the first time they heard about it, as it had already been documented that delaying treatment in infants was lethal.

Midway into the study, in a scenario that was becoming familiar, the DSMB halted the research because the mortality in the delayed treatment group vastly exceeded the mortality in the infants who were treated immediately. The results of the study were predictable and castigating: delayed treatment resulted in four times more deaths in the delayed treatment group compared to those who were treated immediately after diagnosis. The deaths of the infants were unnecessary and unconscionable. When the study results were published in the *NEJM* in 2008, the authors did not reference or discuss the studies conducted five years earlier that had concluded, "The effectiveness of HAART in infants and children to reduce HIV-1-related deaths is at least similar to, or even greater than, that observed in adults" (De Martino et al. 2000).

An additional example of a study that should not have been approved by an IRB was conducted in Thailand and led by Lallemant and associates from the Institut de Recherche pour le Développement in France, Thailand, and Harvard University with funding from NIH and organizations in Thailand and France. The design of the study defied scientific logic, as it sought to determine how little treatment could be given before infants born to HIV-infected mothers became infected. The results were reported in the *NEJM* in 2000 (Lallemant 2000). The study consisted of four cleverly worded research-study arms:

1. "Long-long": Treatment of the mother initiated at twenty-eight weeks of gestation with six weeks of zidovudine administered to the infant [similar to what was deemed standard of care in the United States at that time].
2. "Long-short": Treatment of the mother initiated at twenty-eight weeks of gestation with three days of zidovudine administered to the infant.
3. "Short-long": Treatment of the mother initiated at thirty-five weeks of gestation with six weeks of zidovudine administered to the infant.
4. "Short-short": Treatment of the mother initiated at thirty-five weeks of gestation with three days of zidovudine administered to the infant.

Fortunately, the "short-short" arm was quickly discontinued by the DSMB, but not before it was shown that the HIV infection rate was more than twice as high. This could easily have been foreseen, sparing the infants' lives. Incredibly, the investigators knowingly placed HIV-exposed infants at greater risk of acquiring HIV infection by seeing how little treatment could be given.

It is unclear how the Thai study could have been approved by all of the IRBs involved—French, Thai, and Harvard—and subsequently published in a prestigious medical journal such as the *NEJM*. It was conducted at a time when there was conclusive evidence that early initiation of cART and prolonged treatment of HIV-exposed infants provided the greatest protection from perinatal HIV transmission. The study seemed to be based on scientific curiosity rather than on achieving maximum protection from HIV infection for the infants. Questions were raised of how multiple IRBs could have approved a study to determine how little drug could be given before an infant became HIV infected, risked dying, or required lifelong drugs.

UNFORESEEN OUTCOMES OF INCREASES IN RESEARCH FUNDING

Elisabeth Glaser, pediatric AIDS clinicians, activists, and I had advocated for more than a decade for increased funding for HIV/AIDS. When the increase finally came, it came quickly and was responsible for many of the major advances in prevention and treatment. But the large amounts that subsequently became available in the late 1990s and early 2000s had reached what is often called "absorptive capacity." All of the funds simply could not be used wisely, so abuses were inevitable. Clinical researchers began designing studies in HIV/AIDS in both the United States and low-income countries that many considered unnecessary. By 2012, the combined funds for biomedical research from the NIH and the Organization for Economic Co-Operation and Development (OECD), an organization composed largely of wealthy European-country members, was more than $90 billion. That same year, the NIH budget for HIV/AIDS research alone was more than $30 billion ("Experts Rethinking Billions" 2008).

Large amounts of money for research did not ensure either high-quality research or a prioritized evaluation of new prevention and treatment interventions that could benefit individuals in low-income countries. Even individuals within the academic community acknowledged that such vast amounts of research funding resulted in a proliferation of studies and medical publications that were inaccurate and often completely false. In a highly controversial meeting of the International Congress on Peer Review and Biomedical Publication held in Chicago in 2013, John Ioannidis, an epidemiologist at Stanford University, created a storm of scientific controversy when he stated, "Most publicized research findings are probably false" and suggested that the problem was ongoing (Ioannidis et al. 2014). Others at the meeting suggested that there were practices and perverse incentives in academic research resulting in the publication of questionable studies. They did not spell out what the perverse incentives were, but I assumed that they were referring to the large amount of funding that was being made available for research and awarded to individual researchers and their academic institutions.

It was generally believed that when millions of dollars were spent on a clinical research study in an income-poor country, most of the benefit went to individuals and researchers within the country. This was not the case. In fact, for decades, no overhead was awarded by NIH to institutions in low-income countries where the research was being conducted. US institutions sponsoring the studies extracted 45 percent or more (Harvard University extracted 69 percent) of the total cost of the research study for overhead, which went to paying generous salaries, benefits, and travel expenses for US researchers, support personnel, managers, and administrators and the expansion of infrastructure such as laboratories, offices, and educational facilities. The amount was not trivial. In 2011, the total obtained by twenty of the major universities was more than $7 billion (Ledford 2014). Some institutions, such as Johns Hopkins, even recruited HIV/AIDS researchers who were highly successful in obtaining research grants because of the large amounts of overhead that would then accrue to their university .

The discrepancies between the amounts of money US institutions obtained for overhead and what was given to institutions in low-income countries was a matter of justice and equity. I gained a first-hand glimpse of the distortions when I visited a clinical research site in Uganda, where a successful trial of single-dose NVP to prevent mother-to-child HIV transmission had been performed. The purpose of my visit was to meet with Professor Francis Mmiro, an obstetrician and the lead investigator in the NVP study. I was planning an international conference on Global Strategies for the Prevention of HIV Transmission from Mothers to Infants that was to be held in Uganda in 2001, and Mmiro was one of the organizers and featured speakers. I had the opportunity to visit Mmiro and the obstetrical ward on one of my planning trips to Kampala.

The obstetrical ward was where the NVP perinatal HIV prevention clinical research study was performed and was located at the Makerere University School of Medicine Hospital. The obstetrical ward devoted to HIV research was clean, spacious, and populated with numerous health-care workers. But when Mmiro and I walked back through the general obstetrical ward, the difference between them was striking. It was overcrowded, completely open, and left women with no privacy. They had to dress, undress, and perform basic bodily functions in the open. The infrastructure of the hospital was neglected, as indicated by the number of broken or missing light bulbs, broken hospital beds, and general disrepair. Worst of all, the elevator was broken, and pregnant women in labor had to climb three flights of stairs to get to the general obstetrical delivery ward. I witnessed women in labor pain crawling up the stairs on their hands and knees.

Shaken by what I saw, I asked Mmiro about the hospital's financial situation. Mmiro told me that the hospital was having difficulty covering maintenance costs and even the smallest needs, such as medical journals to keep medical staff up to date. I was surprised and immediately became suspicious, as I was aware that millions of dollars had been funneled into clinical research trials in Uganda and other low-income countries. I asked Mmiro why he was not using the overhead money from the NIH grants to fund his various needs, and I was shocked when he said that he was not permitted to receive any overhead at all. Mmiro explained that US investigators had told him that there was a US rule that prohibited developing countries from receiving any overhead from US research grants, including grants from NIH.

Upon returning to the United States, with the help of Congressman McDermott, himself a physician, I investigated the matter further and learned that no such rule had ever existed. For decades, low-income countries engaged in clinical research supported by the US government had not received overhead and thus had been unable to improve their infrastructure, all because of a presumed rule that someone had invented. It appeared that thousands of clinical research locations in low-income countries had been denied millions of dollars of equitable overhead costs for at least ten years.

To address this injustice, I worked with Greg Gonsalves and other AIDS activists to change a rule that never existed. In spite of our intense advocacy for equal overhead distribution, the NIH agreed to provide only a meager 8 percent while major academic institutions continued to extract 45 percent or more. Unknown to Greg and me at that time was that an intense lobbying campaign had been initiated by academic institutions to prevent equivalent increases in overhead costs. While the 8 percent was helpful, it was undoubtedly not equitable and certainly not sufficient to raise the standards of clinical research and health care.

The lack of adequate overhead support for the Ugandan NVP study may explain why serious questions on the quality of the data were raised when the FDA reviewed the study results. Medical safety specialists, the NIH, auditors, and Boehringer Ingelheim (the company that manufactured the drug) all called attention to administrative irregularities, and the NIH suspended research for a year to review the details of the study.[5] It seemed unlikely that one of the most important lessons of the investigation would be resolved: how could poor countries be expected to conduct research that meets US standards without adequate funding? Overhead costs reimbursed on clinical research studies conducted in low-income countries remain at 8 percent to this day.

By 1998 additional studies of prevention of perinatal HIV transmission were unnecessary. Yet with generous amounts of funding available, the number of studies in low-income countries actually proliferated. By 2000 over seventy-five studies on perinatal HIV transmission were conducted or were in the process of completion in more than twenty countries. In contrast, without any additional studies in the United States, HIV-infected pregnant women were placed on HAART, the standard of care for all HIV-infected individuals, pregnant or not, and HIV infection in infants born to HIV-infected mothers plummeted from two thousand per year to fewer than one hundred per year in just two years (CDC 2006). San Francisco, once the epicenter of HIV and the city where AIDS was first reported in infants, has had no infected infants since 2005.[6]

Some of the studies of prevention of mother-to-child HIV transmission funded by NIH raised serious ethical questions. Between 1995 and 1997, three years after NIH stated that placebo studies for prevention of perinatal HIV transmission were no longer ethical, and at a time when clinical researchers in the United States were declaring that cART could halt disease progression and prevent perinatal HIV transmission, studies using placebo continued in Africa. One study compared the use of three "treatment" arms, which consisted of a single vitamin, multivitamins, and no treatment at all. The "no treatment" (placebo) arm of the study was said to be necessary in order to demonstrate the statistical benefit of one treatment over another. Unsurprisingly, at the end of the study, there was no difference between treatment with a single vitamin, multivitamins, or placebo. There was one deeply disturbing question that was brushed over without acknowledgement of its justification. How could a study have been conducted without giving any of the mothers or infants antiretroviral therapy when ZDV was already known to reduce HIV transmission by 60 percent? Not a single HIV-infected pregnant woman or her infant benefited from the studies. Without treatment, seventy-nine infants became HIV infected and died. Not only had the use of placebos continued, but the women and their infants had also been enrolled in studies that utilized no prior evidence of benefit from studies conducted in the United States or elsewhere—a violation of ethical principles and FDA regulations for research in children. The study results were published in a prestigious medical journal that required the authors to state that the studies had been approved as ethical by their IRBs (Fawzi et al. 1998; Fawzi et al. 2000).

The multiplicity of inconclusive studies on perinatal HIV transmission finally came to an end in 2015, the year that international pediatric researchers were finally forced, by results of studies that they had not performed, to place all HIV-infected pregnant women on lifelong treatment with HAART. The delay cost an estimated 2.2 million lives of women and children and hundreds of millions of dollars spent on research instead of prevention and treatment of HIV (Ammann 2015b).

WHAT DO IRBS REALLY KNOW?

Clinical research must continue if new discoveries in diagnosis and treatment are to benefit those in poor countries, and there is agreement that truly good clinical research must be both scientifically and ethically sound. If a clinical research study is supported by US government funds, it must be approved by a group of individuals referred to as an ethics committee or institutional review board (IRB). The IRBs of the various institutions and organizations that conduct clinical research are theoretically the major gatekeepers to ensuring that unethical studies are not performed in research subjects, including the exploitation of especially vulnerable populations. IRB reviewers are assumed to be free of conflicts of interest and up to date on the most recent scientific advances. They are charged with applying good science and sound ethics to the approval process.

The study of vitamins to prevent perinatal HIV transmission, and other more recent revelations of unethical studies on premature infants approved by IRBs at academic institutions, suggests that many IRBs do not have the scientific and ethical expertise to thoroughly review clinical trials, especially as the number, size, and complexity of clinical trials increase (Carlo, Bell, and Walsh 2013; Sacks and Warren 2015). This places an increased number of research participants at risk. Perhaps it is time to investigate whether some IRBs merely "rubber stamp" clinical research protocols at their own institutions.[7]

With the dramatic proliferation of research studies, many academic institutions do not have the capacity to review research protocols and informed consents in a timely or accountable manner. Nor are there adequate numbers of expert individuals who can serve on IRBs with sufficient knowledge of complex science and international ethics. This often places pressure on universities to employ for-profit institutional review boards, who are hired to review studies and fill in the gaps, further removing research from public scrutiny, as was the case with the HIVIG study published in 2011 that resulted in increased HIV infections in infants (Onyango-Makumbi et al. 2011). When the review boards are for-profit IRBs and not public, they are not required to make the results of their reviews available under the Freedom of Information Act.

An equally important issue with ethical implications is whether all of the research studies approved by IRBs should be conducted and who has the authority and expertise to make that decision. Not every new therapeutic agent is worthy of being evaluated in a clinical research study in humans, especially if there are similar products with high efficacy. Placing vulnerable HIV-infected pregnant women and their infants at risk for adverse effects when a research study is unnecessary should be considered unethical. In most cases, local IRBs would not have an adequate scientific understanding of the countless therapeutic products or studies being conducted by other academic researchers or international organizations in order to determine whether the research studies in question were unnecessary.

Given the many new questions that are being asked regarding international clinical research studies, including scientific value; ethics; exploitation of people to conduct research that is of little to no benefit; the increasing use of research subjects in poor countries using inadequate informed consents; and the increasing potential for conflict of interest among researchers, academic institutions, and IRBs, it is time to call for an independent review of the process of conducting international research and obtain an unbiased scientific and ethical review of clinical research protocols (Ammann 2014a).

HAVE RESEARCH PRODUCT, SEARCHING FOR RESEARCH SUBJECTS

By the mid-2000s, the intended result of increased funding for all medical research, including HIV, was being realized. An almost overwhelming number of potentially exciting therapeutic products were discovered for treating everything from rare genetic and acquired diseases to diseases such as HIV that were affecting millions of people worldwide. The new experimental treatments would require testing in humans to determine if they were useful, as well as to justify the research expenditures to the public. A successful new therapeutic product could mean a major breakthrough in controlling an epidemic of the magnitude of HIV, but it could also result in more research funding, greater publications, greater academic prestige, and perhaps even fulfilling the dream of some researchers to start a new biotechnology company. Just as the ethics of clinical research were changing, so too was the justification of research itself, raising fundamental questions about the purpose of research and discovery and who should benefit most. Discovering a new product for treatment also precipitated an atmosphere of scientific entitlement. Every new product discovered was pronounced as deserving of evaluation for human disease, even if the basic and animal research data was weak, even when superior treatments were already in the works, or even if the new product was estimated to be prohibitively expensive.

The dilemma of having too many products to evaluate without a sufficient number of research subjects became clear to me in January 2013. I was invited to a meeting of international clinical researchers to comment on the science and ethics of a proposed NIH-sponsored pediatric HIV/AIDS study that planned to use a broadly neutralizing monoclonal antibody (BNMAb) to HIV in order to prevent perinatal HIV transmission (Pace and Markowitz 2015; Wibmer, Moore, and Morris 2015). The invitation puzzled me. I called one of the organizers, Bill Snow, an AIDS activist I had known for more than twenty-five years and for whom I had a great deal of respect. Bill assured me that they really wanted me to come and talk about my concerns. "Tell them what you think, ethically and scientifically," he said. Still, I wondered if the purpose of asking me to speak was to quell any future criticism that opposing views had been excluded from the discussion. Some of the meeting organizers knew that I had criticized many of the HIV-prevention research trials for being unethical, for using poor research designs, and for studying experimental products that would never benefit the research-study participants in poor countries.

Even before I was invited to the meeting, I was made aware of the proposed study's controversial plan to use BNMAb in African research subjects. For the last two years, I had received emails and phone calls from clinicians and scientists asking me to intervene and help halt the studies that now included BNMAb. Many of the emails and calls asked that I not identify the person for fear that there would be retaliation through actions such as rejecting research grants, as the people being criticized were often grant-proposal reviewers.

At the Uganda meeting, the product under discussion was a BNMAb selected after an intensive screening of antibodies to HIV. The population selected for the study was once again HIV-infected pregnant women and their infants in Africa, employing a pro-posal which bypassed many of the established requirements of studying a therapeutic product in adults before giving it to infants and children. The meeting was sponsored by the Vaccine Enterprise Group, EGPAF, and NICHD, all organizations with hundreds of millions of dollars invested in clinical research. Individuals from both developed and developing countries participated. They represented academic investigators, NIH researchers, community health-care workers, and what seemed to be a token number of individuals representing HIV-affected communities in poor countries.

Initially, I was told that I would only participate in a discussion group on the ethics of clinical trials using a BNMAb against HIV. By the end of the meeting, however, I was asked to provide my own summary of the scientific issues that needed to be addressed, as well as the ethics of moving ahead with the clinical study as proposed. Although I was not currently engaged in clinical research on monoclonal antibodies, as an immunologist previously at UCSF Medical Center and at Genentech, I had become immersed in the production and evaluation of the therapeutic use of antibodies and the ethical and regulatory guidelines in clinical research studies.

The positive "spin" on the proposed study of the highly experimental BNMAb was perceptible. Lynne Mofenson, Branch Chief of NICHD and the primary force behind the NIH-supported studies for the prevention of perinatal HIV transmission, stated that the primary rationale for performing a study of BNMAb was that there were still more than 300,000 infants infected each year, despite our knowing since 1994 that ART can interrupt HIV transmission. She declared, "New treatments were desperately needed." Her numbers were correct, but the reason for them was wrong.

I had a great deal of respect for Mofenson. She was smart, highly motivated, and her leadership was integral to the development of the important early studies on prevention of perinatal HIV transmission. Mofenson deserved much of the credit for expanding perinatal HIV-transmission studies and for securing the funds to support the studies in the years following the demonstration that ZDV could reduce perinatal HIV transmission. But the ideas that BNMAb was needed in low-income countries because there was no effective therapy or that new treatments costing one hundred times more than existing treatment were needed were absurd and simply not true. Therapeutic denialism was in full force. The real reason there were still 300,000 HIV-infected infants each year was because treating all HIV-infected pregnant women with HAART had not been implemented and was no longer the high priority it had been in the 1994 pediatric HIV/AIDS research community's call for the immediate implementation of known effective interventions.

The inconsistencies in the arguments being presented were apparent. Previously, clinical researchers who were engaged in studies of preventing perinatal HIV transmission had argued that, because countries could not afford HAART, they were justified in performing clinical research studies of inferior treatment that would cost less than standard of care. But then the cost of treatment with generic drugs tumbled from $2,000 to less than $120, yet studies of inadequate treatment still continued. Now the same researchers were proposing to evaluate BNMAb, a research product that, if effective, would cost at least fifty to one hundred times more than HAART and, in addition, would require additional expenditures for a costly infrastructure.

I presented a host of scientific and ethical objections to evaluating BNMAb in impoverished African infants. Cost was a major one; if the cost of a new therapeutic product were unaffordable, then there was no justification for evaluating it in an income-poor setting where it would never be available because of expense. Researchers already knew that the cost of a monoclonal antibody used to prevent respiratory syncytial virus infection in children in the United States was $10,000 per treatment. This greatly exceeded the estimated $120 per treatment for HAART. But there were other issues besides cost. I also wondered why a particular monoclonal antibody had been chosen when there were at least ten other potential candidates and better ones were already being discovered. Were there studies comparing the proposed monoclonal antibody with other candidates, some of which had data suggesting that they would be even more potent? Had researchers found evidence from adult studies in the United States demonstrating that BNMAb was effective in controlling HIV before studying infants in poor countries?

The response to my criticism regarding the cost of BNMAb was met with additional spin. One of the presenters argued that if the monoclonal antibody were effective, the increased use would eventually lead to decreased manufacturing costs. But just one week before the meeting, I had contacted a scientist at Genentech who had performed a detailed analysis of the cost of producing therapeutic monoclonal antibodies. He concluded that in order for the cost of manufacturing a monoclonal antibody to be reduced substantially, it would need to be in widespread use with a large market size and the ability of the health-care provider to purchase the product (Kelley 2009). None of these criteria could be met in an income-poor country.

At the meeting, I felt that many of the investigators and patient advocates did not understand the complexities of the proposed clinical research, not because they lacked the intelligence to do so, but because it was an area completely unfamiliar to them. During one of the discussions, a community activist from South Africa announced, "I don't know what monoclonal antibodies are, and I don't even know how to translate monoclonal antibody to one of my patients." Another stated that she feared that a research study of that magnitude and complexity would interfere with the ability to take care of HIV-infected patients or patients with other equally life-threatening diseases.

She asked if such a study were implemented, would additional financial resources to care for patients be provided, and would the patients receive some form of compensation for their participation in the study? That would, of course, dramatically add to the cost of the study, which was calculated to require three thousand research subjects over a three-year period and cost $30 million—enough money to provide known effective ART to 300,000 HIV-infected pregnant women and their infants, precisely the number of infants estimated to become infected with HIV each year because they lacked access to already existing effective treatment.

At the end of the meeting, I wondered what would happen if the investigators and NICHD, the study's sponsor, were allowed to move forward with the proposed study for the prevention of perinatal HIV transmission. The only BNMAb chosen as the most effective candidate for study several years before was already eclipsed by other more potent monoclonal antibody candidates (Stephenson and Barouch 2016). If therapeutic products with greater potential were discovered after the proposed study had started, would the study be stopped, or would it just continue? With claims that there were insufficient NIH research funds to study new emerging epidemics such as the Ebola and Zika viruses that threaten millions of individuals worldwide, could a $30 million study in Africa with no direct potential benefit be justified?[8] Were all of the safety issues regarding the use of monoclonal antibody in HIV-infected individuals evaluated? I reflected on the unresolved possibility that BNMAb might actually increase HIV infection, an issue that had been ignored in previously conducted studies of vitamins in perinatal transmission as well as in the HIVIG study in Uganda. From my experience reviewing potential therapeutic products in a biotechnology company, I knew that no pharmaceutical or biotechnology company would accept the risk of doing such a study without first having adult data. It was discouraging to think that a publicly funded study would take the risk of conducting research of no value to the research subjects and on a product that was, from the outset, not the most potent but certainly the most expensive.

My efforts to halt what I determined to be an unscientific and unethical study of the NIH VRC01 monoclonal antibody were unsuccessful. In April 2016, NIH announced that, in spite of no evidence of benefit in any study in humans, the VRC01 study was beginning to enroll infants born to HIV infected mothers and more than four thousand adults at risk of acquiring HIV through sexual transmission. The study will include fifteen hundred sub-Saharan African women who will have no assurance that they will receive ARV pre-exposure prophylaxis (PrEP) to prevent them from becoming infected (NIAID 2016). The infant segment of the study was approved by multiple university human-research protection committees (at the research investigators' institutions) and the FDA in spite of its illegality under federal research protection laws (Office for Human Research Protections 2016).

BACK TO ESTHER'S STORY

The story of Esther at the beginning of this chapter illustrates many of the ethical issues that confront clinical research in poor countries today. Understanding who benefits from clinical research requires detailed examination. To begin with, is the purpose of the research study really to benefit Esther and other HIV-infected pregnant women and their infants? Is Esther's consent truly "informed"? Are the health-care workers fully apprised of what standard of care means? Is there a conflict of interest when a clinical research study offers greater financial benefits for those who perform the research than for those who participate? Is it equitable when the greater share of funding is given to the US sponsors of the study than to those in the country where the study is performed? If Esther is enrolled in the research arm that provides inferior treatment and her baby becomes infected, aren't the clinical research sponsors ethically and legally liable for continued care? Why is there no legal representation offered to Esther? Why is there no ombudsman for the HIV-infected pregnant women in the study? Why is a study performed to demonstrate one treatment is better than another without a guarantee that treatment will be made available to Esther and all HIV-infected pregnant women in the country? Why is a study conducted whose primary purpose is to determine the effect of a less expensive but inferior treatment? Is it ethical for the United States to pay for research studies in poor countries when those studies support the financially driven decisions of foreign governments to provide inferior standards of care to their citizens? Are vulnerable individuals in poor countries viewed simply as research objects, akin to laboratory animals, where research is conducted without any obligation to provide benefits to them beyond the research study? Finally, is it justifiable to perform research studies with a research product that has no conceivable immediate benefit and will never be available to individuals in poor countries?

These questions do not mean that clinical research should come to a halt or that new experimental therapies should not be evaluated in poor countries. Clinical research for new methods of diagnosis, treatment, and prevention are necessary, but not at the expense of bending or rewriting established ethical principles to accommodate demands that result from vast infusions of funds from wealthy countries and a surge of new research discoveries of uncertain or no potential benefit. In this context, suggestions to modify ethical guidelines or to even do away with some should always be viewed with suspicion and should never be accepted without review by all those who seek to protect the rights of research subjects, including the research subjects themselves. Leaving these critical questions unanswered will only result in further exploitation of vulnerable individuals in a manner akin to colonialism, where the colonizers justify their exploitation of resources as being, "for the good of humankind," but without the good being realized by those who are exploited.

In the big picture of justice and equity, the risks of research in humans cannot be borne by poor individuals who are viewed as mere chattel, undeserving of direct benefits from their participation in the research.

Misspent Dollars

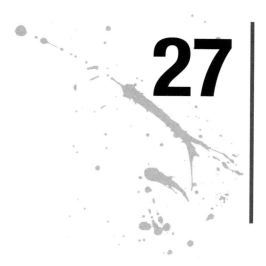

27

FUNDING AT LAST, BUT ABUSES OCCUR QUICKLY

In 1983, the CDC assumed the primary responsibility for the Public Health Services Response to AIDS and began tracking the reports of new cases that were presenting primarily with opportunistic infections and Kaposi's sarcoma (KS). But the CDC itself needed funding and was not a primary agency for funding academic researchers or institutions. Within the CDC, Dr. James Curran took the lead in defining the AIDS epidemic. He was aggressive and intent on fully describing the emerging epidemic in the United States and internationally. He was also the undeserved recipient of much of the criticism for the slow pace at which the US government was responding to AIDS. A turning point in acknowledging the need for increased research funds occurred at a June 30, 1982, meeting of the New York Department of Health—one of the attendees suggested that there might be a close link between AIDS and an infectious agent and suggested that there was an urgent need for the United States to commit at least $1 million to research. The amount was small, but it was a beginning.

One of the many problems within the NIH in shifting its resources to a new epidemic such as AIDS was that its focus had always been on chronic diseases. AIDS was a new disease, and no one knew whether it was an infectious agent or had some other electrifying cause. Another problem was that most research was "institute" directed. The NCI had focused on KS early in the epidemic as a malignancy in AIDS. Initially, they were the "default" institute, until it was later discovered that AIDS was caused by an infectious disease and KS was but one of the many clinical manifestations of AIDS. Regardless of which institute should adopt AIDS as a primary research undertaking, the visibility of AIDS in the media brought with it closer attention to how NIH decided funding priorities and how funds were released for research outside of the NIH. Activists were shocked to learn how long it took to get a grant approved—the time period from requesting grant applications to review and final approval of those applications often exceeded nine months. Just as the activists had been advocating for accelerated drug approval by the FDA, they then began pushing for more rapid funding of research into the cause and treatment of AIDS within and outside the NIH.

In 1982, the two NIH institutes that were receiving funding for AIDS were NCI and NIAID, but the amounts were modest—less than a combined $2 million. By 1984,

233

the amounts for the two institutes had increased substantially but were still modest considering the epidemic's global threat. NCI was getting $17 million and NIAID $20 million. By 1986, NIAID was receiving over $60 million in funding and NCI $45 million.

NIH had been organized to support intramural research (research conducted within the institutes and by investigators fully funded by the institutes) and extramural research (research conducted at academic centers by independent researchers most often affiliated with universities). Because the intramural program's funds were more flexible, it could respond rapidly to the AIDS epidemic, but the response was still modest. The extramural programs were more difficult to fund. The emerging leadership within the NIH was critical of increasing and redirecting NIH research for both intramural and extramural programs. Early research leaders at the NIH were Thomas Waldman at the NCI, who directed immunologic studies; Sam Broder, also at the NCI, who was instrumental in defining the first ARV for the treatment of HIV and for establishing assay methods for screening new drugs; and NCI's Robert Gallo, who along with Luc Montagnier at the Pasteur Institute, discovered HIV as the cause of AIDS in 1983. But it was Anthony Fauci, director of NIAID, who would emerge as the primary force behind the national and international efforts to move the HIV research agenda forward.

HIV activism fundamentally changed not only how research priorities were identified and the speed with which they were funded but also the process of drug development. Within NIH and the academic research community, the debate was between the targeted research approach and the more traditional academic approach of basic research and serendipitous observations. The latter was credited with providing some of the major breakthroughs in past clinical research and chronic diseases, but it was not a means of rapidly giving answers to an epidemic that threatened to overtake the entire world. Activists and HIV-infected patients argued that answers to pressing problems were needed immediately. They suggested that a centralized mechanism was required to decide what research was most important both within and outside the NIH. Analogies were made to the successful coordination of efforts under the Manhattan Project to develop an atomic bomb. Their suggestion was not universally welcomed.

As funding for AIDS research continued to increase, many researchers applying for NIH grants began to include their own fields of interest that had only tenuous associations with HIV/AIDS. It was a nontransparent attempt to gain access to increased funding, whether or not the research was related to AIDS. As the process began to significantly skew research priorities, advocates and activists became concerned that funding for AIDS research would simply be consumed by investigators conducting unrelated research that would not be of immediate benefit to HIV prevention and treatment.

THE LEVINE PANEL INVESTIGATES

In 1993, Congress responded to public concerns about how funding for HIV/AIDS research was being spent by including within the NIH Revitalization Act a requirement that all new funds for AIDS research would be funneled to the central OAR and not to individual institutes. This seemed to be a critically important step in oversight of NIH funding. In 1994, the budget for AIDS research through NIH had reached a level of almost $500 million. By 1995, the funds for AIDS research had increased dramatically through advocacy and activism to a level of $1.4 billion.

Although the funding seemed to come slowly for those who were HIV infected and needed answers quickly, in retrospect, it was in fact the most rapid acceleration of funding for a specific disease in the NIH's history. But questions remained as to the effectiveness of OAR oversight and its ability to ensure that funds were being spent appropriately on the most urgent priorities. Questions about misspending began to increase; in response, William Paul, a leading immunologist within NIH, was appointed as director of OAR in February 1994. To some activists, the appointment of an NIH insider was of concern.

In 1995, one month after his appointment, Paul put together a group of 114 leading scientists representing academics, drug companies, community organizations, and AIDS advocates to investigate how the $1.4 billion had been used and whether an NIH institute devoted specifically to AIDS should be constructed. The panel was chaired by Dr. Arnold Levine of Princeton University (see Chapter 22 for more on the Levine Panel Report). Levine was intent on getting the details of funding, including where it had been spent and how research priorities were established, especially as it was likely that funding for AIDS research would continue to increase dramatically ("Review and Reform" 1996; NIH 1996).

The panel released its findings in March 1996. Disappointingly, but not surprisingly, it concluded that tens of millions dollars had been spent inappropriately, either on studies that had questionable or no relevance to HIV or on administrative expenses that were difficult to identify as being related to AIDS. Of the $1.4 billion total AIDS research budget, 20 percent was categorized as research on clinical trials, with only about half of the amount devoted to high-quality clinical research on treatment for HIV. About one quarter of the funds were for poorly designed or poorly justified studies, and about one quarter was devoted to research that, however meritorious, had little to do with HIV/AIDS. Administrative funds had been used to shore up individual NIH institutes that had insufficient funding; they were using the AIDS-related funds for non-HIV related research and to meet their administrative needs. To some, such a shifting of funds was not surprising, as historically, outside the NIH and within academic research institutions, researchers had become skillful in redirecting funds to their own research goals even when the funds were designated for other diseases.

The report cited specific examples of abuses. For example, Richard Klausner, head of the NCI, was asked where $22 million in AIDS research funds were used within the NCI. The money had been listed under "unspecified personal services," but he could not identify the details of how the funding had been utilized. The National Institute of Alcohol Abuse and Alcoholism stated it had spent several million dollars targeted for HIV/AIDS on issues of alcoholism in general, and $35 million of the AIDS funds were used by the National Heart, Lung, and Blood Institute for development of artificial blood. In spite of the large amount of funding received by the NCI for HIV drug discovery, the Levine Panel noted that the NCI had not discovered any new drug to treat HIV in the eight years since it had pulled ZDV off the shelf of unused drugs and found it to be effective in treating HIV-infected patients. One of the panel members pointed out that of 139 NCI laboratories funded for research in 1994, ninety-two research papers had been published on cancer but only ten papers on HIV/AIDS. Some of the research institutes that had received funding for HIV/AIDS never published a single paper on the topic. Some key multimillion-dollar programs within NIH were judged as a complete failure, producing nothing that could be considered as moving HIV/AIDS treatment and prevention forward. The panel also pointed out that the $100 million that had been devoted to research in developing an HIV vaccine had produced no notable vaccine candidate by the time that the report was issued.[1]

Of considerable concern to the Levine Panel was the general lack of vision about how the increasing HIV/AIDS funding approved by Congress should be spent and what the priorities for research were. This was particularly true for the pediatric AIDS clinical trial group. It also criticized the tendency toward internalization: much of the research funding was directed toward priorities within the various NIH institutes, and submission and funding of research by scientists outside the NIH system was not encouraged.[2]

Meanwhile, scientists working with amfAR and the Pediatric AIDS Foundation were already identifying key research priorities, rapidly reviewing research proposals, and through the foundations, funding promising new research into HIV/AIDS. They had recognized that the contributions of outstanding scientists from all areas of research and around the world would be necessary to overcome an escalating epidemic. Although the research funding provided by these two organizations did not approach the level of the NIH's, they provided seed funding to hundreds of research scientists that allowed them to pursue novel and important approaches to HIV treatment and prevention that could subsequently be funded by the NIH. The ability of these two organizations to move quickly and effectively in identifying new research priorities was a crucial component of the advances that were made in research on HIV/AIDS. It also placed pressure on the NIH to change their process of soliciting and approving research grants to address an epidemic that was expanding beyond what had been predicted.

SERIOUS CONCLUSIONS: A WORRISOME RESIGNATION FOLLOWS

The conclusions of the Levine Panel were widely circulated among the activist community. Laurie Garrett reported them in *Newsday*, and Lawrence Altman reported them in the *New York Times* (Altman 1996). OAR Director William Paul accepted the conclusions, stating, "I believe that AIDS research money must be spent on an open, candid, serious, clear plan that reflects both targeted needs and basic research. And that has not been the case." Paul vowed that "sweeping changes will now be initiated and the future will be clean."[3] To the credit of Paul and the OAR, as well as the NIH directors who were truly engaged in research in HIV/AIDS, the Levine Panel conclusions were accepted and scrutinized, and they resulted in a closer examination of research priorities. The importance of congressional funding for HIV/AIDS was acknowledged, and a discussion on how it should be spent ensued.

Only three years after his appointment as OAR director, Paul announced that he was stepping down: "The time has now come for me to relinquish the responsibilities of this position and return to laboratory science as part of my commitment to the search for a safe and effective HIV vaccine." Paul did not elaborate on the reasons for his resignation. Publicly, he received praise from the current NIH director, Harold Varmus. Paul's most remembered legacy was the ambitious review of the NIH research program in HIV/AIDS under the leadership of Arnold Levine.[4]

Although Paul never enlarged on the reasons for his resignation, it would not be unreasonable to assume that when confronted with the burgeoning bureaucracy of HIV/AIDS research coupled with rapidly increasing funds and mounting difficulties in accountability, he might have perceived that it would be increasingly difficult to maintain accountability through the OAR, an internal NIH office. Perhaps, too, Paul's resignation was prophetic of how difficult it would be to continue the much-needed independent, "outside" review of the NIH's massive spending on AIDS and the increasing problems of conflicts of interest, identifying priorities, and ethical research conduct.

Did the Levine Panel Report prevent future misuse of AIDS research funds? The US government had become the largest funder of HIV/AIDS research in the world, and without the funds we would not have made progress in controlling the epidemic. But, even though the Levine Panel warned against the creation of an HIV/AIDS bureaucracy, the sheer amount of funding available, which totaled billions of dollars, eventually contributed to inefficiency, duplication, inappropriate use of funds designated for HIV, and poor accountability. It is not that there has not been much accomplished with the infusion of massive amounts of funding. Critically important discoveries have been made that have resulted in slowing the epidemic, but much more could and should have been done to use the discoveries to rapidly end the HIV epidemic.

In 2016 the question remains of how NIH funding is being used and who is setting the priorities. By 2015 the NIH budget had become so massive that the budget itself, and not accountability, became the justification for urging Congress to approve their annual increases. The emergence of the Ebola epidemic was blamed on the failure to increase NIH funding. Francis Collins, head of NIH, declared, "Frankly, if we had not gone through our ten-year slide in research support, we probably would have had a vaccine in time for this that would've gone through clinical trials and would have been ready."[5] This statement was made the year the NIH research budget had reached almost $30 billion. Just two years later, university clinical researchers and NIAID have put together plans for several large and costly research studies of VRC01, an "in house" HIV neutralizing monoclonal antibody considered by some scientists as not having sufficient efficacy or safety studies (as discussed in Chapter 26) (Graham 2015; *ClinicalTrials.gov* 2016a; Stephenson and Barouch 2016; Ammann 2013, 2014b). The cost of the proposed NIH-funded study is likely to be in excess of $200 million. Disturbingly, one component of the study included the use of placebo for evaluation of VRC01 in the prevention of HIV infection in fifteen hundred African women at high risk of infection. In a déjà vu of Tuskegee and Guatemala, five hundred women would receive no protection from a much more lethal STI than syphilis or gonorrhea. Perhaps an alternate explanation of whether funds for an Ebola virus vaccine could have been available lay in the lack of strategic flexibility and in who decides public-health research priorities.

The proliferation of funds resulted in their assimilation through the creation of programs that were too often unnecessary, duplicative, and peripheral to the major AIDS priorities or could be performed by groups that already existed. As an example, in the years that followed the Levine Panel Report, the responsibility for the development of drugs and formulations for infants and children shifted from highly experienced pharmaceutical companies to NIH-funded institutes and organizations. The subsequent failure of the academic PPRU, funded by the NIH, to accomplish the task of accelerating drug development for infants and children fulfilled the prophetic warnings from the Levine Panel: there are some tasks that are better accomplished by the pharmaceutical industry than by academic research. Inexperienced investigators, unskilled in conducting pharmacokinetic studies and developing infant drug formulations, took too long to acquire the necessary expertise at a time when lifesaving drugs for infants and children were urgently needed. The PPRU network, of which there were seventeen nationally that were funded with millions of research dollars, represents the type of failure that the Levine Panel suggested avoiding. The PPRU epitaph on their website reads: "The PPRU network sunsetted in 2010 and is no longer active. This information is intended for reference and historical purposes."

PEDIATRIC HIV/AIDS CLINICAL TRIALS ON TRIAL

The large population HIV-infected infants, children, and pregnant women that would need to be recruited for the proposed NIH-sponsored clinical research trials were only available in low-income countries where significant numbers of HIV-infected individuals lived and had little access to HIV prevention and treatment. The ethical conflicts surrounding the use of these vulnerable women and children were significant. On the one hand, their needs were great. Most of the countries were very poor, and HIV was destroying the health of individuals, families, and communities without any foreseeable interventions. Medical infrastructure was inadequate, and trained health-care workers were almost nonexistent. ARVs were either impossible to get or in limited supply. The only way to gain access to HIV prevention and care in countries with failed governments and ministries of health was through clinical research studies. Enrolling in a research study might provide immediate health benefits, such as preventing infants from becoming infected with HIV and halting the progression of HIV to AIDS in a pregnant woman, at least temporarily. Rationalizations from the US sponsors for these studies usually included, "Why shouldn't individuals in poor countries benefit from the research discoveries conducted in wealthy countries?" and, "Why shouldn't people in poor countries be allowed to participate in research for the benefit of 'mankind?' Isn't doing something better than doing nothing?"

On the other hand, the extreme poverty and lack of health care created a captive population vulnerable to exploitation: poor people might volunteer for research as the only means of obtaining a modicum of health care. But would all individuals in the research studies receive benefits for their participation? For poor people without heath care, income, or even sufficient living essentials, the intangible concept of "for the benefit of mankind" would hardly do it. What about providing increased access to health care, immunizations for their children, free transportation, nutritional supplements, etc.?

Some studies randomly assigned research subjects to placebos or to inferior treatment. Individuals enrolled in the studies would not know what treatment, if any, would be of benefit to them. Would the benefits of enrolling be limited to the duration of the study? Would the treatment, if successful, be made available to the study participants and to all HIV-infected individuals residing in the country? What kind of informed consent would be used when many of the research subjects were illiterate or spoke languages that were difficult to translate? How would "recombinant DNA" or "retroviral," for example, be translated into a local language? Would legal protection be provided to the research subjects to be certain that they were not exploited or harmed? Would an impartial ombudsman be assigned to each research project? What level of standard of care would be provided in the comparative research study arms? There were also potential conflicts of interest in decision making when US researchers and the research cosponsors in the countries where the studies would be performed benefited personally. Researchers from wealthy countries could exert undue influence. Who wouldn't want to participate in clinical research sponsored by the most advanced country in the world, and who wouldn't want to get access to funds to support the research when there was both prestige and monetary reward to be gained?

TOO MANY LIVES LOST

Following the successful 1994 study showing that ZDV could prevent HIV transmission from mother to infant, studies on perinatal HIV transmission proliferated. Any research group with funding, whether an academic institution, an international organization, or the NIH-sponsored pediatric HIV/AIDS researchers, could come up with some variation in the approach to preventing HIV transmission, even if it lacked a sound scientific rationale, duplicated previous research studies, or would not help end the pediatric HIV/AIDS epidemic. Rather than taking a coordinated approach to seeking a definitive answer, especially one that provided HAART for all HIV-infected pregnant women, the approach to the perinatal HIV trials was to divide and "not conquer." The sense of urgency for ending the pediatric HIV/AIDS epidemic faded.

Even UNAIDS could not resist the temptation to get into the act. Conducting clinical research trials was not in UNAIDS' mission, but that did not stop it from paying for and coordinating a very large and expensive study on preventing perinatal HIV transmission. The study was called the Perinatal Transmission Study (PETRA), conducted in South Africa, Uganda, and Tanzania. It evaluated various combinations of ZDV, 3TC, and placebo given during the prepartum, intrapartum, and postpartum periods (PETRA Study Team 2002). When the results of the PETRA study were published in 2002, six years after it had been initiated, the disappointing results were predictable. Statistical analysis revealed that the greater the amount of treatment given and the longer the duration, the more likely HIV transmission was prevented—a fact that had been known for at least six years. Another "let's see how little we can give and still prevent infection" study had bitten the dust, but not before 1,765 mother/infant pairs had been subjected to the risks of not getting adequate treatment, having their HIV infection progress, and seeing their infants become HIV infected and die.

Somewhat surprising was what was omitted from the PETRA research study results. In spite of being a large and expensive multicenter study with access to highly sophisticated European laboratories, maternal viral loads were not measured in the various treatment regimens. Like many other perinatal HIV-transmission studies, they used HIV infection and death as end points instead of viral load, which could have ended the study earlier, preventing many of the infant HIV infections and deaths. A critical opportunity had been overlooked to provide further correlation of HIV transmission and viral load under various treatment regimens. The PETRA study, involving large numbers of poor women and infants, failed to contribute to progress in ending the pediatric HIV/AIDS epidemic. Nonetheless, other studies that were already in progress utilizing similar study designs were not halted, but continued and would ultimately fail as well.

Why were so many clinical research studies considered necessary? Why did pediatric clinical researchers reject the data that HAART was most effective in treating HIV infection and reducing viral load? Why wasn't a definitive study initiated in 1998 to evaluate the impact of treating all HIV-infected pregnant women with lifelong HAART to prevent HIV transmission and treat their own infection? If it worked, which it would have, lives would have been saved. What possibly could have been the rationale for performing multiple studies that withheld known potent ART at a time when HAART's success was apparent to HIV experts?

An even more disturbing question was whether the myriad studies actually slowed progress in the prevention of perinatal HIV transmission by delaying provision of lifesaving standard of care. It might be concluded, looking at the large number of highly variable studies that were performed and that failed to reach a consensus for prevention of perinatal HIV infection, that no one really cared. Perhaps it was in the interest of researchers and their academic institutions to perpetuate the research studies by designing their "own" studies as a means of ensuring ongoing support of clinical research per se, rather than as a means of ending the pediatric HIV/AIDS epidemic—a kind of academic entitlement.

Not everyone in the pediatric HIV clinical research community agreed with the approach NIH was using to end the HIV epidemic in children. Several of them contacted me and even suggested that some studies were unethical. Most insisted on remaining anonymous, but a few were outspoken. Dr. Andrew Wiznia worked at the Bronx Lebanon Hospital, where 40 percent of hospitalized patients were in foster care and many were HIV infected, further complicating their access to ARVs. Wiznia recognized the urgency of treating HIV-infected children long before there were formal clinical trials. He had observed the high viral loads in infants born with HIV infection, much higher than that seen in any infected adults. He concluded that with these high levels of virus replicating on a daily basis, early treatment with combination antiretroviral drugs was even more urgent in infants than in HIV-infected adults. Wiznia was ahead of his time.

Ironically, there was little to argue against providing HAART to HIV-infected children in low-income countries. Studies conducted in the United States and Europe showed the long-term benefits in reducing both the complications of HIV and the potential substantial health benefits of HAART. A study performed in Switzerland, a country with a high level of health-care and government infrastructure, documented the short-term increase in health-care costs but the long-term substantial benefits in improving health and reducing health care (Sendi et al. 1999; Erb et al. 2000). Similar studies followed in low-income countries. All concluded that access to HAART in low-income countries would have a much greater benefit to the society at large (Bendavid et al. 2009; Loubiere et al. 2010).

The reality was that more clinical research studies were not needed before implementing HAART in all HIV-infected individuals in low-income countries. In 2013, Drs. Seema Shah and Christine Grady from the NIH wrote a letter to the *NEJM* in response to an article by Drs. Kevin De Cock and Wafaa El-Sadr calling for an urgent new randomized controlled trial in Africa to determine whether ART should be started at higher CD4 counts (De Cock and El-Sadr 2013). I agreed with Shah and Grady's analysis. They articulated what so many people in low-income countries already knew: "Lack of treatment may be due to fiscal constraints and lack of capacity in the health system; implementation research could better identify strategies for earlier linkage to treatment or for building such capacity. Most important, sustainable funding for treating people with HIV who we know require such treatment for their health is more urgently needed than an additional randomized, controlled trial on when to start ART in Africa" (Shah and Grady 2013).

Over time, pediatric clinical researchers chose to ignore the many suggestions and criticisms that additional efficacy research studies were unnecessary. Instead, major efforts were made to select different countries where clinical research could be conducted— Kenya, Uganda, Botswana, South Africa, Swaziland, Malawi, Ethiopia, Nigeria, Thailand, Brazil, etc. The number of academic universities in the United States that sponsored research studies proliferated as well—Harvard, Johns Hopkins, University of North Carolina, University of California, Columbia, University of Alabama, University of Washington, etc. While the precise number of studies that enrolled HIV-infected pregnant women, infants, and children from poor countries is difficult to ascertain, the US Government Clinical Research Study Database does have most of the research studies listed. When I searched the database using various combinations of keywords, I found 630 research studies involving treatment of HIV-infected children and seventy-four for the prevention of perinatal HIV transmission ("HIV/AIDS Clinical Trials" 2015).

For Better or for Worse?

The Pediatric AIDS Clinical Trial Group Expands

28

BENEFIT OR EXPLOITATION?

The lack of an effective HIV vaccine facilitated the exploitation of infants who were born to HIV-infected women in low-income countries by providing researchers with a rationalization for inappropriately using these infants in order to evaluate vaccines of dubious efficacy and even those that had failed in adult clinical research studies. This is illustrated by an article published in 2013 titled "Immunogenicity of ALVAC-HIV vCP1521 in Infants of HIV-1-Infected Women in Uganda (HPTN 027): The First Pediatric AIDS Vaccine Trial in Africa" (Kintu et al). HPTN 027 was an NIH-supported clinical trial designed to evaluate the safety and immunogenicity of the HIV vaccine ALVAC-HIV vCP1452 in sixty infants born to HIV-1-infected mothers with CD4 counts of >500 cells per microliter. Infants were randomized to the vaccine or placebo, once again after placebo studies of HIV in infants and children were declared unethical. While the article indicates that the study was approved by the Institutional Bio-Safety Committees and adhered to the Helsinki Declaration, there was no justification for evaluating the same vaccine that seven years before was reported to have failed in adults and to have no effect beyond a demonstration that it was safe but not sufficiently immunogenic to produce any protective immune response (Jacobson et al. 2006).

The argument to justify using an experimental vaccine in infants that would have no benefit to them went something like this: "A vaccine to prevent HIV infection is needed; some (unrelated) vaccines for other viral infections are known to protect infants; infants are different than adults; just because a vaccine does not work in adults does not mean that it will not work in infants; we need to know what vaccines work and do not work." What was not mentioned in the arguments was that perhaps the only reason for doing the studies was that the funding and the infants were available and could be exploited without opposition from "outside" ethicists and scientists. Ethical guidelines state that conducting research on infants that is of no benefit to them is exploitation, especially when there is no evidence of efficacy from studies in the United States. The HPTN 027 vaccine study seemed to have slipped past all the scientific and ethical committee standards to prevent exploitation of infants and children.

Studies such as these raise many questions about how clinical research studies get approved when they are conducted in infants and children in low-income countries.

There seems to be no consistency in the approval process. Too often, oversight is conducted by poorly informed and inexperienced individuals or committees. A fundamental question is "Why was it so important that a vaccine trial, using a vaccine that had been proven not to work, be conducted in vulnerable infants in Africa, as the title of the study suggests?" Was it just because *something* needed to be done to take advantage of the available funding? This example calls for major revisions in scientific and ethical reviews of research studies conducted in vulnerable populations to prevent both harm and exploitation from clinical trials such as this one, which have no value to the research-study participants or even to science itself.

AT THE CROSSROADS: CHOOSING THE WRONG PATH

The years between 1996 and 1998 marked a crossroads in pediatric HIV/AIDS clinical research. Studies of HIV-infected adults had convincingly shown that HAART was the most effective treatment for controlling HIV infection, reducing morbidity and mortality, improving health, and thereby reducing the long-term cost of the HIV/AIDS epidemic. These advances could have ignited the ending of the pediatric HIV/AIDS epidemic had they been quickly adopted by the PACTG. The short-sighted presentation to the Levine Panel by the director of the PACTG, Stephen Spector, is likely to have contributed to the panel's recommendation to consider reducing the PACTG's funding (NIH 1996). Confronted with the recommendation that funding should be reduced in the United States, the pediatric AIDS research community reached a juncture at which they could choose one of two paths: The first would take the incredible advances in HIV research and apply them to ending the international pediatric AIDS epidemic. The second would deny the validity of the definitive results from research conducted in adults and claim that they did not apply to HIV-infected pregnant women, infants, and children in poor countries. The latter path was chosen—a lethal decision that withheld HAART from those who desperately needed it and facilitated the continuation of the pediatric HIV/AIDS epidemic.

It is important to reflect on why a more aggressive approach to ending the pediatric AIDS epidemic was not the paramount mission of pediatric HIV/AIDS clinical research after 1998. In the United States, the HIV-infected and uninfected community of adult activists was highly informed of research results and well aware of the potential impact of new ARVs on their well-being and, indeed, on their very survival. They rejected the paternalistic approach of "we know what is best for you" presented by academic researchers and government regulators, which would have prevented early access to experimental treatment. Instead, they demanded that they themselves could evaluate the risks and benefits of early initiation of HAART. In the process, they revolutionized the approach to research and drug approval, putting in place the means to rapidly access new lifesaving ARVs. There was no one who dared deny them access to the best treatment available, even while research studies were still being conducted.

Looking back at the beginning of the HIV/AIDS epidemic, it is clear that the activists were correct. Years before drugs received final FDA approval, HIV-infected men and women in the United States gained access to lifesaving drugs. Revolutionary new ARVs were quickly prescribed and not delayed until the results of multiple duplicative or unnecessary research studies were available. The international community of women and children with HIV/AIDS, in spite of its numbers, lacked the activism and advocacy to demand immediate access to lifesaving HAART. Their cause should have been taken up by the pediatric HIV/AIDS researchers, who instead conducted a multiplicity of research studies on ARV efficacy rather than implementation. They had before them evidence that the pediatric HIV epidemic in the United States had come under control—HIV transmission rates to infants had fallen to less than 3 percent by 1996 without any additional perinatal HIV transmission studies beyond the 1994 ACTG 076 ZDV study. The precipitous fall was not the result of additional research studies, but rather the outcome of the universal early implementation of HAART by practicing physicians who believed in the results of research and FDA approval of ARVs.

The US approach to clinical research in low-income countries was, again, paternalistic—"we know what's best for them"—but the citizens of those countries lacked the help from activists to challenge that attitude. The approach was to offer less expensive (in the short term) but inferior treatment for the sake of research that could never have been conducted in the United States and to justify the decisions based on guidelines crafted using dubious science and ethics. After a nearly twenty-year wasteland of unending research studies involving tens of thousands of research subjects in poor countries, in 2015, the pediatric AIDS research community was finally forced to recommend HAART for all HIV-infected pregnant women based on undisputable evidence from the Strategic Timing of Antiretroviral Treatment (START) study evaluating immediate initiation of HAART in HIV-infected adults (Lundgren et al. 2015). The pediatric HIV/AIDS epidemic could have ended by now if the recommendation to treat all HIV-infected individuals had been taken seriously, as was first proposed in 1996.

THE BROKEN PROMISE OF PROMISE

The IMPAACT website (*www.impaactnetwork.org*) states, "The IMPAACT Network is a cooperative group of institutions, investigators, and other collaborators focused on evaluating potential therapies for HIV infection and its related symptoms in infants, children, adolescents, and pregnant women, including clinical trials of HIV/AIDS interventions for and prevention of mother-to-child transmission." The list of research topics that it covers is diffuse, some with tenuous relations to critical priorities of pediatric HIV/AIDS, raising questions of manageability but ensuring a steady stream of funding for a diverse group of investigators and research targets.[1]

The PROMISE study represents the flagship research study of IMPAACT. But it stood out alone in the scientific community for failing to support provision of lifelong HAART for all HIV-infected pregnant women (IMPAACT 2015). In order to conduct the PROMISE study, the research investigators, with the concurrence of IMPAACT leaders, had to consider HIV-infected pregnant women and their infants in low-income countries as less deserving of lifesaving treatment and prevention than individuals residing in income-rich countries. They also had to ignore the overwhelming scientific data that supported the remarkable benefits of early initiation of HAART on life and health. But more than that, immediate initiation of lifelong treatment of HIV-infected women, pregnant or not, had the potential for ending the pediatric HI/AIDS epidemic.

Once a universal standard of care for treating all HIV-infected individuals, including HIV-infected pregnant women, was recommended by every major international health organization, the PROMISE study should have been stopped by the DSMB and all ethical committees responsible for its oversight. Instead, it was allowed to continue with unethical and inferior treatment and misleading informed consents, resulting in harm to the research study participants—progression to AIDS for some women and HIV infection of their infants for others.

The design of the PROMISE study was in violation of the ethical guidelines for research in humans established by the World Medical Association Declaration of Helsinki, *Ethical Principles for Medical Research Involving Human Subjects*, which states in article thirty-three: "The benefits, risks, burdens and effectiveness of a new intervention must be tested against those of the best proven intervention(s)" (WMA 2013). PROMISE was an unethical study because it violated these international ethical principles by continuing to offer less than standard of care to HIV-infected pregnant women and, in the process, sending the wrong message to the governments of poor countries— delivering standard of care need not be a priority for your country. The PROMISE study investigators were indifferent to the HIV research advances and the recommendations of NIH's own panel of experts.

Getting large organizations to change their ethical or scientific views on large and expensive research studies that are already in progress is formidable. In 2013, I wrote to NIAID outlining why the PROMISE study failed to conform to international ethical standards and failed to incorporate recent scientific advances using HAART. I also pointed out that the study failed to adhere to HIV treatment recommendations by IAS and the USPHS to treat all HIV-infected individuals. I suggested that NIH should distinguish itself by performing studies that are directed to ending the pediatric AIDS epidemic, stating, "The NIH should not support clinical research that utilizes comparative study arms that will be abandoned, complicate the ability to conduct the research, are unnecessary, or are considered unethical."

The use of vulnerable HIV-infected pregnant women and their infants in low-income countries for studies that delayed or limited treatment finally ended in 2015. On July 7, 2015, IMPAACT quietly announced: "Because of START [Strategic Timing of Antiretroviral Treatment] results, they'll be offering ART to all mothers all arms in PROMISE" (IMPAACT 2015). Significantly, START had not been conducted by IMPAACT. In fact, it was not designed to examine HIV-infected pregnant women but rather to prove once and for all that early initiation of HAART, regardless of CD4 count or clinical status, should be the standard of care for treating all HIV-infected individuals. The study, conducted by the adult HIV/AIDS community, evaluated 4,685 HIV-infected patients and was stopped early by the DSMB because the results were so significant. Recommendations to treat all HIV-infected individuals—infants, children, men, women, and pregnant women—followed ("Starting Antiretroviral Treatment" 2015; Lundgren et al. 2015). IMPAACT had no option but to follow the recommendations. After more than fifteen years of denying that HIV-infected pregnant women needed to be treated in the same manner as any other infected individual, tens of millions of dollars in research study expenditures, and placing tens of thousands of HIV-infected pregnant women and their infants at risk, they were proven wrong, but this did not stop the IMPAACT/PROMISE network from continuing to pursue research studies in poor countries, costing millions of dollars to evaluate experimental treatment unlikely to be of any benefit (Ammann 2014a).

Turning the Corner

29

WHO WAS PATIENT ZERO? WHAT DOES IT MEAN FOR ENDING THE HIV EPIDEMIC?

Yes, there was a patient zero, but it was not really Gaëtan Dugas. The real patient zero is unknown. But Dugas, the person identified in Randy Shilts's book *And the Band Played On*, and his sexual exploits beginning as a twenty-year-old Air Canada flight attendant from Toronto, remains instructive as to how HIV can spread. Dugas became the center of epidemiologic investigations examining the spread of AIDS in the United States and elsewhere. His physical attractiveness facilitated multiple liaisons; on one occasion, Dugas described himself as the "prettiest one" at a gay bar in San Francisco, where he was a frequent visitor among the gay community. He kept a record of his sexual partners, which subsequently became an early means of contact tracing for many public-health and epidemiology investigators who were tracking the spread of HIV (Shilts 1987).

Dugas did not confine his sexual activity to San Francisco. Taking advantage of his position as a flight attendant, he traveled to Los Angeles, Fire Island, and New York City, continuing to have sexual encounters with multiple individuals in each location. He was allegedly one of the first patients to be diagnosed with KS. Dugas attracted the attention not only of physicians who saw him as a patient, but also of public-health professionals who were trying to understand the spread of HIV; namely, Drs. David Auerbach, William Darrow, Harold Jaffe, and James Curran from the CDC, who published their conclusions in the *American Journal of Medicine* in 1984 (Auerbach et al. 1984). Using charts with circles linking different individuals with Dugas at the center, the CDC investigators identified him as the central figure in their study. He could be linked to a total of forty of the first 248 cases of AIDS in the United States—nine cases in Los Angeles, twenty-two cases in New York City, and nine more in eight other cities. Dugas claimed to have had an average of 250 sexual partners each year, amounting to more than 2,500 sexual partners in the United States and Canada during his lifetime.

But the real patient zero had to be someone who was unknown to the world of epidemiology, because the HIV/AIDS epidemic really began somewhere in the forests of West Africa, perhaps not far removed from northern DRC in the region of the Ebola River where the Ebola virus is believed to have originated in 1976. In fact, HIV may have originated seventy-five years earlier. The most prevalent theories on the origin of HIV suggest that the source was from chimpanzees that inhabited the Cameroon, Gabon, Equatorial Guinea, Congo Brazzaville, Central African Republic, and the DRC. Bush hunters who focused on monkeys as a source of food were likely to have become infected from injuries sustained while hunting chimpanzees. The virus "jumped" from chimpanzees to humans and spread to sexual partners. It is also possible that colonizers facilitated the spread of HIV through the sex trade and the reuse of needles for medical treatment. All of this would have happened during the early 1900s. Human blood samples from 1959 and 1960 from Kinshasa, DRC, were evaluated by scientists, who extrapolated that the virus must have existed in the early 1900s in Africa. AIDS probably did not become an epidemic until the 1970s, when there was a dramatic increase in the number of patients with features characteristic of AIDS—opportunistic infections, KS, and TB—in Kinshasa, the capital of DRC (Pepin 2013; Sharp and Hahn 2010).

Initially AIDS did not spread rapidly. Traveling long distances within a country such as the DRC with few roads, railroads, or airplane flights was difficult to impossible. More rapid spread of HIV required sexual networks that were not present in remote areas. Once outside forested areas, truck drivers, soldiers, and migrant workers were identified as facilitating a more rapid spread of HIV. Studies found that by the 1980s, 35 percent of Ugandan truck drivers were HIV-infected, along with 30 percent of military personnel. Travel of HIV through human carriers may have also been a result of numerous Haitians who were in the Congo to provide "technical assistance." From there, HIV may have traveled to the United States and Europe as well as other countries as a consequence of gay sex tourism (Sharp and Hahn 2010; Pepin 2013).

The long interval between the acquisition of HIV infection and symptoms, six to eight years and more, and the lack of a means to diagnose HIV meant that individuals were unaware that the disease they were suffering from resulted from HIV. Most individuals continued to be sexually active, unknowingly transmitting the virus to their partners. Today, however, HIV can be detected early after infection, and individuals can be educated about how to prevent others from becoming infected or, if uninfected, how to protect themselves from acquiring HIV from a sexual partner.

The very different ways that HIV and the Ebola virus are transmitted, one by sexual contact and the other by direct non-sexual contact, is likely a major factor in why the HIV/AIDS epidemic spread to so many millions of individuals before it was recognized as a worldwide threat compared to the almost immediate recognition of Ebola. The initial infection with HIV results in signs and symptoms that are similar to influenza virus infection and are not fatal, followed by years of being asymptomatic, during which time the virus continues to spread. Eventually, HIV progresses to AIDS with recognizable signs and symptoms. During the asymptomatic period, individuals may not realize they are infected and transmit HIV to sexual partners or, in the case of HIV-infected pregnant women, to their infants. HIV infection's absence of severe outward manifestations contributes to its spread. In contrast, because the signs of Ebola are much more immediate and alarming, the infection is more dramatic, resulting in a more rapid medical response and public-health control of the infection. As a consequence, even though in the past there have been periodic outbreaks of Ebola virus, infection has been contained and restricted to specific regions or countries. However, the 2014 Ebola virus outbreak was different. It was one of the largest ever recorded, resulting in the death of over twelve thousand individuals, which is about the same number as die from HIV every two days (Frieden et al. 2014).

No matter when HIV actually jumped from animals to humans, what is so surprising today are the many slogans that suggest that the HIV/AIDS epidemic can be brought to a halt and HIV eradicated without identifying those who are HIV-infected or providing them with treatment and education to prevent further HIV spread. UNAIDS is especially fond of coming up with slogans that imply the HIV/AIDS epidemic is ending, such as "Getting to Zero," but then failing to achieve the projected results. The most recent UNAIDS slogan is, "90, 90, 90," an ambitious but unachievable target without employing contact tracing—"By 2020, 90 percent of all people living with HIV will know their HIV status. By 2020, 90 percent of all people with diagnosed HIV infection will receive sustained ART. By 2020, 90 percent of all people receiving ART will have viral suppression" (UNAIDS 2014a). These are aspiring goals for an organization that, along with WHO, failed to recommend universal HIV testing, contact tracing, and treating all infected individuals with HAART for almost two decades while the epidemic expanded to infect and kill tens of millions of individuals worldwide.

When one recalls how the HIV epidemic expanded, it seems that its origin has been largely forgotten. If a single individual, the real "patient zero," could have initiated an HIV/AIDS epidemic that ultimately resulted in more than eighty million HIV-infected men, women, and children, it should motivate us all to apply every known means of HIV prevention, no matter where HIV exists or how few patients are infected. It hardly seems plausible that focusing simply on geographic regions with a high percentage of HIV-infected individuals in urban areas will bring about the epidemic's eradication. Of course, a vaccine for HIV is always possible and would certainly result in "turning the corner" in the HIV/AIDS epidemic, but after thirty years of intensive research without an effective vaccine yet in sight, every known means of HIV prevention must be used now to end the HIV/AIDS epidemic, and it must be used worldwide. Contact tracing, no matter how socially uncomfortable or politically difficult to achieve, must be put in place if we are truly serious about identifying 90 percent of HIV-infected individuals and then providing 90 percent with effective antiretroviral treatment. We owe all HIV-infected individuals the right to know that they are infected and the right to lifesaving treatment, not because it's a slogan but because it's the ethical thing to do.

TURNING THE CORNER TOWARD A CURE: A HOPE OR A REALITY?

Like most people who had been tracking possible cures for HIV, I was surprised when I first heard about an infant who may have been cured of HIV. It was something that everyone had hoped for, but there had only been sporadic media and academic reports of potentially cured patients during the past fifteen years. But in 2013, a most convincing report came from Dr. Hannah Gay, a pediatrician at the University of Mississippi Medical Center in Jackson. Her sole patient ignited the HIV world, especially the pediatric HIV/AIDS community, with the speculation that a cure for HIV infection was possible. It was one of the most well-documented cases to be reported since HAART became available and, importantly, the child was followed for the longest period of time without showing evidence of infection, lending credibility to the possibility that HIV could be eradicated (Persaud et al. 2013).

I thought back to the 1998 Think Tank that we organized, sponsored by amfAR. It was there that Ho had precipitated an intense debate with the question, "Is eradication of HIV possible?" At that point in the HIV/AIDS epidemic, it was known that the virus wasn't just circulating in the blood; it was also "hiding" in almost every organ of the body—lymph nodes, spleen, liver, brain, gastrointestinal tract, etc. The first plausible example of a possible cure came thirteen years after the Think Tank and Ho's challenge to the scientists. On March 10, 2010, the details of a single patient (the Berlin patient) were reported in the scientific journal *Blood* (Allers et al. 2010). But this was an extremely complicated HIV-infected patient who had received a bone marrow transplant for leukemia and had been cured of his HIV infection. The bone marrow came from a donor who had a genetic mutation that prevented HIV from infecting cells. The transplant procedure was complex and, although it brought hope for a cure, the process was complicated and expensive and could not be universalized.

Katherine Luzuriaga and her coworkers in Wooster, Massachusetts, reported tantalizing evidence for a cure in 2000 (Luzuriaga et al. 2000). At follow-up, infants whose treatment with ART was initiated at less than three months of age lacked plasma viremia, and HIV could not be cultured from their blood cells. An additional suggestion that HIV might be "functionally cured" came from a 2012 report of fourteen HIV-infected adults in France (Landau 2013). Similar to the pediatric patients reported by Luzuriaga, treatment had been initiated with ARVs soon after infection. The patients stopped taking ART after three years, which usually results in resurgence of HIV infection. However, the HIV viral levels remained low for an average of seven years.

Gay's patient was an infant born to a woman who had no prenatal care. The mother's CD4 count and viral load were both abnormal but not in the range that would have been treated in many low-income countries that adhere to the faulty WHO guidelines for initiating ART during pregnancy. US guidelines would have recommended waiting to see if the infant was HIV-infected, using a sensitive test for the virus in the baby's blood and delaying treatment for weeks. Nevertheless, Gay initiated HAART in the infant at thirty hours of age, prior to a confirmed diagnosis of HIV infection. What Gay did that was so different from the faulty dogma of the time, but consistent with what every infectious disease pediatrician is trained to do, was start lifesaving treatment immediately and then plan to stop the treatment if the infant was not infected.

Blood samples from the infant that had been obtained before treatment was started confirmed that the infant was infected; therefore, HAART was continued. By twenty-nine days of age, HIV was undetectable in the infant. Between eighteen and twenty-three months, the mother missed several clinical follow-up appointments. The child returned to the clinic at twenty-three months of age, at which time the mother reported that she had stopped HAART when the infant was eighteen months of age. Amazingly, in subsequent follow-up visits at twenty-three and twenty-four months of age, blood tests on the infant showed no detectable virus.

Gay's patient was simultaneously reported in the media and at the Conference on Retroviruses and Opportunistic Infections in Atlanta on March 3, 2013. This single patient report generated remarkable worldwide enthusiasm that perhaps, at last, an infant had been "cured" of HIV. The circumstances were unusual, but retrospectively it was something that could have been discovered sooner in many more HIV-infected infants. It took someone who was not part of the "established" research community to take the courageous and decisive step to administer HAART to prevent HIV infection in an infant not yet two days old.

During an interview conducted by Michael Krasny on *Forum* on March 5, 2013, Anthony Fauci, head of NIAID and a leader in the fight against HIV, and I discussed the implications of Gay's patient. Fauci pointed out that the circumstances of the infant receiving HAART so early after birth would not happen in low-income countries, but the observations were of critical importance for future research into a possible cure for HIV. I took the opportunity to point out that we didn't have to wait for future research before implementing what we already know and have immediately available—providing HAART to all HIV-infected individuals including pregnant women to block transmission to their infants. Countless lives could be saved with what was already available ("Child Cured" 2013).

In June 2014, I called Gay to ask how she made her decision to treat aggressively and early. As the story unfolded, Gay recounted several observations that had resulted in her decision to treat immediately. The most important was that she viewed the circumstances that confronted her as an instance of PEP, not just preventing perinatal HIV transmission. She reasoned: if the most potent ARVs are used for women and girls who are raped, or for health-care workers who were accidentally inoculated with HIV, and they then do not get infected with HIV, why would it be any different for her infant patient? Unencumbered by limited and scientifically rigid US and WHO guidelines for treating HIV-exposed infants, Gay pulled out all the stops—she gave the most potent ARVs she had to the infant even before she knew the infant was HIV-infected. By using the best available treatment, she did what responsible health-care professionals most often do.

The optimism regarding the potential cure of HIV infection continued for more than two years. But on Friday July 11, 2014, Gay emailed me that the child had "relapsed" and now had detectable levels of HIV. HAART was restarted as Gay and others reflected on the disappointment and began to ask questions about what this all meant and what should be done next. Certainly, there was a vast difference between a possible cure and a "functional cure" when the virus could not be detected but was not eradicated. But this remained as one of the few, if not only, clear documentations that early treatment of an infant could keep HIV at bay for more than two years without treatment. There were implications for early treatment of HIV-exposed or infected infants in low-income countries—not having to treat an infant for the first two years of life could simplify the child's care and take the child past the most vulnerable phase of HIV infection. It was also possible that infection would be more easily kept under control or that some form of immunity would develop that would eventually drive the virus back into obscurity. The story is not yet completed.

ELIMINATION OF PERINATAL HIV TRANSMISSION: HIV IN CUBA (AND ELSEWHERE)

On June 30, 2015, it was announced that Cuba had become the world's first country to eliminate perinatal HIV transmission. The conclusion was based on the fact that only two infants were born with HIV infection in 2013, fulfilling the goals of a program initiated by the Pan American Health Organization/WHO (PAHO/WHO) to eliminate perinatal HIV and syphilis in the Americas. Elimination was defined as a reduction in transmission of HIV and syphilis to such a low level that it no longer constituted a public-health problem. The definition was problematic, however, considering the story of patient zero and the history of HIV as having in all likelihood originated with a single infected patient somewhere in Africa. Nevertheless, achieving control of HIV transmission to such low levels was a milestone, and Cuba's being the first income-poor country to do it caused many to ask exactly what they had done that was not being done in other low-income countries. This is not to say that elimination of perinatal HIV had not occurred in wealthy countries such as the United States and Canada, where elimination by the WHO definition had occurred decades earlier after implementing the lifelong treatment of HIV-infected women, pregnant or not, with HAART.

Exactly what did Cuba do? Although the guide for implementation developed by PAHO/WHO for the Americas was used by Cuba, they employed a more aggressive and integrated approach to prevention and treatment. Cuba viewed both HIV and syphilis as STIs rather than as WHO's medically incorrect characterization of "HIV and sexually transmitted infections," which contributed to siloed approaches to HIV prevention and treatment. Cuba also conducted a more cohesive approach to eliminating HIV by incorporating it into a universal health-care system in which maternal and child health programs were integrated with HIV. They also focused on an often-neglected aspect of the HIV epidemic—the disproportionate impact of HIV on adolescent girls and young women. In what seemed to be a form of contact tracing, their partner notification program identified individuals who did not know they were infected with syphilis, HIV, or both, who were then provided with treatment. (Incongruously, PAHO/WHO recommended identifying and testing of sexual partners only if syphilis were diagnosed.) Apparently, this was accomplished without coercion or compromising human rights principles.

In spite of a more than a fifty-year embargo by the United States, Cuba provided an example to the world that perinatal HIV could be eliminated by adhering to fundamental principles of prevention and treatment; integrating HIV into a universal health-care system; implementing treatment with HAART as soon as a diagnosis was established; ensuring equity in prevention and treatment for women; treating HIV as an STI with similar diagnostic, treatment, and public-health approaches for control; and conducting contact tracing while maintaining fundamental health-care rights.

PART 5 Ending the Pediatric HIV/AIDS Epidemic

They fancied themselves free, and no one will
ever be free so long as there are pestilences.

Albert Camus, *The Plague*

What Went Well

30

IT WILL END

On July 28, 2007, I was in Jinja, Uganda, standing on a grassy field surrounded by more than three hundred orphans waiting for Hope Walks to begin. Hope Walks was an event organized by Global Strategies and held in various cities to raise awareness and funds to support AIDS orphans in poor countries. The walk in Jinja was not a fundraiser but an event to call attention to the vast AIDS orphan crisis. In Uganda, where orphans remain largely invisible, there was a rare chance to make them seen and known. My Ugandan friends and Mary Ann McCoy from Children of Grace, an NGO supporting orphan education and care, planned the details of the walk.

The orphans stood ready to march with Hope Walks/Jinja T-shirts covering remnants of their school uniforms and with faces revealing both awe and anticipation. Just before the walk was to begin, the sky began to darken, and an impending storm threatened to rain on the parade. I watched as the dark clouds increased in intensity. Then I heard the thunder roll and wondered if the walk would be canceled by something entirely out of our control.

The rain came—not a sprinkle, but a downpour. Within seconds, we all scattered to find whatever shelter we could. I found myself huddled together with several of the orphans underneath a corrugated metal roof, wondering if all of the planning and excitement would come to naught. As the rain continued to pound, I leaned down to one of the orphans and asked, "Do you think the rain will stop?" Without hesitation and with a smile of confidence, the child replied, "It will stop." And stop it did.

The parade started and wove through the streets of Jinja with hundreds of onlookers, first hearing the sounds and then seeing the orphan children and, perhaps for the first time, the extent of the orphan crisis that had been precipitated by the HIV/AIDS epidemic. We all hoped that what would be most remembered was that the epidemic could and must stop.

In the years that followed Hope Walks, advances in HIV prevention and treatment proliferated, and there was evidence that the HIV/AIDS epidemic was slowing. During that time I was asked many times whether I thought the HIV/AIDS epidemic would stop. I would recall the words of the orphan child in the midst of the thunderstorm—"It will stop." I believed then that the pediatric HIV/AIDS epidemic would stop, and I still believe today that it can be stopped. The remarkable scientific and clinical research studies performed by some of the most brilliant scientists and clinicians in the world provided all of the answers needed to end pediatric HIV/AIDS. The scientific community had shown their ability and tenacity in discovering the cause of AIDS and treatment for HIV infection and finding solutions to end one of the worst epidemics in the world. What faltered was not the scientists who made the incredible research discoveries but the implementation of the research results.

SOME OF THE MOST IMPORTANT ADVANCES IN HIV/AIDS

Some of the most important advances in HIV/AIDS are outlined in the Appendix, "Timeline of Pediatric HIV/AIDS Milestones." Advances in the HIV/AIDS epidemic were not the result of a single discovery by a single individual. Rather, the progress made is an example of a long series of investigations and discoveries by many individuals over a period of decades. The many discoveries converged to create one of the most amazing stories of how research contributes to medical progress when confronted with a new disease. HIV existed somewhere in remote regions of Africa devoid of even the basic rudiments of health care decades before AIDS was described by Gottlieb in 1981. It spread from one individual to another through sexual transmission, causing a wasting disorder as a result of unrecognized opportunistic infections. It was soon labeled "slim disease," a catchall for anyone with severe loss of weight—whether related to AIDS or to malnutrition or TB or any other infection that could not be diagnosed but caused dramatic weight loss. For decades the virus continued to spread without anyone identifying the cause of the wasting disorder, all the while traveling with individuals across Africa and eventually reaching the United States. By the time AIDS was recognized in 1981, the immunologic and virologic tools developed for research of other diseases were available to define the syndrome now known as AIDS.

THE DISCOVERY OF AIDS

Michael Gottlieb is credited with putting together the unusual occurrences of opportunistic infections in young gay men with impaired immune systems and reporting AIDS in 1981, alerting the worldwide medical community to the existence of a new disease. Gottlieb was a faculty member and immunologist at UCLA. His report stemmed from his observations of patients who had CMV infection, PCP, KS, and mucosal candidiasis (CDC 1981b). Rock Hudson and Elizabeth Glaser were among his other patients. Gottlieb's contacts with the entertainment industry, especially Elizabeth Taylor, resulted in making the newly identified syndrome of AIDS visible not only to the world of medicine and public health but also to the entertainment industry. Gottlieb facilitated collaboration among these groups and individuals, thereby accelerating AIDS recognition. After his first description, additional reports followed from distant geographic regions with similar clinical findings, primarily in young homosexual men. The discovery that AIDS was associated with a unique pattern of immunodeficiency—markedly decreased CD4 cells, a subpopulation of immune cells called T-cells, and elevated antibodies called immunoglobulins—led to the identification of AIDS features in other populations: women, infants, intravenous drug users, and individuals who had acquired the disease from blood transfusions (Curran 1985). Gottlieb's keen observations led to the

AIDS epidemic's early identification. Although the disease is likely to have been in Africa decades earlier, vaguely labeled as "slim disease," its recognition in the United States lead to accelerated research into the cause, prevention, and treatment, which has benefited the entire world.

DISCOVERING THE CAUSE OF AIDS AND A TEST TO DIAGNOSE INFECTION

In 1983 the critical discovery was made that a retrovirus, subsequently called human immunodeficiency virus (HIV), was the cause of AIDS. This pivotal discovery catapulted basic and clinical research into defining the HIV/AIDS epidemic and developing tools for diagnosis, prevention, and treatment of the infection. Montagnier and his associates at the Pasteur Institute in France first reported the virus's description (Barre-Sinoussi et al. 1983). Later, two US investigators—first Gallo at the NIH and later Levy at the UCSF Medical Center—described a similar retrovirus associated with AIDS (Gallo et al. 1983; Levy 1984). All three viruses were subsequently called human immunodeficiency virus type I (HIV-1). Once the virus was discovered, a diagnostic test to detect antibodies to HIV quickly followed. In 1985, the US FDA approved the first such blood test, known as an enzyme-linked immunoassay (ELISA).

The importance of the ELISA test lay in its ability to identify HIV-infected individuals and the modes of HIV transmission—sexual, exposure to infected blood including transfusions, intravenous drug use, transmission from HIV-infected mothers to their infants, and transmission by breastfeeding. Additionally, HIV antibody testing was used to map the worldwide distribution of HIV and to identify populations at risk of acquiring HIV infection.

LOW-COST RAPID HIV TESTING

Performing the ELISA test required a venipuncture using a syringe and needle, expensive equipment and supplies, and laboratory technicians with special training. An additional requirement was an equally complex confirmatory test called the Western blot. All this added up to an expensive diagnostic test that limited its usefulness in low-income countries. A simpler, easier to use, and less expensive HIV antibody test was needed. In 1992, a new approach was introduced: rapid HIV testing, which could be performed on finger-stick blood samples, saliva, or urine. The test was stable at room temperature and was significantly less expensive, costing less than two dollars per test compared to more than forty dollars for ELISA testing. Because of ease of use and the minimal training necessary to conduct the test, it could be administered by mid-level health-care workers in remote and rural regions. Results were available in less than two hours, meaning patients could wait for the test results before departing the clinic. This resulted in an increased number of individuals who could be informed of their results, educated on how to prevent HIV infection if they tested negative, and informed of treatment options if they tested positive.

An additional advance in the use of rapid HIV testing resulted from solutions that originated within low-income countries that could not provide the extensive pre- and post-test counseling largely imposed on them by income-rich countries as a condition for providing funds. They developed an "opt out" procedure in which patients were told that they would be tested for HIV and told the results the same day unless they voluntarily chose to decline. In 1999, the Institute of Medicine issued a report titled *Reducing the Odds: Preventing Perinatal Transmission of HIV in the United States* that recommended universal voluntary "opt-out" testing for pregnant women (Stoto, Almario, and McCormick 1999).

MEASURING IMMUNITY

Two assays were used for diagnosing immunodeficiency in AIDS—one measured the function of the immune system, and the other measured the number of TDL and TDL subsets that represented cell-mediated immunity. "T" stands for thymus, the organ that produces the immune cells that travel through the body, protecting an individual from bacterial, viral, fungal, and protozoal infections. Advances in measuring TDL included the ability to differentiate between T-helper cells and T-suppressor cells. T-helper cells could be identified using a monoclonal antibody, OKT4, resulting in renaming the T-helper cell CD4 (cluster of differentiation 4). These cells were crucial for protecting individuals from infection but were also the target of HIV. Because of its greater simplicity and reduced cost, measuring TDL rather than immunologic function became a standard for defining the degree of immunodeficiency in HIV-infected individuals. Following the implementation of ART, measuring TDL also became the primary means of determining how much recovery of the immune system had occurred.

Numerous clinical studies confirmed the association of CD4 cell deficiency and the susceptibility to opportunistic infections and other complications of HIV infection (El-Sadr et al. 2006; Govender et al. 2014). CD4 counts, expressed either as a percentage or total number of CD4 cells/mm3, were used by the CDC, WHO, and health-care providers to stage the severity of AIDS. Subsequently, the level of CD4 cells was used as a surrogate marker of immunologic recovery. The primary utility of measuring CD4 cells, however, was not in staging HIV infection, but as a cost-effective means of determining the response to ART. With the recent recommendation to treat all HIV-infected individuals regardless of CD4 counts, initiating ART based on CD4 determinations is no longer considered standard of care.

VIRAL LOAD ASSESSMENT

Antibody tests to detect HIV infection often did not become positive until four to eight weeks after infection. This "window period" was of great concern to blood banks, as an individual could be HIV-infected but would not be identified by routine antibody testing for up to eight weeks. Donation of blood from an HIV-infected donor during this time would transmit HIV to a blood recipient or even to multiple blood recipients if the blood were divided into red blood cells, platelets, and plasma. A sensitive test to detect the virus rather than the antibody was needed and was eventually provided by the PCR assay.

PCR techniques that measured HIV RNA were used to measured viral particles in the blood (viral load). Determination of viral load was indispensable for determining whether ART was of benefit in a HIV-infected individual—only effective drugs lowered the viral load ("Report of the NIH Panel" 1998; Blaser et al. 2014). Many clinical studies utilized both CD4 counts and viral load to predict the course of HIV infection once treatment had been initiated. The correlation with viral load was so great that in 1997 the FDA approved the viral load assay as a surrogate marker for efficacy of ARVs. Viral load is expressed as HIV RNA copies/mL, but often expressed simply as the number of copies of HIV.

Measurement of the viral load was a major advance in understanding the course of HIV infection and obtaining rapid approval of efficacious drugs to treat HIV infection. Precipitous decreases in viral load in patients treated with combination ARVs predicted the long-term benefit in decreasing mortality and long-term complications of HIV, allowing the patient to remain healthy without having to wait years for the clinical markers of advancing HIV disease or death to appear. The viral load was also used as an indicator of the development of HIV drug resistance. An increasing viral load in patients on long-term ART was an indicator that they were becoming resistant to one or more ARVs, signaling the need to change treatment.

The viral load assay would have been ideal for use in low-income countries for early detection of HIV, especially in infants born to HIV-infected mothers, where antibody to HIV reflects the mother's infection but not the infant's. However, current assays are expensive, requiring elaborate equipment and special laboratory facilities to prevent contamination of blood samples. PCR methodology for use in low-income countries is likely to be limited until less expensive and easier to use assays become available. Additionally, caution should be exercised in recommending viral load assays as a requirement for initiation of HAART to avoid viral load becoming an obstacle, such as occurred with CD4 counts, to starting lifesaving treatment in HIV-infected individuals.

TREATMENT OF HIV INFECTION

The first major breakthrough in treatment of HIV was reported by Fischl and coworkers in 1987 in the *NEJM* under the title "The Efficacy of Azidothymidine (ZDV) in the Treatment of Patients with AIDS and AIDS-related Complex: A Double-blind, Placebo-controlled Trial" (Fischl, Richman, Grieco, et al. 1987). The importance of the ZDV study was that it broke through a barrier of scientific skepticism that a non-toxic drug could be found to control a virus that integrated itself into human cells. HIV uses reverse transcriptase to convert its genetic RNA into the host DNA, which then produces more RNA copies of HIV. Detailed molecular virology studies identified additional targets for designing drugs that were effective in controlling HIV replication and preventing HIV from entering CD4 cells, the major target of HIV infection, and other cells susceptible to viral entry. In 1995, the FDA approved the first of a new class of drugs, Invirase (saquinavir), a PI. Two additional PI drugs, RTV and indinavir, were approved in record time in 1996. Also in 1996, NVP, the first of the new class of drugs called non-nucleoside reverse transcriptase inhibitor (NNRTI) drug, was approved by the FDA. The new classes of drugs were shown to be highly effective in controlling HIV and, equally important, were shown to be dramatically more effective in reversing the course of HIV infection when used in combination. The use of highly active antiretroviral therapy began to be called HAART, and by 1998 their dramatic impact on reducing mortality and the complications of HIV was convincing. There were striking decreases in HIV mortality and HIV transmission from mothers to infants. Unfortunately, these early results were largely confined to the United States and Europe. Delays in implementation of HAART occurred in low-income countries where, paradoxically, 95 percent of the epidemic existed. The delays were primarily the result of WHO failing to incorporate lifesaving advances in their treatment guidelines, developing treatment recommendations based on economics rather than standard of care, and the pediatric AIDS research community delaying implementation of treatment and prevention in HIV-infected pregnant women and their infants in order to conduct additional research studies.

Beginning in 2003, three additional new classes of drugs were approved—integrase inhibitors, entry inhibitors, and fusion inhibitors. By 2014, the armamentarium for the treatment of HIV infection increased extensively to more than thirty individual and combinations of drugs. With the evidence that HAART was more effective than a single or two drugs used together, HAART became standard of care. Additional advances in treatment were the result of placing ARVs together in a single pill and developing formulations that could be administered only once a day. Fortunately, pharmaceutical companies producing the ARVs overcame some of the patent issues that could have prevented combining drugs made by two different manufacturers. They worked collaboratively to develop and test the most effective drug combinations. The vast array of drugs available for treatment of HIV infection brought optimism that the impact of the HIV/AIDS epidemic could be controlled as the HIV community and public-health officials watched the number deaths from HIV decrease dramatically. But the slow implementation of HAART in low-income countries tempered the optimism that treatment could decrease mortality and HIV transmission comparable to that observed in income-rich countries.

PREVENTION OF MOTHER-TO-CHILD TRANSMISSION (PMTCT)

In 1994 it was discovered that when ZDV was given to HIV-infected pregnant women, followed by a six-week course of ZDV prophylaxis for the infant, there was a 60 percent reduction in HIV transmission. It was the most important discovery in HIV prevention for several decades (Connor et al. 1994). It catapulted the HIV-prevention community into thinking about how perinatal HIV transmission might be reduced and whether ARVs could also prevent HIV transmission from an HIV-infected sexual partner to an uninfected partner. A 1999 clinical study in Uganda revealed that a single dose of NVP given to an infected pregnant woman during labor and a single dose given to her infant resulted in a 50 percent reduction in HIV infection, even when breastfeeding was continued (Guay et al. 1999). It was the first time that an inexpensive treatment (less than two dollars) was available for prevention of mother-to-child HIV transmission in low-income countries. In addition to the low cost of NVP, a single dose of the drug could easily be administered to the mother and infant by mid-level health-care workers and birth attendants.

HAART's dramatic impact in adults, demonstrating an increase in CD4 counts and a decrease in viral load, often to undetectable levels, coupled with reversal of progression to AIDS and dramatic reduction in complications of HIV infection, suggested that HAART should replace ZDV for preventing HIV transmission from infected mothers to their infants, as it would be more effective than one ARV. In fact, surveillance studies by the CDC in the US documented that the widespread use of HAART was associated with HIV transmission rates to infants plummeting from greater than two thousand per year to fewer than one hundred ("Perinatal HIV Down as Treatment Increases"

1997; CDC 2006). Tragically, the international pediatric AIDS research community stubbornly refused to accept any of the studies performed in HIV-infected adults and even dismissed the results of their own studies showing perinatal HIV transmission rates of less than 2 percent with HAART. The outcome was unfortunate—millions of HIV-infected pregnant women progressed from HIV infection to AIDS, and millions of infants became HIV-infected and died.

POST-EXPOSURE PROPHYLAXIS (PEP)

If treatment of HIV-infected pregnant women with ARVs could prevent the transmission of HIV to their infants, then it seemed probable that ARVs could also prevent HIV infection of individuals exposed to HIV, either as a result of accidental inoculation of blood from an HIV-infected individual or following rape by an HIV-infected perpetrator. Animal studies with viruses similar to HIV had shown that early administration of ARVs could prevent infection. Additional uncontrolled studies in humans indicated that providing ARVs within seventy-two hours of HIV exposure also prevented HIV infection (Gerberding and Katz 1999). Given the life-threatening consequences of HIV infection and the requirement for lifetime treatment with ARVs, recommendations were made to provide ARVs within the first seventy-two hours following exposure to HIV following accidental inoculation of HIV-infected blood or following rape. As more potent ARVs became available, prophylaxis with HAART within seventy-two hours of exposure was recommended, continuing treatment for four weeks. In spite of the known efficacy of PEP, many low-income countries with high rates of HIV infection and rape against women and girls fail to provide PEP to prevent fatal HIV infection. If the mother becomes both HIV infected and pregnant following rape, she may also transmit HIV to her infant.

PRE-EXPOSURE PROPHYLAXIS (PREP)

The concept of treating sexually active HIV-infected individuals with HAART to prevent HIV transmission to uninfected sexual partners was an extension of the successful use of HAART in HIV-infected pregnant women to prevent their infants from becoming HIV infected. If it worked in the latter circumstance, why would it not also work in the former circumstance, especially since all evidence pointed to a link between HAART's ability to reduce viral load and transmission of HIV? Unlike PEP, which was a thirty-day course of ARVs taken after high-risk exposure to HIV, PrEP refers to the daily use of ARVs by individuals without HIV infection who have unprotected sexual intercourse with an HIV-infected sexual partner. Initial studies showed a 40 to 60 percent reduction in HIV transmission (Grant et al. 2010). Maximum effectiveness required strict adherence to taking ARVs on a daily basis. It is anticipated that the use of PrEP will significantly reduce the number of new HIV infections worldwide. Possible problems in expanded use of PrEP include the development of ARV resistance, changes in behavior that increase unprotected sexual activity, increase of other STIs, and long-term expense compared to the use of condoms and/or abstinence (Baeten and Celum 2012).

TREATMENT AS PREVENTION

Studies on perinatal HIV transmission convincingly demonstrated the association of combination ARVs, reduction in viral load, and decreased HIV transmission. The key observation, derived from treatment with HAART, was the correlation between the degree of viral load reduction and subsequent transmission of HIV. Definitive proof that treatment with a combination of ARVs could indeed prevent transmission of HIV between sexual partners came from the NIH-supported HPTN 052 study (Cohen 2010; Cohen et al. 2011). The study was conducted in several countries by Cohen and collaborators, who reported that early initiation of HAART resulted in a 96 percent reduction in HIV transmission from HIV-infected sexual partners treated with HAART to their uninfected partners. The implication of this study was far reaching and provided justification for the aggressive early treatment of all HIV-infected individuals with HAART, which would simultaneously control the consequences of HIV infection and also reduce the number of newly infected individuals, an affect that could result in significant control of the HIV/AIDS epidemic by decreasing the number of new HIV infections transmitted heterosexually, the major means of HIV transmission. The START study results, reported in 2015, which initiated HAART in all HIV-infected individuals whether symptomatic or not and regardless of CD4 count, confirmed the earlier results reported by Cohen and collaborators and resulted in the universal recommendation to immediately treat all HIV-infected individuals with HAART (Beyrer et al. 2015).

PREVENTION OF OPPORTUNISTIC INFECTIONS

Often people assume that highly technical and expensive solutions are required to have a widespread impact on disease prevention. Low-tech and low-cost solutions are frequently ignored or remain untested. Such was the situation with CTX, which was first introduced as an antibiotic in the mid-1960s to treat respiratory, gastrointestinal, and urinary tract infections in children and adults. Subsequently, CTX was discovered to have antiprotozoal activity and was used for the prevention and treatment of PCP in children and adults with primary and secondary immunodeficiency.

Because CTX is a generic drug, the annual cost of CTX prophylaxis is less than six dollars per patient for an entire year of treatment. Unlike ARVs, CTX is readily available, can be stored without refrigeration, and can be easily administered by mid-level health-care workers in rural hospitals and clinics. Its availability preceded the HIV/AIDS epidemic by years, as it was used for the treatment of other infections in children and adults. The universal availability of CTX, its low-cost, and its minimal side effects had a profound impact on the health of HIV-infected individuals who were not receiving ART. After a long delay, WHO and other international organizations issued overdue guidelines in 2004 for the routine use of CTX for prophylaxis of opportunistic infections in HIV-infected adults and children (UNAIDS, WHO, and UNICEF 2004)

CIRCUMCISION

Circumcision, conducted primarily for religious reasons for centuries, has been associated with a number of benefits, including reduced risk of urinary tract infection, genital ulceration, STIs, and penile cancer, as well as a possible reduction in transmission of human papilloma virus (HPV), which is associated with cervical carcinoma. Aaron Fink published the first suggestion on a possible protective effect of male circumcision (MC) on HIV acquisition in 1989. The most compelling data came from two NIH-sponsored controlled clinical trials, one conducted in Kenya and one in Uganda, reported in 2006. Both studies showed an approximate 50 to 60 percent reduction in HIV acquisition (Lawoyin and Kehinde 2006; O'Farrell et al. 2006).

Following the announcement of the results of the NIH studies in Kenya and Uganda, NIAID Director Anthony Fauci stated, "While the initial benefit [of male circumcision] will be fewer HIV infections in men, ultimately adult male circumcision could lead to fewer infections in women in those areas of the world where HIV is spread primarily through heterosexual intercourse" (NIAID 2006). Several studies calculated that the implementation of MC could avert as many as 1.5 million new HIV infections and 300,000 deaths in ten years and prevent an additional 2.7 million infections and 2.7 million deaths over the next ten years. More than two decades after Fink's groundbreaking observations and six years after the definitive studies of Auvert et al. (2001) in South Africa that MC was associated with a decreased transmission of HIV, WHO incorporated recommendations for circumcision in their 2007 guidelines. Recommendations for circumcision were also included in the 2014 revisions of the IAS's prevention and treatment guidelines. Using modeling studies of male infant circumcision, some have suggested that male infant circumcision could result in cost savings for HIV prevention in high to moderate seroprevalent regions (Vermund and Hayes 2013).

BEHAVIORAL CHANGES

During the HIV/AIDS epidemic, there were many skeptics who argued that behavioral changes in sexual practices were not possible or would not have a widespread impact on decreasing HIV infection. However, convincing evidence that sexual behavior could be changed first originated in Uganda. In the late 1980s, the Ugandan government addressed the escalating HIV/AIDS epidemic by conducting an intensive media campaign that included HIV transmission and prevention discussion in government agencies, public meetings, education facilities, and churches, emphasizing abstinence and "zero grazing" (i.e., fidelity to a sexual partner). It was followed by an emphasis on ABC: Abstinence, Be faithful, Condoms. By the mid-1990s, a reduction in the seroprevalence of HIV was reported from fifteen to five percent. Behavior change occurred on a population basis, but there were questions as to how long it would last (Murphy et al. 2006). Recently, the Ugandan government acknowledged that the impact of the ABC campaign has waned, and the number of HIV-infected individuals is increasing.

Attributing a significant decrease in the population seroprevalence of HIV to a single method of prevention or behavior change would be incorrect. The number of new HIV infections began to stabilize in the United States in 1992 and has been consistent ever since. Similarly, a much later but still highly significant decline in the worldwide number of new HIV infections was reported by UNAIDS. New HIV infections declined from 3.4 million each year globally in 2001 to 2.3 million in 2012. An epidemic of the magnitude of HIV requires considering every means of preventing HIV transmission. It is doubtful that the contribution of any single means of prevention can be precisely calculated in the context of the multiple prevention methods available. What remains important is that, no matter what method is invoked, behavior change will be required if the HIV/AIDS epidemic is to be brought under control.

EXPANSION OF ACTIVISM AND ADVOCACY

There was another important advance, not scientific but involving a myriad of emotions, direct engagement, negotiating skills, and organization—activism and advocacy. The difference between activism and advocacy is not in their ultimate goal but in their intensity in reaching the goal. The activism of the HIV/AIDS epidemic originated with those who were HIV-infected and those who were most closely involved with the pain, suffering, stigma, and indifference associated with it. At the beginning of the epidemic, denial, ignorance, blame, and discrimination flourished. As HIV/AIDS expanded, no group of individuals was immune from the epidemic's impact—men, women, children, rich, poor, educated, uneducated, powerful, or disadvantaged. Early activists most often represented the "why" of the HIV/AIDS epidemic: Why was research so slow? Why was the public and government response to the epidemic not immediate? Why were drugs to treat HIV infection approved so slowly? Why were the benefits of research and drug development not made immediately available to all of those who were HIV infected, including individuals in low-income countries?

Not everyone approved of their methods, but in the end everyone had to acknowledge the activists' impact on altering the status quo for the benefit of many, even those with diseases other than AIDS. Previously secluded meetings of government and nongovernment organizations, whether congressional, NIH, FDA, medical subspecialties, international conferences, or foundations, were likely to be attended by, and even interrupted by, activists who demanded greater attention to the emerging HIV/AIDS epidemic. Those who are tempted to dismiss the activists' concerns as self-serving need only look across the United States and around the world to observe the results of activism and to agree that these people were needed to help control an ever-expanding HIV/AIDS epidemic.

HIV activism was unique. Perhaps for the first time in any epidemic, those who were affected the most sat alongside decision-makers and even participated in determining what type of scientific, industry, or government response was needed to solve their health needs. Their access was face-to-face as they questioned the why and how of developing solutions. Individuals immersed in other diseases learned from the HIV/AIDS activists how to keep those in power and control from ignoring their concerns. Whether the cause was breast cancer, malignancies, rare diseases, research investment, directing or redirecting public funding—activism was acknowledged as necessary for getting the attention of individuals and government entities who needed constant prodding and reminders of their duties to those in need.

PEPFAR to the Rescue

31

PEPFAR: A SURPRISING PROPOSAL TO THE US CONGRESS

The proposal came as a surprise to many: appropriate $15 billion over five years to combat the HIV/AIDS epidemic—the largest amount ever requested by anyone within the US government for global health. The person who made the proposal was also a surprise: President George W. Bush, who many in the activist/advocacy community presumed was unsympathetic to the global HIV/AIDS epidemic. Bush may have been partially politically motivated. One story holds that in 1998 Condoleezza Rice suggested to Bush that if he won the presidency his foreign policy should focus on Africa. It may also have been a result of his emphasis on "compassionate conservatism," viewing the needs of low-income countries such as those in Africa and the HIV/AIDS epidemic as likely targets. No matter the reasons, here was a Republican president testing whether or not Congress would approve the largest proposal for funding HIV programs that the world had ever seen.

Congress accepted the challenge and in 2003 approved Bush's proposal, which became known as PEPFAR (the President's Emergency Plan for AIDS Relief) (PEPFAR 2009). Those who were experienced with the US government's international funding were concerned about how such a large amount of money would be spent and who would receive it. They knew that it was not unusual for funds to either "disappear" or for government organizations to take such a large share of the funds that little was left to implement lifesaving interventions for individuals who needed them. In order to avoid repeating such problems, the Global AIDS Act, under which PEPFAR was funded, specified goals accompanied by measurable outcomes that were required by law to be accomplished within a specific time period. The legislation also established the State Department Office of the Global AIDS Coordinator (OGAC), along with a newly created position of US Global AIDS Coordinator to oversee all international AIDS funding that fell under PEPFAR's umbrella.

When PEPFAR began, fifteen countries were designated as "focus countries," including Botswana, Côte d'Ivoire, Ethiopia, Guyana, Haiti, Kenya, Mozambique, Namibia, Nigeria, Rwanda, South Africa, Tanzania, Uganda, Vietnam, and Zambia. It did not mean, however, that other countries were excluded from receiving smaller amounts of support, but exactly why certain countries were chosen and others excluded was an ongoing mystery. The OGAC was responsible for distributing the funds through a number of government agencies, including USAID, HHS, the CDC, the NIH, and the Health Resource and Services Administration (HRSA). From 2003 to 2008, Congress dedicated an estimated $18.8 billion to PEPFAR, including commitments to the Global Fund, UNAIDS, International AIDS Vaccines Initiative (IAVI), and NIH research, as well as all of PEPFAR's bilateral country and regional programs for HIV/AIDS and TB.

During the first five years, PEPFAR focused on establishing and expanding prevention, care, and treatment programs. In one of the many reviews of the initial years of implementation, it was estimated that PEPFAR provided "treatment to more than two million people, care to more than ten million people—including more than four million orphans and vulnerable children—and prevention of mother-to-child treatment services for nearly sixteen million pregnancies" (PEPFAR 2009). After five years of implementation and evaluation, PEPFAR was generally deemed a success, both within the United States and internationally (Abrams et al. 2012). As a result, in 2008 an appropriation of $48 billion was committed to PEPFAR for an additional five-year period, including $39 billion for PEPFAR's bilateral HIV/AIDS programs, US contributions to the Global Fund, $5 billion to the President's Malaria Initiative, and $4 billion for TB (PEPFAR 2009).

PEPFAR continued as the United States' keystone effort to address major global health issues on a scale acknowledged as the largest in the history of global health. But both its scope and the amount of funding would change during the Obama administration, a surprise to many who felt that Democrats were more sympathetic to the global HIV/AIDS epidemic than Republicans were. In May 2009, a Global Health Initiative (GHI) was launched with PEPFAR as an integral component of an even larger effort in terms of scope, but it did not include the promised increased funding. To oversee this expansion, Eric Goosby was sworn in on June 23, 2009, as an ambassador and the United States' global AIDS coordinator.[1]

I was invited to attend Goosby's official State Department swearing-in ceremony in Washington, DC, with Secretary of State Hillary Clinton presiding. Eric was surrounded by his family, and in the audience were the many friends and collaborators with whom Eric had worked through decades of deep involvement in the HIV/AIDS epidemic. Also present were representatives of government and non-government organizations that had received PEPFAR funding in the past and certainly were making their presence known to express their interest in future funding. Clinton knew the importance of PEPFAR and had visited many of the most hard-hit regions of Africa along with Goosby, including regions where Global Strategies had established programs in the DRC and Liberia. In fact, following the swearing-in ceremony, Clinton told me that she would never forget the women she had met at HEAL Africa in Goma, DRC, who had suffered from so much physical and sexual violence.

Goosby was well-known and well-liked in the international HIV/AIDS circle, especially in San Francisco, where he had received his initial training and was first immersed in the HIV/AIDS epidemic. He had been the director of the National AIDS Policy and the Ryan White Care Act under President Clinton, and from 2001 to 2009, he was the CEO and Chief Medical Officer of Pangea Global AIDS Foundation. When Goosby accepted the position as the global AIDS coordinator, the worldwide economy was in jeopardy, and there was concern that funding for PEPFAR would also be in jeopardy; Goosby was not assuming an easy task (Goosby et al. 2012)

Under Goosby's leadership, PEPFAR's accomplishments continued. One tangible way to measure success is to examine the numbers provided by the US government's report on PEPFAR-funded programs. Numbers should be considered approximations, keeping in mind the difficulty in verifying their accuracy when data is obtained in income-poor settings. Nevertheless, the accomplishments are impressive. The PEPFAR website lists the following accomplishments as of September 30, 2013:

> In Fiscal Year (FY) 2013, PEPFAR supported HIV testing and counseling for more than 57.7 million people, providing a critical entry point to prevention, treatment and care. Of those receiving PEPFAR-supported HIV testing and counseling, more than 12.8 million were pregnant women. PEPFAR provided 780,000 of the women who tested positive for HIV with antiretroviral medications to prevent mother-to-child transmission (PMTCT) of the HIV. As a result of PEPFARs support, 95 percent of the babies were born free of HIV. By the end of 2013, PEPFAR reached the President's 2011 World AIDS Day goal of directly supporting 4.7 million voluntary medical male circumcision (VMMC) procedures. PEPFAR supported 17 million people with care and support, including more than 5 million orphans and vulnerable children, in FY 2013. (*www.pepfar.gov*)

PEPFAR'S IMPACT

Was PEPFAR a success? Yes. Massive increases in funding and the launch of programs to deliver ARVs made ART widely available, saving millions of lives worldwide and significantly reducing the mortality associated with HIV infection. Kimberly Scott of the Institute of Medicine, who completed an evaluation of the PEPFAR program, said, "This is a remarkable story that the American people should know about" (Sepúlveda et al. 2007).

In November 2013, Goosby stepped down from his position as the global AIDS ambassador to return to his alma mater, the UCSF Medical Center. He agreed to lead a new center on implementation sciences, perhaps related to frustration over not seeing implementation move more quickly under PEPFAR. Interestingly, he also returned to seeing patients on Ward 86 at San Francisco General Hospital, where he had seen some of the first patients with AIDS at the beginning of the epidemic (Bleicher 2014). Ambassador Goosby joined the Global Strategies board of directors in January 2014.

In an interview conducted by UCSF, Goosby was unusually candid about some of the difficulties encountered by PEPFAR. He acknowledged that one of the major flaws was that the established system of care was not sustainable. Too much funding went to approaches that had failed (Bleicher 2014). A particular disappointment for me, confirmed as I listened to Goosby during one of his lectures, was PEPFAR's failure to make tangible progress in the number of HIV-infected children who were placed on ART. It is not known whether this was because PEPFAR did not establish strong follow-up programs as a part of perinatal HIV-transmission prevention, because of the pediatric AIDS research community's overemphasis on research studies, or because of the fatalistic political or cultural attitude on the part of governments and communities concerning the vast numbers of infants and orphans requiring treatment and care. Whatever the cause(s), the result was a tragic loss of infants' and children's lives due to untreated HIV infection.

During his tenure as the global AIDS ambassador, Goosby was a strong supporter of HIV prevention and treatment of mothers and children. He incorporated lifetime treatment of HIV-infected women into PEPFAR's perinatal HIV transmission programs, known as Option B+, giving full credit to Malawi for developing the concept and increasing by an extraordinary 700 percent the number of pregnant or breastfeeding women who had been placed on ART.[2]

REFLECTIONS ON PEPFAR FUNDING FROM A VERY WISE NIGERIAN PHYSICIAN

In May 2014, I met with Dr. Chris Isichei from Faith Alive, a faith-based hospital and clinic in Jos, Nigeria. I hadn't spoken with Isichei at length for many years. We met for the first time in person in 2003 in California, where we planned a workshop for birth attendants at Faith Alive. It was one of the first-ever workshops to be conducted in a country with one of the highest numbers of HIV-infected individuals in Africa. In the years that followed, everything that Chris and his coworkers had hoped for happened: the HIV program that had started with only a handful of birth attendants grew to one that, by 2008, was caring for more than nine thousand HIV-infected individuals.

The funds for the expansion of HIV prevention, treatment, and care for thousands of individuals came to Chris and Faith Alive from the United States through PEPFAR and generous donations from US faith-based groups, such as Bayside Church in Sacramento, that provided volunteers and donated more than $1 million for expanding the HIV/AIDS programs. These funds allowed for greater laboratory resources, the provision of ARVs to prevent perinatal HIV infection, and treatment of thousands who were already HIV-infected. As his programs expanded, Chris and his coworkers came to rely on the PEPFAR funds.

Unfortunately, the infusion of PEPFAR funds removed Nigeria's own obligation to consider its responsibility for sustaining the programs. In addition, as much as 40 percent of the funding, which went through US-based academic and non-profit organizations, remained in the United States or went to expatriates working to implement programs in Nigeria. Nevertheless, Chris and his coworkers were grateful for what they were given—without it, the HIV/AIDS epidemic would have languished in a country that had the wealth to help but was seemingly indifferent to the suffering of its own people and saw no moral obligation to do anything about it.

In the years since our first meeting, Chris and I had communicated by email periodically, especially when Chris wanted me to review one of the manuscripts that had resulted from his studies on HIV-infected patients. Now I was sitting with Chris in California, just as I had done in 2003, but instead of planning a workshop for preventing perinatal HIV transmission, I was talking to him about his views on what should have been done to control the HIV/AIDS epidemic in Nigeria.

Before we began, as was true in so many of my greetings with my African friends, Chris initiated the conversation by asking me about my family, remembering each family member by name, and then thanking me, telling me that the very first infant who had received NVP to prevent perinatal HIV transmission in 2004 in a rural village, following Global Strategies' first workshop for traditional birth attendants, was now thirteen years old, well, and healthy. He was the pride of the family and the village, as was Hauwa Kadima, the birth attendant trained at the 2004 workshop who had administered the first dose of NVP. Deep inside, I felt the emotion that accompanies the realization that a life has been spared the ravages of HIV infection—here was a child whose future had forever been altered by a simple and inexpensive drug. That effect needed to be multiplied a thousand fold.

We moved the conversation from individuals to a more global issue—what should have been done differently to bring the HIV/AIDS epidemic under control in Nigeria and throughout the world? Isichei's perspective was important for a number of reasons. He had devoted his life to helping others through preventing HIV infection and acquiring the lifesaving drugs that were needed for those already infected. He had also worked tirelessly to prevent the stigma associated with AIDS and for communities to accept HIV-infected individuals within their midst, establishing vibrant HIV support groups and community-based treatment programs. Building a sustainable program for HIV prevention and treatment in an income-poor country required funding, and Chris had experience in getting funds from a number of different sources. In a country that "officially" had an HIV seroprevalence rate of 3.1 percent and 3.5 million individuals living with HIV infection, this was a formidable task.

The question of what should have been done differently was particularly relevant for Chris at this time. He had been informed just six months before that he would be losing the PEPFAR funds that had supported him for the previous ten years. PEPFAR was Chris's major source of financial support, and without it he was at a loss for funding continued treatment for the over nine thousand patients he saw each month. Fortunately, he was not completely abandoned, as funds continued to come from many faith-based groups in the United States.

There was eagerness in Chris's voice as we spoke. Initially, he told me that there were five major points, but when we completed the conversation almost two hours later, there were nine. As we concluded our discussion, I went over each one of the points with him again to be certain I understood them all. Here is what Dr. Isichei, living in the midst of one of the largest epidemics of any African country, struggling daily to sustain programs to meet the prevention and treatment needs of his people, told me:

1. HIV programs should have been integrated into the general health-care system of hospitals and clinics rather than put in place in a "parallel" program as required by the US funders. The implementation of a parallel HIV program was duplicative, expensive, and required separate infrastructure, separate laboratories, separate drug tracking, separately trained health-care workers, and separate hospital records.
2. Sustainable technical interventions that were low cost and simple to use but with high impact should have been implemented. Laboratories established by funders to monitor patients with HIV were furnished with complex and costly equipment that could not be maintained or repaired without outside support. Alternative readily available and less expensive approaches to monitoring HIV-infected patients were abandoned in favor of high-cost approaches requiring importation.

3. Rather than relying on imported capacity that would end when funding ended, local capacity to address the epidemic should have been built. Building local capacity should have included the education and training of local health-care and community workers and extending their education beyond HIV to include the diagnosis and treatment of other diseases that they were likely to encounter, such as malaria, TB, malnutrition, chronic kidney disease, and intimate partner violence. Program planning should have included not only local health-care workers but also individuals infected with HIV who could most intimately identify the needs.

4. HIV programs should have been designed with the input of local health-care and community workers. Funders who came from US government agencies, WHO, and academic universities imposed their programs on the Nigerians without asking for their opinions and without first identifying the needs viewed from their perspective.

5. The pediatric HIV/AIDS treatment program should have been started sooner. The two- to three-year delay in providing treatment and ARVs formulated for infants resulted in the premature death of thousands of HIV-infected infants and children.

6. Local ministries of health should have been informed of changes in funding well in advance of when the changes actually occurred, which would have allowed sufficient time to obtain replacement funds from the national government.

7. Treatment and care of patients should have been prioritized above research and time-consuming data gathering that used up too many of the financial resources and too much time that was desperately needed to improve the quality of patient care.

8. As soon as funding became available, plans should have been put in place to manufacture HIV-testing and treatments within the country rather than importing them from outside the country. Importation of desperately needed technology, supplies, and drugs insured non-sustainability once funding was discontinued.

9. Programs should have been incorporated in both urban and rural regions as soon as funding was granted. As much as 30 percent of the HIV/AIDS epidemic was afflicting rural regions where a reservoir of HIV remained, ensuring ongoing and future HIV transmission.

Here was a roadmap of solutions to ending the global HIV/AIDS epidemic.

WHITHER PEPFAR NOW?

The fate of PEPFAR was decided neither by the recipients of its benefits nor, in all likelihood, by those who devoted all of their energies to trying to make it a success. Its fate was decided as it began: at a presidential level, initiated with President George Bush's establishment of the largest health-related program in the world and realigned with President Obama's creation of the GHI. As stated on the *ghi.gov* website, the intent of the GHI was to "broaden the United States' involvement in global health." Broadening did not mean, as many in the HIV/AIDS community expected, maintaining PEPFAR's funding. What it meant for HIV was a proposed reduction of more than $500 million. Such a substantial funding cut would have caused an uproar and an avalanche of demonstrations by US activists if it had been for programs in the United States, but the response was muted, surprising even the most ardent activists and advocates (Jervis 2012). Those who would suffer the consequences could only conjecture what should've been done differently.

Dr. Isichei and I concluded our conversation with continued reflections on why the lives of so many of the poor and suffering hang in the balance of decisions made by people and governments they do not know. Would it have been different for women and children in remote villages and in the crowded cities of Africa who never got treatment or learned how to prevent HIV, if prevention and care programs had not been imported from wealthy countries but instead had been established collaboratively with health-care communities in both poor and wealthy countries, viewing them as equal partners in the battle against the HIV/AIDS epidemic?

Solutions

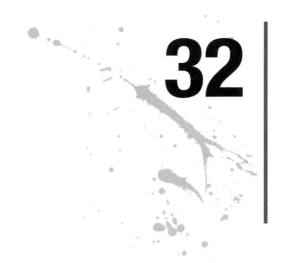

THE PEDIATRIC HIV/AIDS EPIDEMIC SHOULD HAVE ENDED

All the scientific advances, tools, and knowledge necessary to begin the process of eradicating HIV in infants and children were in place by 1996. The pathway to ending the pediatric HIV/AIDS epidemic should have started then. Was it possible?—Yes!

Physicians in the United States, without self-interest, government, or bureaucratic interference, did what should have been done in low-income countries. In the late 1990s, they treated their HIV-infected patients, including pregnant women, with HAART. As a result, for the first time since the beginning of the epidemic, the number of deaths from AIDS dropped substantially (23 percent) across the United States. In 1997 clinicians reported a 60 to 80 percent decline in death and hospitalizations in patients treated with HAART. By 1998 the HIV transmission rate from infected mothers to their infants had plummeted to less than 2 percent. Fewer than one hundred infants were born HIV infected each year (CDC 2006; Del Rio and Hernandez-Tepichin 1996). The CDC attributed these dramatic changes to the widespread use of HAART. Physicians and health-care providers in the United States had done what they always do with other infectious diseases—treat immediately with drugs proven to control infection. In this instance, it was HIV and treatment with HAART, drugs for which activists successfully fought to get early access to treatment and which the FDA had approved in record time so that HIV-infected individuals could immediately be given lifesaving treatment (FDA 2014). Individuals in low-income countries deserved no less.

Meanwhile, the number of those infected by HIV and dying in poor countries continued to increase into the millions. More unnecessary research and inferior treatment guidelines were not what they needed. They needed access to the same medical advances that had changed HIV infection in the United States from an acute and fatal disease to a chronic and manageable one, saving hundreds of thousands of lives. They needed fundamental principles of public health applied to their circumstances, including finding those who were HIV infected and getting them on ART. And equally important, they deserved the respect and dignity of their lives being viewed as important as the lives of those in income-rich countries.

My goal in this book is to discuss the remarkable achievements that occurred during the early decades of the HIV/AIDS epidemic, but also to identify what went wrong and resulted in an epidemic that, after more than three decades, continues at an alarming rate. This book does not conclude with pessimism, nor does it fail to acknowledge the efforts of thousands of individuals who strove to accomplish the goal of ending pediatric HIV/AIDS. Importantly, success in ending the pediatric HIV/AIDS epidemic can still be achieved if known solutions are implemented—not some new slogan, not as part of some millennium goal over the next ten years, or five years, or even the next two, but immediately.

PRIMARY PREVENTION—STOP IT BEFORE IT BEGINS: FOCUSING ON UPSTREAM SOLUTIONS

To end the pediatric HIV/AIDS epidemic, the focus must be on upstream solutions— stopping HIV transmission before it can spread. For too many decades, public-health approaches have been working downstream, after HIV infection has already occurred. It seems intuitive that if you want to prevent an infectious disease from spreading, you must place a high priority on preventing the infection in the first place. This is called primary prevention, and it is logical to conclude that the pediatric HIV/AIDS epidemic would no longer exist if women were protected from getting HIV infection to begin with.

Just talking about primary prevention as a priority is not enough. Given the destruction inflicted by HIV, it is not surprising that the rhetoric from influential individuals to end the HIV/AIDS epidemic has been strong. In 2000, former South African President Nelson Mandela warned, "AIDS is clearly a disaster, effectively wiping out the development gains of the past decades and sabotaging the future." Dr. Kim Jim Yong Kim, outgoing head of WHO HIV/AIDS was quoted in the *Boston Globe* in 2005 stating, "4.9 million new infections [annual HIV infections worldwide] is a castigation of global efforts to do prevention. We have failed, failed, failed." Former Secretary of State Colin Powell declared in 2001, "It is increasingly clear that few issues are as threatening to global economic prosperity and development, international security, and our common humanity as the threat presented by HIV/AIDS." UN Special Envoy for HIV/AIDS in Africa, Stephen Lewis, also proclaimed in 2001, "We are dealing with a kind of contemporary apocalypse."[1] All of these declarations occurred more than a decade ago, yet the HIV/AIDS epidemic has still not ended. Rhetoric without action did not and will not end the pediatric HIV/AIDS epidemic. In the "war against AIDS," it is as if there have only been multiple skirmishes while the global war to end HIV rages on. Wars are expensive, and HIV is no exception. The expense in human lives seems to have been tolerated because the public somehow became desensitized and forgot about the HIV/AIDS epidemic's devastation of individual lives, families, and communities, especially those in geographically isolated regions of the world.

Since 1985 we have known every means of HIV transmission and how to prevent it. Today we can say the same thing. Although we do not have a vaccine to prevent HIV, many of the known prevention measures are as effective as vaccines for other diseases. While we wait for a vaccine, we must use what we know is effective—prevention of perinatal HIV transmission, condoms, abstinence, reducing the number sexual partners, circumcision, HIV testing of blood products, PEP following rape and accidental inoculation, needle exchange for drug users, contact tracing, and treatment as prevention— these are known effective methods for primary prevention, and they are available now.

Without primary prevention, the current rate of more than 600,000 new HIV infections of women and children each year is likely to continue. The new infections will be added to the thirty-five million existing infections, all of which require lifelong treatment. As HIV becomes a chronic treatable disease, the budgets of even the most advanced developing countries will come under stress, and given the emergence of new infectious disease epidemics such as the Ebola and Zika viruses, along with the proliferation of other chronic noninfectious diseases that require treatment, such as hypertension, diabetes, and cancer, there is the risk of HIV funding diminishing greatly. The requirement for chronic treatment of HIV will eventually bring about drug resistance, triggering the need for even more potent and expensive ARVs and adding new demands on an already inadequate health-care infrastructure in poor countries. To preclude these outcomes, primary HIV prevention is a necessity.

If the pediatric HIV/AIDS epidemic is to come to an end, upstream solutions must become a priority—preventing women from becoming infected in the first place.

DO ASK, DO TELL

It's simple. HIV infected? Let your sexual partner know. In fact, is there anyone who would not want to be informed that he or she is being exposed to a potentially lethal viral infection?

An important means of protecting women and eventually children from HIV infection is the following: Do Ask, Do Tell. "Do Ask" is asking a sexual partner if he or she has been tested for HIV and, if so, asking for the result. Every individual has the right to be protected against a fatal infection. "Do Tell" is telling a sexual partner if you have been tested for HIV and then disclosing the result. All who know that they are HIV infected have an ethical obligation to warn their sexual partners. Do Ask, Do Tell is integral to the success of universal HIV testing, stopping HIV transmission, and ending the HIV/AIDS epidemic.

As with many other aspects of the HIV/AIDS epidemic, it is incongruous that the recommendation for universal HIV testing should have taken so long. Almost all public-health agencies now recommend it but have not also emphasized the equally important need to notify sexual partners of the test results. The ability to test for HIV first became available in 1985 when the HIV blood test was approved. Calls for expanding HIV testing to all individuals at risk for HIV were initially defeated based on arguments that there was no value in letting someone know they were HIV-infected unless treatment was available, and expanding HIV testing would cause testing to become mandatory, leading to increased discrimination against those who were infected. From a public-health point of view, many of the arguments were erroneous—identification of HIV could have resulted in providing HIV-infected individuals with drugs to prevent opportunistic infection and treatment following approval of ZDV. Knowing the HIV status of an individual could also have resulted in education on how to prevent HIV transmission to uninfected sexual partners, sparing them from an unwanted infection.

Just how urgent is Do Ask, Do Tell? The number of individuals who do not know they are infected is likely to be more than 200,000 in the United States and more than nineteen million worldwide (Branson et al. 2006). Imagine the lives that could be saved if all of those people got tested, knew their HIV infection status, and if infected, warned their sexual partners to protect themselves from HIV infection. Imagine, too, how many of those identified as already infected could then benefit from early treatment, transforming a uniformly fatal infection into one that can be controlled.

In an epidemic that has gone on far too long and has been too costly in terms of human suffering and premature loss of life, it is imprudent to believe that we can ignore identifying all those who are HIV infected and those who are unknowingly being exposed to HIV infection and still claim to be able to bring the HIV/AIDS epidemic under control. It is time to insist that the HIV prevention message declare that it is all individuals' responsibility—indeed, their moral duty—to protect themselves and others from HIV infection. Further, in an epidemic that disproportionately infects women and children who are kept from the knowledge that they are being exposed to HIV, it is unconscionable to ask them to continue bearing the burden of undisclosed HIV infections. Do Ask, Do Tell is an essential means to end this tragic injustice and the epidemic itself.

CONTACT TRACING: THE RIGHT TO KNOW

Do Ask, Do Tell addresses an individual's responsibility to prevent the transmission of HIV. Contact tracing addresses the public-health responsibility to control an HIV/AIDS epidemic that is not ending.

No infectious disease epidemic has ever come under control without either a vaccine to prevent infection or contact tracing to control the spread of infection. Smallpox was controlled with vaccination. Ebola was controlled by contact tracing. Used for more than one hundred years to control the spread of infectious diseases such as polio, measles, TB, SARS, and STIs such as syphilis and gonorrhea, contact tracing is an essential public-health tool for ending infectious disease epidemics. In 2016, there is no valid reason to not employ contact tracing as a means of controlling the spread of HIV to millions of individuals each year. Indeed, it is disingenuous for organizations such as WHO, UNAIDS and the USPHS to imply that the HIV/AIDS can be brought under control without contact tracing.

In 2014, the entire world focused on the sweep of the Ebola virus from one country to another as contact tracing was utilized to contain its spread. Thomas R. Frieden, director of the CDC, stated it bluntly: "Three core interventions have stopped every previous Ebola outbreak and can stop this one as well: exhaustive case and contact finding [tracing], effective response to patients and the community, and preventive interventions" (Frieden et al. 2014). Important questions must be asked at this point. Why was contact tracing so readily called for and applied to contain the Ebola epidemic but has not been used for HIV? How can public-health officials call for contact tracing for an epidemic that has killed twelve thousand individuals yet remain silent about contact tracing for an epidemic that has continued for over three decades, infected seventy-eight million people, and killed thirty-nine million men, women, and children? Multiple outbreaks of Ebola have been contained, but HIV has never been contained. The societal issues of contact tracing are the same for both epidemics—confidentiality, stigma, and protecting uninfected individuals from a lethal virus infection.

HIV remains the only STI where contact tracing has not been used to control the spread of infection. In a review of over 150 medical publications, addressing the issue of how to end the HIV/AIDS epidemic, contact tracing was mentioned only twice. Why are public-health officials so vocal about the use of contact tracing for Ebola and many STIs but mute about HIV, one the world's deadliest epidemics?

Early in the HIV/AIDS epidemic there seemed to be good reasons for not implementing contact tracing. Before 1987, there was no treatment for HIV infection, stigma and discrimination against HIV-infected individuals were severe and sometimes violent, and there were no laws to protect individuals against these unacceptable outcomes. There were sobering reasons for adopting a cautious approach to contact tracing and preventing undesired repercussions, but they were not sufficient to prohibit its use. In fact, the failure to perform contact tracing has now resulted in a new form of discrimination, one that is lethal to a much larger number of individuals, because when women and children are denied prevention measures and life-saving treatment, they are denied their fundamental right to health.

An argument frequently invoked against contact tracing states that identifying a woman as HIV infected might result in increased violence against her. This ignores the evidence that intimate partner violence (IPV) and HIV are closely linked, suggesting that HIV is yet another manifestation of violence against women, one that without diagnosis and treatment has a greater likelihood of ending in death than a bruised body or a fractured bone (Dunkle et al. 2004). Rejecting contact tracing because of theoretical negative repercussions is disingenuous and does not protect millions of women from HIV infection or from stigma. The solution to protecting women from theoretical violence associated with HIV disclosure is not to avoid contact tracing but to develop community support systems through education and strengthen local, national, and international laws that protect women from all forms of violence, including HIV infection.

Those who call for an end to the HIV/AIDS epidemic while simultaneously refusing to implement contact tracing are obligated to explain how the HIV/AIDS epidemic can otherwise be stopped when an estimated nineteen million-plus individuals worldwide do not know they are infected, and millions more continue to be exposed to HIV without their knowledge. When UNAIDS states that their 2020 goal for the HIV/AIDS epidemic is, "90 percent of all people living with HIV will know their HIV status, 90 percent of all people with diagnosed HIV infection will receive sustained antiretroviral therapy, and 90 percent of all people receiving antiretroviral therapy will have viral suppression," they must be called on to defend their continued failure since the beginning of the HIV/AIDS epidemic to openly include contact tracing as a means of controlling the spread of HIV and to explain exactly how their goals can be achieved without this important tool. It is unrealistic and misleading to talk about ending the HIV/AIDS epidemic when there are vast pockets of individuals who are HIV infected, untreated, and unaware of how to protect themselves and others from infection. In 2015, after more than thirty years of an uncontrolled HIV/AIDS epidemic, CDC Director Thomas Frieden became the first major public-health official to call for applying fundamental public-health principles, including contact tracing, to the epidemic by urging "systematic partner notification [contact tracing] and follow-up" (Frieden, Foti, and Mermin 2015).

TREAT ALL

All HIV-infected individuals worldwide should be treated with ARVs as soon as a diagnosis is made. This is a scientifically and ethically sound means of dramatically slowing the HIV/AIDS epidemic. If it were to be applied universally in low-income countries for HIV-infected pregnant women, it would, as happened in the United States, virtually eliminate the global HIV/AIDS epidemic in children.

Thirty-five years have passed since the AIDS epidemic was first described. Twenty-eight years have passed since the first drug (ZDV) to treat HIV infection was approved. The continued gap between HIV-infected individuals who are treated and those who are not is striking, with an estimated twenty-one million (59 percent of) HIV-infected individuals still not on any treatment (UNAIDS 2016). This testifies to the fact that, despite the lengthy amount of time that potent ARVs have been available and the vast amount of research proving the effectiveness of ARVs, HIV is the only major infectious disease where treatment was withheld or remained unavailable until infected individuals reached advanced and often irreversible stages of the disease. The delay in recommending that treatment should be initiated immediately following diagnosis is both puzzling and inexplicable. Evidence for treating all HIV-infected individuals with HAART was presented at the 1996 IAS Conference in Vancouver, which was attended by thousands of expert scientists and clinicians. At the meeting, Dr. Julio Montaner, the conference chair, stated: "HAART has since evolved as the standard of care in HIV disease." Montaner also led a campaign on "Treatment as Prevention," a concept that proved to be true and would later revolutionize the approach to preventing new HIV infections (Montaner et al. 1999).

But even before the Vancouver conference, HIV experts such as Doug Richman and Diane Havlir called for treating all HIV-infected individuals, and in 1995 Dr. David Ho from the Aaron Diamond AIDS Research Center in New York published a commentary in the *New England Journal of Medicine*, titled "Time to Hit HIV Early and Hard," that was based on these scientific advances (Richman and Havlir 1995; Ho 1995). Ho, a cautious and brilliant investigator, based his conclusions on carefully designed studies that suggested that HAART could eradicate HIV infection. In the years that followed, incontrovertible evidence was published that early treatment of HIV-infected individuals with HAART resulted in dramatic immediate and long-term health-care benefits.

In spite of mounting evidence that showed the vast benefits of early initiation of HAART, it took several decades before "treat all" became the standard of care recommended by the major HIV/AIDS organizations, a delay that was impossible to justify considering the number of lives lost to HIV infection and the number of new HIV infections that resulted. In 2012, the IAS and the US Public Health Service, together representing more than sixteen thousand scientists and clinicians, health-care workers and advocates, published their recommendations to treat all HIV-infected individuals (Thompson et al. 2012; Ammann 2012). At the 2012 International AIDS Conference in Washington, DC, Global Strategies launched a "Treat All" campaign, calling on a still recalcitrant WHO and the NIH-supported pediatric HIV/AIDS community to update their HIV treatment guidelines to reflect the standard of care that was now being universally recommended.[2]

At last, on May 17, 2015, following the results of the undeniable benefits of immediately treating all HIV-infected individuals with HAART, based on the clinical trial called "Strategic Timing of Antiretroviral Treatment (START)," NIH announced that all people with HIV should be put on ARVs as soon as they learn they are infected (McNeil 2015). WHO followed suit (Cohen 2015). IMPAACT/PROMISE pediatric researchers had no option but to follow the recommendations. Appallingly, the delays in initiating HAART were costly in the number of lives that were lost to HIV and the number of new HIV infections that could have been prevented. The HIV/AIDS research studies and WHO recommendations to withhold treatment are likely to have resulted in a conservative estimate of more than seven million unnecessary HIV-related deaths of men, women and children over the twenty years that lifesaving HAART was denied to them (Ammann 2015b, 2016).

PROTECT WOMEN FROM SEXUAL VIOLENCE AND HIV INFECTION

HIV infection of women is a downstream manifestation of a long series of interrelated factors, including gender inequality, disregard for the dignity of women, denial of equal rights to health, educational and economic disparities, and sexual violence perpetrated with impunity. In this milieu, HIV is like an opportunistic infection waiting to take advantage of circumstances that provide a haven for its persistence and continuation. HIV exploits the weaknesses of social, cultural, political, and religious views about women that create a vulnerable population unable to protect themselves from HIV infection, while also fostering barriers to prevention and treatment. While many solutions for ending the pediatric AIDS epidemic can be implemented immediately, solutions to ending violence against women are more difficult to achieve.[3]

Gender-based violence (GBV) and HIV are synergistic on their impact on women. GBV refers to violence that establishes, maintains, or attempts to foster unequal power relationships based on gender. IPV, also relevant to HIV infection of women, refers to physical, sexual, or psychological harm, including rape, that occurs in an intimate relationship. (More detailed definitions of violence against women are provided by WHO and are included in the endnotes.)[4]

When the HIV/AIDS epidemic was first described in 1981, 95 percent of individuals with AIDS were male. In 1998, WHO reported that for the first time the HIV/AIDS epidemic had shifted from a majority of men to a majority of women. Currently, women account for over 58 percent of the epidemic in sub-Saharan Africa, and young women aged fifteen to twenty-four are twice as likely as males to be living with HIV. According to WHO, HIV is the leading cause of death in women between the ages of fifteen and forty-four worldwide.

The increased seroprevalence of HIV infection in women has several explanations. For each sexual act, the likelihood of an uninfected woman becoming infected from an infected man is eight times more than that of an uninfected man becoming infected from an infected woman. This is probably the result of HIV's exposure to the large surface area of the vagina and the presence of other STIs. Young girls are particularly susceptible to HIV, as their vaginal epithelium is thinner than older women's. Other factors include cultural and religious practices of early marriage, wife inheritance, sexual cleansing, sexual intercourse with older HIV-infected men seeking "safer sex" with virgins and younger girls, and sexual intercourse with men who have multiple sexual partners.

Studies by Kristin Dunkle, Rachel Jewkes, and their cohorts reported extensively on IPV and concluded that men who are physically violent to their partner are significantly more likely to have HIV and that women who experience sexual violence are more likely to be HIV infected (Dunkle et al. 2004; Jewkes et al. 2010). Other studies conclude that women who report IPV are 1.5 to three times more likely to be HIV-infected (Townsend et al. 2011). These observations raise important public-health and ethical issues about how HIV infection of women is viewed. Basically, HIV infection of women can be interpreted as yet another manifestation of gender-based violence, albeit one that invariably results in death without treatment. GBV against women and the HIV epidemic can be considered as two parallel epidemics that together contribute to the ongoing HIV/AIDS epidemic in women and, because the majority of women who are infected are of child-bearing age, to the ongoing epidemic of HIV infection in infants and children.[5]

Proposed interventions to end GBV in low-income countries must take into account differences in cultural norms and the lack of infrastructure and resources to support approaches that require sustainable legal protection. It is not surprising that interventions encouraging the prosecution of rapists may increase stigma and violence because they require identification of the person who has suffered GBV. Exporting solutions that have worked in developed countries that are supported by a network of advanced legal and social mechanisms may not only fail to be effective in low-income countries, but it may also have unanticipated negative repercussions. In her book *The Invisible Cure: Africa, the West, and the Fight against AIDS*, Helen Epstein suggests that the denial, silence, shame, adverse gender roles, and stigma about HIV may have been amplified by Western-initiated donor funding (2007). The insistence on extreme confidentiality in the absence of family and community support and without access to health care resulted in denial of health care to the most vulnerable populations, primarily women and children with no legal or social recourse. HIV was given a sanctuary of silence by "outsiders" when it was responsible for the death and destruction of individuals, families, and communities.

Surprisingly, the implementation by international organizations of programs to prevent and treat HIV infection do not always take into account the impact on gender inequality. The rapid and strong worldwide promotion of condoms and MC contrasts with the much slower and weaker promotion of effective interventions that could greatly benefit females, such as "test and treat," "treat all HIV-infected individuals," "test and tell," and contact tracing (Wagner and Blower 2012; Wong et al. 2009). The latter interventions bypass many of the roadblocks to equalizing health-care access by utilizing routine annual HIV testing and immediate treatment if a person is found to be infected. Such approaches to HIV prevention and treatment are now known to reduce the number of new HIV infections, reduce the progression of HIV to AIDS, dramatically increase the number of individuals tested for HIV, and at the same time reduce the stigma associated with HIV infection.

Advocacy groups, international organizations, and research studies have identified ending impunity as one of the most important factors for stopping violence against women—whether intimate partner violence, non-partner violence, or violence during conflict. Enactment and strengthening of national and international laws and legislation coupled with strong enforcement could have the most immediate impact. Legislative approaches to reducing GBV are in place in over 120 countries but are plagued by lack of enforcement and a failure to address many of the social, religious, and cultural norms that contribute to gender inequality. Although the solutions to ending GBV are complex, difficult to implement, and perhaps even in some instances unknown, this is no excuse for truncated or delayed responses. Sufficient information from discussions, international conferences, and meetings has been compiled, printed, and distributed, fully describing the extent of GBV and its association with HIV. Now is the time to act on the information. Long-term solutions to ending the synergy of GBV and HIV infection must have as their foundation not only an end to gender inequality but also the understanding that the right to health and human rights are integrally linked.

STOP THE SPIN: A SUSTAINABLE RESPONSE TO THE EPIDEMIC THROUGH TRUTH TELLING

In a global epidemic of HIV's magnitude, we should not tolerate even a hint of "spin" on the facts, nor should we tolerate compromised truth telling—not by scientists, not by researchers, not by activists, not by international health organizations, and not by politicians. When misguided researchers say they have a cure for HIV when they don't, or organizations responsible for controlling the HIV/AIDS epidemic ask for yet another $10 billion but fail to acknowledge that they have repeatedly been unsuccessful in controlling the spread of HIV, they are spinning the truth. The HIV/AIDS epidemic has ravaged humanity for over three decades, and the destruction it has left in its wake makes it clear that we must continue to take HIV seriously. While the progress in HIV discovery and implementation has been extraordinary as a result of basic and clinical research and the application of ways to prevent and treat HIV infection, the advances have failed to reach many regions of the world. Public confidence in health and medicine has always been an essential component of acquiring the economic and political support needed to bring an epidemic under control, including HIV. The truth about the HIV/AIDS epidemic must be told, even if the news is bad or if specific goals have not been achieved. Only then can real solutions be devised.

When the AIDS epidemic was first recognized in 1981, the communication between scientists, clinicians, public-health officials, and the media was intense, but it was also characterized by responsible documentation of facts and careful attention to neither overstating nor understating the epidemic's seriousness. Checking and double checking numbers, verifying information, and accurately reporting new discoveries was considered part of responsibly handling an epidemic that would soon evolve into one of enormous historical proportions. Media and science reporters such as Randy Shilts, Larry Altman, Laurie Garrett, and Jon Cohen became well known for their integrity and accuracy in chronicling the HIV/AIDS epidemic, including both the successes and failures.

One example of spin was committed by WHO, which sought to convey the impression that their efforts were successful in treating the majority of HIV-infected individuals who needed treatment. The truth was that WHO ignored the treatment recommendations of the most recognized scientific experts to initiate early HAART in all HIV-infected individuals, and in 2002 they redefined those who needed treatment as only the sickest individuals, denying treatment to millions of HIV-infected individuals who were merely observed as they progressed to advanced stages of disease and death. It was an unprecedented maneuver that allowed WHO to publically claim that they were treating the majority of those who "needed" treatment. It also dismissed more than a half century of infectious-disease principles, which should have evoked outcries from physicians and activists involved in infectious-disease treatment. WHO hinted that their recommendations were because ARVs were too costly, but even when costs dropped from $5,000 per year, per patient to less than $120 per year, per patient, they failed to quickly change their guidelines to include treating more HIV-infected individuals. The medical journal *Lancet* refused to participate in this deceptive spin and uncompromisingly commented on WHO's failure to achieve its goals, writing, "2005 is likely to be remembered more for the three million deaths and almost five million new infections [than for its success]" ("Maintaining Anti-AIDS Commitment" 2005).

There also were attempts to spin the response to the HIV/AIDS epidemic as a public health victory. Shortly after reading the sobering 2012 statistics on the global HIV/AIDS epidemic, which indicated that there were still more than two million new HIV infections each year (including more than 50 percent women and children), I was stunned when I picked up the June 6, 2013, issue of the *NEJM* and saw an article titled "Response to the AIDS Pandemic—A Global Health Model," written by Peter Piot and Thomas Quinn. As I read their article, the statistics of the current HIV/AIDS epidemic kept intruding—thirty-four million people living with HIV, still only 30 percent of those needing treatment receiving it, and still almost three hundred thousand new infections in children each year. Was it not audacious, after more than thirty years of a continuous epidemic, to refer to the response to the HIV/AIDS epidemic as a public-health "model"? It seemed disingenuous as well as dishonorable to talk of success in light of the millions of individuals who had contracted HIV infection and died.

Alan Brandt, PhD, from the Department of History of Science at Harvard University, attempted to put the brakes on the spin that presented the global HIV/AIDS epidemic as a model of success. In the same June 6, 2013, issue of the *NEJM*, he stated, "Many historians would consider it premature to write the history of the HIV/AIDS epidemic. After all, more than thirty-four million people are currently infected with HIV. Even today, with long-standing public health campaigns and highly active antiretroviral therapy (HAART), HIV remains a major contributor to the burden of disease in many countries." I agreed and would add that we should all be cautious in the premature declaration of victory or in claiming that our approach has been a model of success when we are still dealing with millions of new HIV infections each year—numbers that were unimaginable in 1981 when AIDS was first discovered.

A stark reminder that we are in the middle, not at the end, of the HIV/AIDS epidemic comes from Southern Africa, where some refer to the HIV/AIDS epidemic as a hyper epidemic. The overall prevalence of HIV in adults in Swaziland is 31 percent, in Botswana 25 percent, and in South Africa 17 percent. In Swaziland, 54 percent of women between the ages of thirty and thirty-four are infected with HIV, and in KwaZulu Natal Province in South Africa, 40 percent of pregnant women are HIV-infected in this decade ("HIV and AIDS in sub-Saharan Africa" 2013).

It must be acknowledged that there was real progress in identifying the cause of AIDS and devising prevention and treatment strategies that initially slowed the HIV/AIDS epidemic. However, the failure to fully control the global HIV/AIDS epidemic was not in medical or scientific discovery, which occurred rapidly and was rich with solutions to end the epidemic. The failure was putting the discoveries into place rapidly and efficiently enough to end the HIV/AIDS epidemic. Distorting failures by spinning them as successes neither honors the millions who suffer the consequences of HIV infection nor accelerates the ability to conquer this epidemic that has gone on far too long. The truth must be told. The deficiencies of the model(s) must be ascertained and acknowledged, and every known means to overcome them must be implemented.

BRING BACK THE ACTIVISM

Activism during the AIDS epidemic brought about dramatic changes in how research priorities were decided, how research was performed, when results were implemented, and how government agencies conducted their business of protecting individuals from discrimination while insuring that they had full access to lifesaving treatments. Today, ending the pediatric HIV/AIDS epidemic quickly requires renewed activism that defends vulnerable women and children in low-income countries. US activism was carried forward by those most affected—HIV-infected individuals from the gay community. Internationally, the much-needed activism for ending the pediatric HIV/AIDS epidemic must include women who are HIV-infected as well as women who experience physical and sexual violence. They know best the need to defend their right to protection from violence and the need for a universal standard of care that provides them and their infants with all of the prevention and treatment methods available. HIV-infected women must "sit at the table," not in the audience, with the decision makers. Because the majority of HIV-infected women now reside in low-income countries where the rights of women are severely compromised, it is not an easy task to develop a community of women, organized, directed, and controlled by women, who can call into accountability international, national, and community establishments to protect their rights and those of their children. Essential for achieving equity is an activist community to overcome paternalistic attitudes that demean women's value and deny them an equal voice in health-care decisions.

Activism is an essential ingredient for change. Without it, large international organizations, governments, and ministries of health are likely to ignore the needs of ordinary individuals and minority populations or even exploit them for personal gain. Organizations may listen momentarily only to relapse into indifference when initial confrontations cease. It is what happens after the meeting is over that counts. Politicians and bureaucrats listen to the powerful, favor the status quo or move imperceptibly toward responding to pressing health-care needs. Activism unsettles complacency. Dr. Martin Luther King Jr. recognized the hazard of silence when he said, "The greatest tragedy of this generation which history will record is not the vitriolic words of those who hate, or the aggressive acts of others, but the appalling silence of the good people." He recognized, too, in a speech to the Medical Committee for Human Rights in 1966, that this applied to health care: "Of all the forms of inequality, injustice in health care is the most shocking and inhumane" (King 2004).

Both activism and advocacy are essential for achieving change. Advocacy seeks to accomplish change through established mechanisms and the use of consensus. Advocacy, in most instances, is "polite and patient." It also takes time that individuals dying from a fatal disease do not have. In contrast, activism evolves from frustration when established mechanisms for invoking change, including advocacy, are ineffective for developing solutions for specific issues. Activism refuses to accept the status quo and may use aggressive methods such as demonstrations, disruptions, and confrontation to accomplish goals. The early decades of the HIV/AIDS epidemic illustrated how activism altered the course of an epidemic. HIV activists (primarily in the United States) helped to overcome many of the obstacles facing HIV, ranging from accelerating the discovery of the cause of AIDS to increasing funding for research, treatment, and prevention. Activists in the United States irrevocably altered the drug approval process by insisting on accelerated drug approval and early access to drugs. They helped to implement laws to protect HIV-infected individuals from stigma and discrimination, devised legislation to provide medical and social support for HIV-infected individuals, and demonstrated to the public in general that those with a specific disease could influence research and treatment priorities and accelerate access to experimental drugs.

Not everyone agreed with the tactics used by the HIV activist community, but few will deny their effectiveness in revolutionizing the interaction between the research and academic communities, drug development by pharmaceutical companies, and government involvement in funding research and delivering health care. The activist community was composed primarily of young gay men, many of whom were HIV-infected, who had the political and economic power to demand that they be heard. They accomplished many of their goals by inserting themselves into every component of the HIV/AIDS epidemic to influence the outcome of HIV prevention and treatment, as well as to change how the public, government organizations, industry, and the US Congress viewed the issues surrounding the HIV/AIDS epidemic. Importantly, many of their own lives were at stake.

Prominent among the early activist organizations were ACT UP (AIDS Coalition to Unleash Power), TAG (Treatment Action Group), GMHC (Gay Men's Health Crisis), Project Inform, and TAC (Treatment Action Campaign, South Africa). All greatly influenced the course of the HIV/AIDS epidemic, and without them, millions more people would have become infected or succumbed to HIV infection without treatment. Within the organizations were individuals who dedicated their lives to achieving lasting change. Conspicuous among them were Mark Harington, Peter Staley, Martin Delaney, Gregg Gonsalves, Elizabeth Glaser, Brenda Lien, Terry McGovern, and Larry Kramer. There were others who used their celebrity status to influence the course of the HIV/AIDS epidemic, persuading the US Congress, wealthy donors, and corporations to support efforts to control the HIV/AIDS epidemic. They were celebrities who were recognized worldwide—Magic Johnson, Bono, Elton John, Greg Louganis, Elizabeth Taylor, and Sharon Stone. Others became celebrities because their HIV-infection status was presented before the media and the government, turning their tragedy into activism for children. Among them were Ariel Glaser, Nkosi Johnson, and Ryan White.

Activism is essential to ending the pediatric HIV/AIDS epidemic. Greg Gonsalves was one of the few US activists who continued to confront the HIV/AIDS epidemic internationally in women and children. His words from a 2011 interview still ring true: "My greatest fear is that we've made all of these successes—ten years ago we started this new phase where it seemed finally the whole world is backing the effort to eradicate HIV. All of a sudden the political will has evaporated. We need a new infiltration of religious leaders, activists, and doctors . . . to say, 'No, you can't write us off.'"[6]

A renewed activism composed of strong and truly representative groups of HIV-infected women and their supporters, thoroughly schooled in their legal and ethical rights to standard of care and equitable prevention and treatment measures, is a necessary prerequisite for quickly ending the pediatric HIV/AIDS epidemic.

INTEGRATION OF HEALTH-CARE ACCESS AND DELIVERY

Health-care access and delivery in low-income countries, most of which lack adequate infrastructure, must be integrated into primary health care to ensure progress and provide maximum benefit and sustainability. Integration of health care may be defined in different ways, but in general it is understood to mean the sharing of resources and infrastructure, including health-care services; clinic space; health education; pharmacy, laboratory, and diagnostic services; and training of health-care workers. In the broadest sense, it also shares logistical support, such as maintenance of patient records and databases. For the patient, it may mean "one-stop shopping" (Coetzee et al. 2004; Pfeiffer et al. 2010; Tudor Car et al. 2011). This is in contrast to the disease-focused approach to delivering health care, which came to characterize the HIV/AIDS epidemic, largely imposed by income-rich funders driven to a greater degree by research than by the goal of ending the epidemic through integrated health-care delivery. The delay in integrating HIV/AIDS care into primary care is surprising, given the many advantages that integration offers to low- and middle-income countries by providing individuals with both traditional and holistic approaches to health care.

There were many reasons why HIV prevention and treatment was not integrated into primary care. One was that it was more convenient for wealthy funders to impose a highly sub- specialized approach to HIV health care. During the first fifteen years of the epidemic, most of the basic research and clinical advances came from wealthy countries, especially the United States. The drugs that were used to treat HIV infection were new and complex and, in a somewhat paternalistic attitude, were felt to require advanced education and complicated and expensive laboratory tests before they could be used. There were also many research questions specific to the HIV/AIDS epidemic in low-income countries that involved both new drugs and laboratory tests. Research often required separate patient records and health-care workers dedicated exclusively to HIV care. However, the clinical research that dominated studies in low-income countries was not necessarily directed toward how to best implement lifesaving treatment and prevention discoveries, but rather toward questions that were of greater interest to the scientific community. In many instances, the research would bring prestige and increased funding that was of greater benefit to the researchers and their institutions than to the research subjects in income-poor countries.

As funding from international organizations increased, even more individuals from income-rich countries were employed to establish and oversee programs and to work side-by-side with indigenous health-care workers. These individuals began to dominate the decision-making process, seeking to replicate what had been successful in the United States. In Abigail Zuger's review of Helen Epstein's book *The Invisible Cure*, she summarizes Epstein's views of the response to the African HIV/AIDS epidemic as "painting an unforgettable nuanced portrait of Western efforts in Africa: well-meaning, vitally necessary, and yet often so misguided. Well-financed Western research projects seduce health-care workers from other important work. Western bureaucracy lurches and stalls. And Western money sometimes bypasses the people who need it most, nourishing consultants and middlemen rather than patients."[7]

From the onset of introducing HIV prevention and treatment programs in low-income countries, local health-care professionals, with decades of experience dealing with other diseases (including those common to HIV-infected individuals), were bypassed and told that HIV health-care delivery must exist with its own separate group of experts, separate health-care facilities, and separately trained health-care personnel, a process that diverted much-needed health-care workers from caring for patients with other diseases.

Fortunately, there is increasing recognition that integration of health-care services is not only desirable but necessary if the HIV/AIDS epidemic is to be brought under control. There are too many missed opportunities to provide education on HIV prevention and to diagnose HIV infection when HIV is viewed as the "property" of a few highly sub-specialized individuals. Many of the studies documenting the improved outcome of integrating health care come from regions where the HIV seroprevalence is the highest. For example, studies from South Africa and Zambia document the benefits of integrating ART for HIV-infected mothers into antenatal care rather than relying on separate stand-alone programs for prevention of perinatal HIV transmission (Pfeifer et al. 2010; Herlihy et al. 2015). Integration of HIV services into antenatal care provides an opportunity to address other health issues that coexist in pregnant women, such as malaria, immunizations for mothers and infants, control of STIs, family planning, and early detection of diabetes and hypertension. Integration of health-care services for HIV and TB, which often coexist in the same individuals, reduce duplication of services and underutilization of staff and increase the survival of HIV-infected patients as a result of improved access to care (Kerschberger et al. 2012; Louwagie et al. 2012; Medley et al. 2015).

Integration of HIV into primary health care is a necessity, given the issues of sustainability that exist in low-income countries. As the HIV/AIDS epidemic continues, and as the impact of treatment with HAART prolongs lives, the number of people living with HIV will increase. HIV-infected individuals are living longer and are developing chronic diseases associated with aging such as diabetes, hypertension, and cardiovascular disease. Low-income countries cannot afford to have separate health-care delivery programs for each of these diseases but must, if the health of their citizens is to improve, look to integration as a means of addressing the future expanding needs of primary health care.

USE CREDIBLE ECONOMIC ANALYSES: VALUE-BASED HEALTH CARE

An inappropriate or misguided economic analysis of health-care costs can profoundly influence the selection of health-care priorities and the amount of funding directed to each priority. It may result in an excess of funds being directed to a disease that has a minimal impact on public health or benefit a limited number of individuals, or it may result in underfunding a disease that has significant long-term consequences for a large number of people. In the United States, for example, there has been a recent emphasis on the potential of stem-cell transplantation for diabetes, a costly approach to treatment, while tens of thousands of poor people are increasingly unable to access insulin, a less expensive standard treatment used since the 1920s. When international organizations and research groups used costs to justify delaying HIV treatment or using inferior treatments, it was based on a single factor—the short-term cost of drugs to treat infection. Instead of factoring in the broad benefits of treatment, such as decreased hospitalizations, fewer opportunistic infections, and prolonged life expectancy, which could reduce the number of AIDS orphans (a far more costly outgrowth of the HIV/AIDS epidemic), treatment was delayed while ministries of health watched the devastation expand and researchers performed studies on less costly but also less effective treatments.

Economic analyses are necessary. Health-care interventions require data analyses to determine their efficacy. But increasingly, as a result of rising health-care costs, they also demand economic analyses. There are a number of different economic analyses used— cost-effectiveness analysis, cost-benefit analysis, and cost-utility analysis. As the cost of health care increases worldwide and collides with limited financial and infrastructure resources, the economic analysis for health-care delivery has included what is termed "value-based health care" (VBHC). While not perfect, VBHC focuses not only on cost but also on health-care quality and both short-term and long-term health outcomes. The term is increasingly used to argue for universal health-care coverage, not as a cost, but as an investment in the future health of individuals as well as in the health of a community and/or country. It emphasizes that short-term, less expensive health care does not always deliver the best quality care for an individual or a population and almost certainly is not in the best interest of reducing long-term costs.

Providing HIV prevention and treatment for HIV-infected pregnant women to prevent an estimated 300,000 newly infected infants each year and ARVs to treat an estimated one million HIV-infected children is not an overwhelming economic cost in the context of other global health issues. But in the absence of effective advocacy and activism, many economic analyses have gone unchallenged and, in some instances, have delayed or displaced issues of high priority for delivering standard of care to vulnerable populations.

A fundamental problem in most economic analyses is that economists are not qualified to make the types of value judgments that are an integral part of the decision-making process unique to patients and their physicians, yet their analyses are highly influential in making government and institutional decisions. Economic analyses can identify cost and obstacles to implementation, but they are not very good at making value judgments, in spite of increasing demands for "value-based health care." Many ethical issues are embedded in the debate about what economic analyses' objectives should be. To begin with, there is the issue of whether health-care systems' objectives are related to efficiency (maximizing interventions subject to resource constraints) or related to equity (being fair or impartial). These are not merely theoretical debates— they have a significant impact on who receives treatment and what kind of treatment they might receive.

The marked contrast between the United States and low-income countries as to who gets treated and when they get treated has much to do with activism and advocacy, but an important factor in the equation is who is regarded as having the authority to make health-care decisions based on economics and what analysis should be used. During the HIV/AIDS epidemic in low-income countries, the decision-making process was wrested from health-care professionals and, in the absence of forceful activism, was placed in the hands of large international organizations such as WHO and UNAIDS and national ministries of health with myopic views of long-term health-care benefits. The result is what is sometimes referred to as "territorial equity," in which allocation of health-care resources among countries and even regions within a country is determined by health-care authorities who fail to take into account differing clinical needs that determine short- and long-term benefits to HIV-infected individuals.

It is not surprising that women and children suffered the greatest discrepancies in accessing life-saving ARVs. They lacked strong advocates in the international community, and their very vulnerability, created by poverty and lack of political influence, prevented them from intervening in the decisions that affected their destiny. Inadvertently, some economic analyses even exacerbated the discrepancies by focusing on technological interventions that could be implemented in urban areas but were either unaffordable, unavailable, or of little benefit to delivering health care in impoverished areas. They calculated unnecessary costs and, much worse, concluded that interventions to prevent perinatal HIV transmission should not be performed until certain high-cost technologies were in place.

Inappropriate application of economic analyses can have disastrous consequences, as exemplified by the HIV/AIDS epidemic. WHO employed shortsighted and outmoded approaches to define economic costs of health-care delivery in developing their 2002 HIV treatment guidelines. While it is difficult to ascertain precisely what economic variables WHO used to conclude that denying treatment until HIV had advanced to the most severe forms of the disease was of greater benefit than immediate treatment, there is published evidence that WHO/UNAIDS utilized truncated economic analyses, and in some instances dismissed alternative conclusions, rather than employing data generated from value-based health-care analyses supported by scientific data.

Short-term and truncated economic analyses kept HIV prevention and treatment from millions of women and children and in the long run contributed to perpetuation of the HIV/AIDS epidemic and, paradoxically, to escalating treatment costs. Economic analyses cannot, and should not, replace the gatekeeper role of the health-care professional in protecting the patient from inequitable health-care availability. Primary prevention and providing HAART for all HIV-infected women and children should not be considered a cost but an investment and a desirable and necessary goal for achieving an end to the pediatric HIV/AIDS epidemic. The dignity of those affected by HIV must be acknowledged, and their needs must be determined by a partnership between patients and the health-care professionals who care for them.

CONDUCT AN INDEPENDENT REVIEW OF ETHICAL STANDARDS FOR CLINICAL RESEARCH AND TREATMENT IN LOW-INCOME COUNTRIES

It is almost unthinkable. Could some of the well-conducted and well-meaning clinical research studies directed at ending the pediatric HIV/AIDS epidemic have actually delayed achieving the goal? How will historians of medicine and science view the research conducted in low-income countries and WHO's recommendations to withhold treatment from the majority of HIV-infected individuals, which led to the death of millions?

Inevitably, comparisons will be made with two infamous research studies, conducted decades ago, that also withheld treatment from research subjects. The names of Tuskegee and Guatemala are etched in the archives of medical history as unethical US-approved and funded research studies. The Tuskegee study, conducted between 1932 and 1972, withheld penicillin treatment for syphilis from African American men and their sexual partners while the course of untreated infection was observed. The Guatemala study, conducted between 1946 and 1948, experimented on prisoners, prostitutes, soldiers, children, and mentally ill individuals, who were deliberately infected with syphilis and gonorrhea but whose adequate treatment was not documented in 75 percent of the research subjects. Both studies resulted in strengthening ethical guidelines for clinical research with the anticipation that similar studies would never be performed in the future (Katz et al 2008; Semeniuk and Reverby 2010; Reverby 2011; Mays 2012). It remains an enigma why clinical research studies conducted during the HIV epidemic that exploited the vulnerability of an exponentially larger number of women and children in income-poor countries has not been met with outrage.

There are haunting parallels between Tuskegee, Guatemala, and several of the US-sponsored research studies to prevent and treat HIV. In addition, the WHO guidelines to withhold treatment from the majority of HIV-infected individuals was without medical precedent and resulted in millions of infected individuals going untreated. The Tuskegee, Guatemala, and more recently proposed studies on HIV prevention that once again will use placebos and inferior treatment to conduct research of no significant benefit to the research subjects were all approved as ethical within academic institutions (*ClinicalTrials.gov* 2016a).

The Tuskegee and Guatemala research studies were considered necessary, even though they withheld treatment that had been proven to be exceedingly effective for treating syphilis and gonorrhea. The Guatemala studies, and many of the HIV/AIDS studies, could not have been conducted in the United States, either because there were inadequate numbers of research subjects or because it would not have been considered ethical to withhold known effective treatment in the United States. All of the studies involved sexual transmission of infection, yet none of them required identification, testing, or treatment of sexual partners or infants born to them. In most instances, sexual partners were unaware that they were being repeatedly exposed to a preventable and treatable infection. The informed consents used for the studies were in some instances absent and in others inadequate or misleading. The research subjects were often placed at high risk for infection but received little to no benefit for their participation, suggesting the research subjects' exploitation because of economic, social, gender, age, political, racial, or legal inequities. The Tuskegee and Guatemala studies' design seems destined to be repeated in a new NIH-funded study of HIV with much larger numbers of vulnerable African women placed at risk for infection (*ClinicalTrials.gov* 2016a).

Most disturbing is the inability of advocates to halt research studies that exploit vulnerable populations. In April 2016, the NIH embarked on a clinical research study (VRC01) reverting to the use of placebo and comparing it to an experimental monoclonal antibody of no known benefit (in essence, a double placebo study) in individuals at high risk of acquiring HIV infection. The study will enroll more than four thousand research subjects: 2,700 men who have sex with men (MSM) and 1,500 vulnerable women in sub-Saharan Africa who are HIV uninfected but will have sexual intercourse with HIV-infected partners. The men in North and South America, but not the women in Africa, will be provided with free ARV PrEP during the study. The study also includes the administration of the monoclonal antibody to infants born to high-risk HIV-infected mothers without assurance that the infants will receive standard of care ARVs to prevent their infection. Mothers will be asked to sign a fourteen-page informed consent while they are in labor, with those who are illiterate placing an X on the consent page acknowledging that they understood they will not benefit from their research participation (NIAID 2016).

It seems that the lessons of Tuskegee and Guatemala were quickly forgotten, as this US government-sponsored study will place the lives of thousands of individuals at risk for acquiring an STI, without the assurance that they will receive known effective standard of care. The VCR01 study is likely to be the single largest and most expensive phase 2 clinical research study in both dollars and lives to evaluate a research product of no documented benefit for HIV prevention. No pharmaceutical company would consider it. Importantly, it is an example of how both the complexity of science and the global ethics of research, in an atmosphere of billions of dollars of publically funded research, have systemically overtaken the ability of university ethical review committees, the NIH, and the FDA to understand the intricacy of rapidly expanding science and universally accepted ethical principles of protecting vulnerable subjects from exploitation.

A major difference in the Tuskegee, Guatemala, and HIV studies was the number of individuals who were placed at risk for disease progression and death. The Tuskegee study followed 439 untreated African American men, the Guatemala study involved over 1,300 research subjects, but the HIV/AIDS research studies and WHO recommendations to withhold treatment are likely to have resulted in an unimaginable over thirty million unnecessary HIV-related deaths and fifty million unnecessary new HIV infections in men, women, and children over the last two decades of the HIV/AIDS epidemic.[8]

WHO guidelines were first fully published in 2002, and subsequent revisions inexplicably excluded the majority of HIV-infected individuals from treatment, even though treatment with ARVs had been shown to reverse the course of HIV infection, prevent the complications of HIV, and prevent HIV transmission. Their defense was that there was insufficient evidence to treat all HIV-infected individuals. However, one could argue that it was WHO that lacked evidence to support its recommendation that withholding treatment had any benefit for HIV-infected individuals or for the long-term outcome of the epidemic itself. For the first time in medical history, a major public-health agency recommended withholding known effective treatment from a progressively fatal infection, even as the HIV/AIDS epidemic was expanding worldwide at the rate of millions of new infections and deaths each year. A surge in multiple-drug resistant TB accompanied untreated HIV infection, and the complications of HIV advancing to AIDS resulted in increased clinic visits and hospitalizations, as well as expensive drugs to treat opportunistic infections. The long-term cost of caring for the increased number of untreated individuals who advanced to AIDS and the increased number of AIDS-related orphans would far exceed the cost of early treatment with HAART and would in the long term jeopardize the ability to control the global HIV epidemic.

The pediatric HIV/AIDS community also claimed that there was insufficient evidence to treat all HIV-infected pregnant women and infants with HAART in low-income countries, in spite of unambiguous evidence to the contrary. They also insisted that separate studies of ARVs in HIV-infected pregnant women and their infants were necessary, in spite of being informed by the FDA that separate efficacy studies were in fact unnecessary. The consequence of their decision was dire. Had HAART been initiated for the prevention of perinatal HIV infection worldwide when first recommended by HIV/AIDS experts in 1996 and again in 1998, it is likely that there could have been an estimated eight million fewer HIV-infected infants over the last twenty years.

In order to defend their positions, WHO and the pediatric HIV/AIDS research community employed a diluted definition of standard of care that allowed them to utilize only what was available in the poorest country, not the best-known standard of care utilized in the United States and Europe. With the concurrence of US academic IRBs, the universally accepted WMA definition of standard of care was altered to accommodate research in low-income countries that could not be conducted in wealthy countries (WMA 2013).

There have also been calls for the dissolution of the ethical imperatives to require informed consent for some research studies (Faden, Beauchamp, and Kass 2014). Informed consent is one of the central tenets for protecting individuals from unlawful and unethical research abuses. The requirement for informed consent was one of the most important outcomes of investigations into the US-sponsored Tuskegee and Guatemala studies. When properly administered, informed consent allows research subjects to determine whether they are receiving the best standard of care, the risk they may incur, and the benefits they may receive.

A 2015 consensus statement from the International AIDS Conference in Vancouver, British Columbia, made it clear that for the prevention and treatment of HIV, only a universal standard of care is acceptable. The consensus stated:

> Rather than waiting for immune deterioration [as WHO had recommended and as many US government-sponsored research studies had done], immediate antiretroviral (ARV) treatment more than doubles an individual's prospects of staying healthy and surviving. Offering immediate ARV access is further supported by studies showing antiretrovirals can prevent transmission from people living with HIV to their negative partners. And data shows ARVs can effectively protect people at risk of infection through prophylactic use. Medical evidence is clear: All people living with HIV must have access to antiretroviral treatment upon diagnosis. Barriers to access in law, policy, and bias must be confronted and dismantled. (Beyrer et al. 2015)

The Vancouver Consensus established a universal standard of care, but new questions were put in place: "Science has delivered solutions. The question for the world is: When will we put it into practice?" I would add, "Who will now provide the resources to put the recommendations into practice?" After almost two decades of delaying life-saving treatment and training health-care workers to make the difficult decisions on who should be excluded from treatment, who will now retrain them to treat all HIV individuals and provide the resources to do it? Will WHO and the US government accept the responsibility as theirs?

The history of the pediatric HIV/AIDS epidemic has taught us that clinical research is essential for solving the great public-health issues of our time. But it has also taught us that we must guard against abuses related to the scientific and ethical conduct of research, especially when it involves increasing numbers of vulnerable individuals in low-income countries. The continued proliferation of new treatments as the result of research will require identifying large numbers of untreated individuals for studies to prove efficacy, further increasing the risk of exploitation of vulnerable populations, especially women and children (Ammann 2014a). Past ethical abuses, the potential for future abuses, and the continued denial by some clinical researchers and their institutions that unethical research has been and will continue to be conducted demand an examination of the ethical and scientific proficiency of academic IRBs and a thorough review of existing ethical standards by experts and advocates who lack conflicts of interest and with the full participation of those most at risk of exploitation.

CONCLUSION

This chronicle is drawing to an end, and this seems to be the
moment for Dr. Bernard Rieux to confess that he is the narrator.
But before describing the closing scenes, he would wish anyhow
to justify his undertaking . . . His profession put him in touch with a
great many of our townspeople while the plague was raging, and he
had opportunities of hearing the various opinions. Thus he was well
placed for giving a true account of all he saw and heard. But in doing
so he has tried to keep within the limits that seem desirable . . . All
the same time, following the dictates of his heart, he has deliberately
taken the victim's side and tried to share with his fellow citizens the
only certitudes they had in common—love, exile, and suffering. Thus
he can truly say there was not one of their anxieties in which he did
not share, no predicament of theirs that was not his.

Albert Camus, *The Plague*

The story told in this book is one of hope and caution. Never before in the history
of modern medicine have such extraordinary advances been made so quickly in the
prevention and treatment of an infectious disease as they have been in the HIV/AIDS
epidemic. The epidemic taught us that remarkable progress can be made when those
affected by a disease engage, support, and challenge scientists, health-care professionals,
community workers, government agencies, and international health organizations. But
the story told here also highlights the tragic consequences of hubris and a lack of public
accountability in global-health policy making and research.

I have taken great pains throughout the book to accurately document the repeated
decisions by government bureaucracies, policy makers, and clinical researchers to create
clinical guidelines and policies that incorrectly recommended withholding lifesaving
treatment to HIV-infected individuals until severe disease progression and even death.
Their decisions were justified by claims of insufficient scientific evidence for early treatment. Their flawed arguments had lethal consequences that were borne by disadvantaged
women and children in income-poor settings. By 1996, only fifteen years after AIDS was
first described, the capacity to inexpensively diagnose infection, to monitor the amount
of virus in the blood of infected individuals, and to treat infection with triple combinations of ARVs was so effective that the disease was transformed from an acute and
fatal illness to a chronic one. In the period following the 1996 announcement of the

effectiveness of combination antiretroviral treatment, the US FDA approved more than twenty ARVs for the treatment of HIV, more than for any other viral infection. Further, the agency declared repeatedly that separate efficacy research studies for these drugs were not needed in all populations infected with HIV and that viral load, determined by a simple blood test, could be used as a surrogate marker for drug efficacy, making the use of disease progression and death as research endpoints unnecessary.

The aggressive use of antiretrovirals and diagnostics in high-income countries like the United States led to a marked decline in the number of HIV-related deaths, drastically fewer new HIV infections, decreased clinical and hospital visits, and fewer opportunistic infections. For HIV-infected pregnant women, the outcome was control of their infection and decreased HIV transmission to their infants, resulting in the virtual elimination of HIV infection in infants in the United States and Europe. During this period, evidence also continued to mount that delaying treatment could have severe negative and irreversible health effects due to unchecked viral replication. Early in the new treatment era, groups of HIV experts and advocates repeatedly called for early antiretroviral treatment of all infected people. In recent years the early initiation of ART has been shown to decrease sexual transmission of HIV to uninfected partners by more than 90 percent compared to delayed treatment.

In 1997, the US NIH publicly announced that, in response to the call to hit early, hit hard, HAART would become the new standard of HIV care ("A Timeline of HIV/ AIDS" 2015). In 1998, an NIH-commissioned panel of over twenty-five clinicians, basic and clinical researchers, public-health officials, and community representatives defined eleven principles of treatment that included providing early HAART to all HIV-infected individuals and giving all HIV-infected women optimal ART, regardless of pregnancy status ("Major Report" 1996).

In what I have termed "therapeutic denialism," this evidence and these recommendations were largely ignored by many in the larger research community and by WHO and UNAIDS, which instead issued calls for additional research and persisted in recommending delayed antiretroviral treatment in its policy guidance for low-income countries. This policy of withholding known effective treatment for an infectious disease until it has progressed to advanced stages is without precedent in the history of public health control of infectious disease epidemics. It has taken almost two decades for clinical guidelines and policy recommendations in low-income countries to reflect the substantial evidence of the effectiveness of early treatment. As a result, for almost twenty years, HIV continued to spread in low-income countries, claiming the lives of millions of men, women, and children each year. During this period, HIV-infected pregnant women in low-income countries, many of them poorly educated, were placed on inferior HIV treatment regimens in research studies aimed at finding more cost-effective perinatal prevention solutions.

So what explains the stubborn refusal of WHO, UNAIDS, and HIV/AIDS pediatric researchers to heed the evidence that early HAART for all HIV-infected individuals (including pregnant women) is the most effective and ethical way forward in tackling the disease? Political and economic forces, self-interest, excessive personal and academic institutional gain, conflicts of interest, and flawed intellectual paradigms may have all played a part.

A climate of fiscal austerity may have reduced the political will to mobilize resources for large-scale treatment and, in turn, may have caused a misguided reliance on short-term cost-effectiveness rather than on HAART's long-term benefits in preventing new infections and reducing costly complications of HIV and eventual death. Regardless, the dominance of short term cost-effectiveness criteria in global HIV/AIDS policy making was particularly harmful because, due to colonial histories and legacies of racial injustice that are embedded in the institutions in which we work, such calculations require a modicum of indifference and demean the value of the lives of disadvantaged women and children from low-income countries, calling into question the use of these criteria for making critical public-health and clinical-research decisions. An additional factor may have been the poor scientific and ethical oversight of billions of dollars of public funds available for HIV/AIDS research and the excessive overhead fees charged by participating institutions, which may have created incentives for many small but inconclusive perinatal HIV transmission studies over a period of several decades, when a single large study that could have been completed in several years would have sufficed. Integral to all these explanations was the acceptance of a unprecedented public health policy that a major infectious disease epidemic could be controlled by withholding treatment from the majority of those who were infected and only treating those with the most advanced disease.

Finally, unlike the circumstances in the United States and Europe, truly representative advocates for HIV-infected pregnant women and children from low-income countries had little access to the policy making arena; their questions about research risks and benefits and the long-term impact of withholding effective treatment could not, therefore, break through the academy's walls or the WHO's bureaucracy. Too many scientific and ethical concerns were ignored, perhaps because they emanated from poor, under-educated, and politically powerless women, and life-and-death decisions were made in isolation, without public scrutiny and without mechanisms for seriously considering outside opinions.

In 2015 the last of the global health and research organizations finally capitulated to the overwhelming evidence that early treatment of all HIV-infected individuals was the right thing to do both clinically and ethically. Yet more is required to end the HIV/AIDS epidemic than simply redrafting guidelines, expanding treatment, and crafting clever slogans. Accountability demands acknowledging that something went wrong in the public-health response to the epidemic, something that must be corrected before the unnecessary loss of additional lives. Importantly, it must never be repeated. Accountability also demands that such acknowledgements must come from those who for decades imposed complex and lengthy guidelines, unimaginably complicated flow-charts, and pages of tables with unnecessary AIDS classifications (all of which seemed aimed at keeping most individuals off treatment), when a simple "treat all HIV-infected individuals" would have sufficed. The obligation and cost of retraining thousands of health-care professionals in the new treatment recommendations must now be assumed by the organizations responsible for first training them incorrectly.

This acknowledgement and stocktaking is important for the future of public health and clinical research. It remains to be seen whether WHO guidelines to withhold treatment and the many duplicative and largely unnecessary perinatal HIV research studies coupled with deficient and misleading informed consents will be retrospectively judged as on par with the infamous Tuskegee and Guatemala studies, which also withheld known effective treatment from participants and either failed to obtain informed consents or used deceptive consents. Warning signs are again in place that the lessons of Tuskegee and Guatemala have been forgotten. In spite of clarion calls from NIH itself that "HIV science has spoken" and prevention and treatment can no longer be withheld, clinical researchers, with the approval of NIH and the support of hundreds of millions of NIH dollars, are moving down the path of exploitation, once again proposing the use of placebo-controlled clinical trials on poor and disadvantaged women who will be selected because of their vulnerability to HIV infection (Fauci and Marston 2015; Smith 2015; Graham 2015). Some of the proposed research will be conducted in Zimbabwe, a country with desperate health-care needs but a questionable human-rights record and substantial economic decline. The unethical use of placebo and comparisons with unproven treatment will be rationalized on the basis of scientific expediency and efficiency that will bring benefit to the United States but not to the women participating in the study, who are likely to be abandoned once the study is completed (*ClinicalTrials. gov* 2016a; Graham 2015). The unanimous approval of such studies by US IRBs raises concerns regarding conflicts of interest and their ethical and scientific proficiency.

The dire consequences of WHO's treatment guidelines and US government-supported clinical-research events in low-income countries during the HIV/AIDS epidemic cost the lives of millions. At the very least, this should cause us to raise questions about exploitation and the accountability and oversight of global health interventions and research programs. At this point in the HIV/AIDS epidemic, it would be a dishonor to the women and children who succumbed to HIV to not carefully examine why known effective treatment was delayed for so many decades, allowing the HIV/AIDS epidemic to expand. Our historical reckoning should examine how the decisions were made, who decided on standards of care for research and program implementation, what economic models were considered, whether advocates and activists from the most affected communities were engaged, whether protections of the human right to health were considered, whether institutional review boards were fully informed of the risks and benefits of research that took place in an environment of poverty and inadequate resources, whether the insular atmospheres of the academy and the creators of guidelines fostered conflicts of interest, which legal safeguards were in place to protect the most vulnerable populations, and importantly, whether outside independent reviewers engaged in overseeing research and public-health programs.

To honor individuals who have fought so valiantly to make HIV/AIDS treatment for all a reality and to protect the health of our global community, we must accomplish what we set out to do when AIDS was first recognized in 1981—prevent all HIV infections and identify and treat every HIV-infected individual. As John F. Kennedy said in 1963, "We have technology, we have the manpower, we have the resources to remove hunger from the face of the earth. All we lack is the will." In 2017, we can say the same of HIV.

TIMELINE
Pediatric HIV/AIDS Milestones and Events

Pre-1981

Back calculating from studies of HIV mutations, the virus may have originated as early as 1900. HIV likely originated in Cameroon and traveled to Congo by Bush hunters.

1981

June 5. Gottlieb first reports AIDS in *Morbidity and Mortality Weekly Report* (*MMWR*). Young gay men with pneumocystis pneumonia are reported in Los Angeles and New York.

July 3. Kaposi's sarcoma in gay men is described in eight cases in New York (*MMWR*).

August 4. Ammann, Conant, Greenspan, Volberding, and Wara conduct the first meeting on AIDS at the University of California Faculty Club, and form an ad hoc group on AIDS.

First presentations by Ammann on mother and infants with AIDS, suggesting transmission from mother to infant, at University of Alberta, Edmonton, Canada.

July 3. First article in *New York Times* on AIDS: "Rare Cancer Seen in 41 Homosexuals," by Lawrence Altman.

Elizabeth Glaser receives blood transfusion contaminated with HIV.

US statistics: US Centers for Disease Control and Prevention (CDC) reports 159 cases of AIDS.

1982

December 10. First case of blood-transfusion AIDS reported by Ammann (*MMWR*).

December 17. Ammann, Oleske, and Rubinstein report infants with AIDS from New Jersey, New York, and California (*MMWR*).

Lymphadenopathy syndrome (LAS) described.

CDC identifies four risk factors for AIDS—homosexuality, Haitian origin, hemophilia, and intravenous drug use—and publishes a working definition of clinical features to define AIDS.

The name *acquired immunodeficiency syndrome* (AIDS) is agreed upon by AIDS healthcare professionals.

First case reported in Africa.

US statistics: 771 cases of AIDS reported to date. 618 deaths.

1983

Dr. Luc Montagnier of the Pasteur Institute in France isolates lymphadenopathy-associated virus (LAV) as the cause of AIDS.

Dr. Robert Gallo of the US National Cancer Institute identifies HTLV-III as the virus that causes AIDS.

CDC defines individuals at risk for AIDS to include sexual partners of AIDS patients, sexually active homosexual or bisexual men with multiple partners, Haitian immigrants, drug abusers, patients with hemophilia, and sexual partners of individuals at increased risk for AIDS.

First World Health Organization (WHO) meeting on AIDS in Denmark.

Ammann presents Pediatric AIDS at the Banbury Conference in Cold Spring Harbor, New York, attended by Gallo and Montagnier.

Willie Brown, California Assembly Speaker, acquires funds for AIDS research at University of California.

Ammann reports on Pediatric AIDS at the New York Academy of Sciences, Scripps Research Institute in San Diego, and the Pediatric Immunology Conference in Erice, Sicily.

Pediatric AIDS is reported by Ammann in the *Lancet* in April and by Oleske and Rubinstein in two different articles in the May *Journal of the American Medical Association* (*JAMA*).

AIDS Medical Foundation started by Krim, Sonnabend, and others.

US statistics: 2,807 cases of AIDS reported to date. 2,118 deaths.

1984

US Department of Health and Human Services (HHS) announces Gallo has found that a retrovirus causes AIDS.

June. Gallo and Montagnier hold a joint press conference announcing the discovery that a retrovirus (identified as HTLV-III by Gallo and LAV by Montagnier) causes AIDS.

US statistics: 7,239 cases of AIDS reported to date. 5,596 deaths.

1985

Food and Drug Administration (FDA) approves the first enzyme-linked immunosorbent assay (ELISA) test for antibodies to HIV.

First International AIDS Conference held in Atlanta. Hosted by HHS and WHO.

The US Public Health Service (USPHS) issues the first recommendations for preventing transmission of HIV from mother to child.

Ryan White, an Indiana teenager with AIDS, is banned from classes.

Rock Hudson announces he has AIDS and dies in the same year.

President Reagan publicly mentions AIDS for the first time.

WHO adopts its own definition of AIDS, known as the Bangui definition.

Transmission by breastmilk confirmed.

First AIDS case in China is reported.

American Foundation for AIDS Research (amfAR) is established by cofounders Krim and Gottlieb and national chair Elizabeth Taylor.

US statistics: 15,527 cases of AIDS reported to date. 12,529 deaths.

1986

Gallo's HTLV-III and Montagnier's LAV are found to be the same virus and both are renamed Human Immunodeficiency Virus (HIV).

Second International AIDS Conference is held in Paris, France.

Ricky Ray, a nine-year-old hemophiliac with HIV, is barred from his Florida school.

Chicago AMA meeting is held to address revising AIDS guidelines.

AIDS Treatment and Evaluation Units are established by NIH.

FDA establishes mechanism for rapid review of drugs.

NIH initiates Zidovudine (ZDV) clinical trial.

US statistics: 28,712 cases of AIDS reported to date. 24,559 deaths.

1987

FDA approves ZDV in record time as first antiretroviral drug (ARV). Study shows that one patient in the treatment group died versus nineteen in the placebo group.

WHO Global Program on AIDS is developed and approved by WHO Assembly.

ZDV is reported by Fischl et al. in the *New England Journal of Medicine* (*NEJM*) to be the first drug to control HIV infection.

Randy Shilts publishes *And the Band Played On.*

Duesberg publishes a scientific paper that questions both the theory that viruses cause cancer and the link between HIV and AIDS.

Home of HIV-infected hemophiliac Ricky Ray is burned by arsonists.

April 6–8. Surgeon General Koop holds a workshop on HIV in children.

AIDS Clinical Trials Group (ACTG) established by the NIH's National Institute of Allergy and Infectious Diseases (NIAID).

Third International AIDS Conference is held in Washington, DC.

US statistics: 50,378 cases of AIDS reported to date. 40,849 deaths.

1988

December 1. First World AIDS Day: "Join the worldwide effort."

Ammann meets with Gottlieb and Glaser to plan the Pediatric AIDS Foundation (EGPAF).

Fourth International AIDS Conference held in Stockholm, Sweden.

NIH establishes the Office of AIDS Research (OAR) and Dr. Anthony Fauci is named acting-director.

The Joint United Nations Programme on HIV/AIDS (UNAIDS) reports that the number of women living with HIV/AIDS in sub-Saharan Africa exceeds that of men.

Ruprecht receives an amfAR grant to test whether ZDV can prevent mother-to-infant transmission of an HIV-like virus in monkeys. (See under 1994, "ACTG 076 perinatal HIV transmission study halted. . . .")

US statistics: 82,362 cases of AIDS reported to date. 61,816 deaths.

1989

Fauci, Head of NIAID, endorses a parallel track policy, giving those who do not qualify for clinical trials access to experimental treatments.

June 16. The CDC issues the first guidelines for preventing Pneumocystis carinii pneumonia.

Fifth International AIDS Conference held in Montreal, Canada.

The number of reported AIDS cases in the United States reaches 100,000.

US statistics: 117,508 cases of AIDS reported to date. 89,343 deaths.

1990

Over 1,000 orphaned children in Romania are believed to have been infected with HIV as a result of reuse of needles.

FDA approves use of zidovudine (ZDV) for pediatric AIDS.

Jonathan Mann resigns from WHO/UNAIDS. Under his leadership the UNAIDS program had become the largest AIDS program in WHO's history.

Sixth International AIDS Conference held in San Francisco, CA.

The number of women infected with HIV estimated to exceed that of men.

Genentech begins studies of gp120, the first vaccine tested in humans to prevent HIV. It does not work.

California AIDS leadership conference pushes for routine HIV testing of all pregnant women, including making it mandatory for doctors to offer the test.

US statistics: 160,969 cases of AIDS reported to date. 120,453 deaths.

1991

The CDC reports that one million Americans are infected with HIV.

WHO estimates that nearly ten million people are infected with HIV worldwide.

The AIDS Clinical Trial Group is informally split into the AACTG (adult studies) and PACTG (pediatric studies).

Kimberly Bergalis is reported to have acquired HIV from a dentist.

Magic Johnson announces he is infected with HIV.

High HIV transmission through breast milk reported. WHO urges continued breast-feeding, fearing high mortality from discontinuing breastfeeding in poor countries.

Duliege reports that a first-born twin is more likely to be infected, leading to recommendations to perform Cesarean sections to reduce HIV infection of infants.

US statistics: 206,563 cases of AIDS reported to date. 156,143 deaths.

1992

FDA passes rules allowing for surrogate markers other than death, clinical endpoints, or long-term clinical outcomes for determining ARV efficacy.

First rapid HIV test approved. Results available in less than thirty minutes.

The first combination drug therapies for HIV are introduced and shown to be more effective than ZDV alone and to slow the development of drug resistance.

Terry McGovern sues HHS to include cervical cancer and candidiasis in AIDS definition on behalf of disadvantaged women.

Clinton establishes a White House Office of National AIDS Policy.

Eighth International AIDS Conference, originally scheduled to be held in Boston, is moved to Amsterdam due to US immigration restrictions on people living with HIV/AIDS.

US statistics: 254,147 cases of AIDS reported to date. 194,476 deaths.

1993

NIH State of the Art Expert Panel on HIV concludes that all HIV infected individuals with CD4 counts of 500 cells/mm3 or less should be treated with available zidovudine.

CDC officially expands definition of AIDS to include cervical cancer and new opportunistic infections as AIDS-defining events in HIV-infected individuals with CD4 counts less than 200/mm3.

ZDV resistance reported.

US Congress enacts the NIH Revitalization Act, giving OAR primary oversight of all NIH AIDS funding.

Ninth International AIDS Conference held in Berlin, Germany.

Perinatal HIV transmission falls in the US even before the clinical trial ACTG 076, studying the effect of ZDV on perinatal HIV transmission, is completed. The decline is attributed to early use of ZDV to treat HIV infected pregnant women even before research results were obtained.

US statistics: 360,909 cases of AIDS reported to date. 234,225 deaths.

1994

ACTG 076 perinatal HIV transmission study is halted after showing a 60 percent reduction in HIV transmission from mothers to infants treating mothers and infants with ZDV. Fewer than five hundred mother-infant pairs were enrolled in the study.

US Public Health Service recommends use of ZDV by pregnant women to reduce perinatal HIV transmission.

Public Citizen, a Washington-based advocacy group, says placebo use is unethical.

Clinton convenes the President's National Drug Task Force meeting on HIV drugs.

A European study on mother-to-child HIV transmission shows that Caesarean section halves the rate of transmission.

Tenth International AIDS Conference in Yokohama, Japan.

Kassebaum introduces the Better Pharmaceuticals for Children Act to the Senate, and Greenwood introduces it to the House of Representatives. The Act later gets renamed the Best Pharmaceuticals for Children Act (BPCA).

December 3. Elizabeth Glaser dies.

US statistics: 441,528 cases of AIDS reported to date. 270,870 deaths.

1995

Split of ACTG into PACTG and Adult ACTG made official.

Ammann proposes that perinatal HIV transmission could be reduced to less than 2 percent in five years using highly active antiretroviral therapy (HAART).

CDC announces that in the US, AIDS has become the leading cause of death among all Americans aged twenty-five to forty-four.

FDA approves saquinavir, the first of a new class of ARVs called protease inhibitors (PI).

HAART use impacts perinatal HIV transmission in US.

US statistics: 513,486 cases of AIDS reported to date. 319,849 deaths.

1996

The HHS Expert Panel on Clinical Practices for the Treatment of HIV-Infected Adults and Adolescents concludes that combination antiretroviral treatment (HAART) should be offered to all patients who have acute HIV syndrome, are within six months of seroconversion, present symptoms ascribed to HIV infection, or have CD4 counts of 500 cells/mm3 or less. Pregnant women should be treated the same as non-pregnant women.

The number of new AIDS cases diagnosed in the US declines for the first time since the beginning of the epidemic.

For the first time the number of Americans dying from AIDS declines, dropping 23 percent, attributed primarily to HAART.

Between 1992 and 1996, the number of mother-to-infant HIV transmissions in the US dropped by two-thirds with increased use of ART.

HIV transmission rate in US reduced to 3.4 percent in infants, as use of HAART increases.

Combination therapy is made available to HIV/AIDS patients for the first time, leading to a dramatic decline in AIDS-related deaths.

Eleventh International AIDS Conference in Vancouver, BC. Ho and Shaw report ten billion HIV virions/day in HIV-infected individuals. Mellors reports viral load and CD4 count predict clinical course. Montaner, Markowitz, and Gulick independently report that combination ART (HAART) is able to control HIV infection and disease progression.

Within one year following the eleventh International AIDS Conference, an estimated 75,000 HIV infected individuals are placed on HAART.

Sperling reports significant association of viral load and transmission from ACTG 076 ZDV study.

FDA approves nevirapine, the first non-nucleoside reverse transcriptase inhibitor.

FDA approves two new protease inhibitors drugs in record time—ritonavir and indinavir.

Amplicor viral level test approved by FDA to determine HIV-1 RNA in human plasma (viral load).

Levine Committee calls for overhaul of NIH AIDS research.

PACTG reviewed by the Whitley-Feinberg Panel.

Ho advocates for "hit early, hit hard," using HAART, and is subsequently named *Time*'s "Man of the Year."

A new Joint United Nations Programme on AIDS formed (UNAIDS).

US statistics: 581,429 cases of AIDS reported to date. 362,004 deaths.

1997

New HIV infections remain stable in the US at forty thousand per year since 1992.

Globally, 2.3 million people die of AIDS in 1997—a 50 percent increase over 1996. Nearly half of those deaths are women, and 460,000 are children under age fourteen.

The United States Agency for International Development (USAID) said it believed that forty million children in developing nations will lose one or both parents to AIDS by the year 2010.

In separate *NEJM* articles, Hammer et al. and Gulick et al. report a 60 to 80 percent decline in death and hospitalizations in patients treated with HAART.

FDA accepts viral load as a surrogate marker for clinical event.

US Congress enacts the FDA Modernization Act, codifying the accelerated approval process.

NIH states, "In response to the call to hit early, hit hard, highly active antiretroviral therapy (HAART) becomes the new standard of HIV care."

The CDC reports AIDS-related deaths in the US declined by 47 percent compared with the previous year, due largely to the use of HAART.

US statistics: 641,086 cases of AIDS reported to date. 390,692 deaths.

1998

The HHS Expert Panel on Clinical Practices for the Treatment of HIV-Infected Adults and Adolescents defines principles of HIV treatment including immediate treatment of all infected men, women, pregnant women, and children and administration of HAART to achieve viral suppression and prevent resistance. The pediatric international clinical researchers reject the conclusions of 1993, 1996, and 1998 panels of HIV experts as they related to HIV-infected pregnant women and children in poor countries and embark on a research agenda that withheld recommended treatment to thousands of HIV-infected pregnant women and infants in income poor countries. After almost two decades they capitulate and accept the 1996/1998 treatment recommendations.

Global Strategies for HIV Prevention founded as a 501(c)(3).

CDC, NIH, and the University of Pennsylvania Health System issue the first national treatment guidelines for the use of antiretroviral therapy in adults and adolescents with HIV. Eleven principles of treatment are incorporated, including early treatment of HIV-infected individuals and HIV-infected pregnant women.

Guidelines developed by National Pediatric Resource Center National Health Resources and Services Administration (HRSA) and NIH recommend treating all HIV-infected infants regardless of CD4 count, viral load, or clinical features, and warn against delaying treatment.

CDC reports that perinatal HIV transmission in US is less than 2 percent, attributed to increased use of HAART.

WHO reports that the worldwide incidence of HIV infection has peaked at about three million new infections per year.

San Francisco starts a pioneering post-exposure prophylaxis (PEP) program, giving HIV drugs to people that might have been exposed to HIV through sexual contact or needle sharing.

Combination of caesarean delivery and ZDV reduce the risk of HIV transmission from a mother to her baby to less than 1 percent.

Twelfth International AIDS Conference held in Geneva.

First case of a patient being infected with a strain of HIV resistant to the most powerful new antiretroviral drugs reported in San Francisco.

Seventy percent of people infected with HIV during the year are in Sub-Saharan Africa.

South Africa President Thabo Mbeki claimed that the anti-HIV drug ZDV was toxic and could be a danger to health.

Ugandan Ministry of Health starts a voluntary door-to-door HIV screening program using rapid tests.

African Americans account for 49 percent of all US AIDS-related deaths, a mortality rate ten times that of whites and three times that of Hispanics.

US statistics: 688,200 cases of AIDS reported to date. 410,800 deaths.

1999

NIH HIVNET 012 Uganda-US study reports that a single oral dose of nevirapine given to an HIV-infected mother and a single dose to the infant reduces HIV perinatal transmission by 50 percent.

Investigators at the Global Strategies Montreal Conference report exclusive breast feeding is associated with reduced perinatal HIV transmission; perinatal HIV transmission is correlated with viral load; less than 2 percent HIV transmission occurs with HAART treatment of HIV infected pregnant women.

The Institute of Medicine issues a report calling for universal voluntary "opt-out" testing for pregnant women.

By the end of 1999, UNAIDS estimated that 33 million people around the world are living with HIV/AIDS, and that 2.6 million people worldwide died of the disease in 1999, more than in any other year since the epidemic began.

HIV-infected mother loses a court case and is not allowed to breast feed her baby.

Researchers at the University of Alabama claim to have discovered that a particular type of chimpanzee, once common in West Central Africa, was the source of HIV.

US statistics: 733,374 cases of AIDS reported to date. 429,825 deaths.

2000

There are fewer than one hundred new cases of HIV infection in infants in the United States.

To counter the comments made by President Mbeki, over five thousand scientists around the world sign the "Durban Declaration," affirming that HIV is the cause of AIDS.

Thirteenth International AIDS Conference held in Durban, South Africa.

Meeting on ARV safety in infants in Washington, DC.

Garcia reports significant association of viral load and perinatal HIV transmission in the US Women and Infants Transmission Study (WITS) cohort.

More than 95 percent of all HIV-infected people are reported to live in developing countries that also experience 95 percent of the AIDS deaths.

Women account for 23 percent of AIDS cases in the United States as opposed to 7 percent in 1985. In sub-Saharan Africa, 55 percent of HIV-infected individuals are women.

The Clinton administration formally declares HIV/AIDS to be a threat to US national security.

US Institute of Medicine releases a report that sharply criticized the Clinton administration for failure to develop a comprehensive and effective plan to combat the disease.

CDC reports that for the first time, the rate of AIDS diagnoses among black and Hispanic gay men has overtaken that of white gay men.

US Ambassador Richard Holbrooke declares AIDS an international security issue because it threatens social, economic, and political structures worldwide.

US statistics: 733,374 cases of AIDS reported to date. 429,825 deaths.

2001

Ministers meeting at the WTO conference in Doha, Qatar, agree on a new declaration on intellectual property rights, making it easier for the governments of developing country to license the production of drugs against AIDS and other diseases without having to get permission from patent holders.

China admits that HIV/AIDS threatens its public health and economic security.

India's generic drug manufacturer Cipla offers to produce and sell ARVs for less than $1 per day.

Fourteen percent of individuals who are newly infected with HIV exhibit resistance to at least one drug.

US pharmaceutical companies withdraw the lawsuit to block implementation of the South African law that permits the import and manufacture of generic antiretrovirals.

US statistics: 816,149 cases of AIDS reported to date. 462,653 deaths.

2002

WHO publishes the first guidelines for providing antiretroviral drugs for HIV infection in resource poor countries. It also releases a list of twelve essential AIDS drugs.

Fourteenth International AIDS Conference held in Barcelona, Spain.

In a survey, 50 percent of Americans believe that HIV can be contracted by casual contact.

The number of children orphaned by HIV/AIDS has risen three-fold in six years to reach an all-time high of 13.4 million.

FDA approves the first rapid antibody HIV test.

USAID announces it is adopting a new approach to preventing sexual transmission of HIV that would be known as "ABC": Abstinence, Being faithful, and Condom use.

Perinatal HIV transmission decreases to fewer than one hundred fifty per year in the United States from two thousand per year in the 1990s.

De Martino and associates report from data in Italian registry that the effectiveness of HAART in reducing death among infants and children is at least equal to, or greater than, that among adults.

Global fund to fight AIDS, tuberculosis, and malaria is established.

US statistics: 886,000 cases of AIDS reported to date. 501,669 deaths.

2003

Bush proposes US appropriation of fifteen billion dollars over five years to combat HIV internationally during his State of the Union address, to be known as the President's Emergency Plan for AIDS Relief (PEPFAR).

William J. Clinton Foundation obtains price reductions for ARVs from generic manufacturers to help developing nations.

Botswana and Swaziland acknowledge HIV seroprevalence of over 35 percent.

CDC proposes making HIV testing a routine part of medical care and putting more resources into partner tracing.

Belgian researcher announces that HIV-2 was probably transferred from sooty mangabeys to humans in Guinea Bissau during the 1940s.

Just over 1 percent, or about 50,000 people, have access to ARVs in resource-poor countries.

WHO announces a "3 by 5" initiative directed at providing three million people in resource-poor countries with ARVs by 2005.

SIMBA ("stopping infection from mother to child via breastfeeding in Africa") perinatal HIV transmission study performed in Uganda and Rwanda shows only 2 percent of infants became HIV infected when their mothers and infants were treated during pregnancy and breast feeding with combination ARVs.

US statistics: 930,000 cases of AIDS reported to date. 524,060 deaths.

2004

HIV seroprevalence reduced by 70 percent in Uganda due to "ABC" program.

Brazil reaches an agreement with pharmaceutical companies to reduce drug prices.

The Bill and Melinda Gates Foundation donates $150 million to Global Fund for HIV, tuberculosis and malaria.

FDA approves the first generic drug for HIV. PEPFAR can now use the drug.

Globally, fifteen million children lost one or both parents to HIV/AIDS by 2004.

Fifteenth International AIDS Conference held in Bangkok, Thailand.

CDC announces that one million people are living with HIV. Twenty-five percent do not know they are infected.

New HIV cases are stable at about forty thousand per year.

ZDV goes off patent.

US statistics: 940,000 cases of AIDS reported to date. 529,113 deaths.

2005

WHO reports that AIDS deaths peaked at about 2.3 million deaths per year but prevalence continues to increase.

WHO's "3 by 5" plan failed to achieve its goal——of the three million people targeted fewer than half received ARVs. "All we can do is apologize. I think we just have to admit we've not done enough and we started way too late" (Dr. Jim Yong Kim).

An editor of the journal *Lancet* writes, "2005 is likely to be remembered more for the three million deaths and almost five million new infections."

International Maternal, Pediatric, Adolescent AIDS Clinical Trials Network (IMPAACT) is started.

Eliza Jane Scovill, daughter of HIV denialist Christine Maggiore, dies suddenly and unexpectedly at the age of three years and five months amid controversy about whether she had HIV.

Worldwide annual statistics: 38.6 million living with HIV; 4.1 million new infections; 2.8 million died of AIDS. (Note: WHO and UNAIDS report worldwide statistics midyear. Here and in future statistics the numbers reflect estimates from the previous year (e.g. the 2005 report would reflect the epidemic in 2004).

2006

CDC announces that perinatal HIV transmission in the US is less than 2 percent.

CDC recommends that all adolescents and adults be routinely tested for HIV.

June fifth marks twenty-five years since AIDS was first reported.

The FDA approves the world's first three-drug-combination anti-HIV drug taken once per day as a single pill (Atripla).

NIH reports that the risk of HIV transmission is reduced by 60 percent in two African trials of male circumcision.

Sixteenth International AIDS Conference held in Toronto, Canada.

Worldwide annual statistics: 39.5 million living with HIV; 4.3 million new infections; 2.9 million died of AIDS.

2007

Study reported in *NEJM* finds those who received early treatment (CD4 count 351 to 500 and higher) have a significantly better survival rate.

Several studies from Africa demonstrate less than 5 percent HIV transmission to infants even when breastfeeding is continued if the mother is treated with combination ARVs.

FDA approves maraviroc (Selzentry), a drug known as an HIV entry inhibitor.

FDA approves raltegravir (Isentress), a drug known as an integrase inhibitor.

Worldwide annual statistics: 33.2 million living with HIV; 2.5 million new infections; 2.1 million died of AIDS.

2008

President Bush calls on Congress to reauthorize PEPFAR at $30 billion over five years and on July 31 signs legislation reauthorizing PEPFAR for $48 billion over five years.

Swiss publish a study that reports HIV-infected individuals taking effective ARVs are less likely to transmit HIV.

WHO and UNAIDS recommend that "male circumcision should always be considered as part of a comprehensive HIV prevention package."

Seventeenth International AIDS Conference held in Mexico City, Mexico.

Nobel Prize for medicine split between Françoise Barré-Sinoussi and Luc Montagnier of the Pasteur for discovery of HIV.

First HIV "cure" performed, using a bone marrow transplant from a donor with a genetic mutation that makes the donor cells resistant to HIV infection.

WHO announces stabilization of HIV epidemic. Thirty-three million living with HIV, down from forty million. Deaths down from 2.2 million to 2 million.

Study conducted by Violari and associates in South Africa is halted by the DSMB after increased deaths and HIV infection occur in infants whose treatment is delayed.

Nearly 70 percent of people in low- and middle-income countries who need antiretroviral therapy do not have access to treatment.

Worldwide annual statistics: 33 million living with HIV; 2.7 million new infections; 2 million died of AIDS.

2009

May 5. President Obama launches the Global Health Initiative (GHI), a six-year, US-led, $63-billion effort to develop a comprehensive approach to addressing global health in low- and middle-income countries. PEPFAR will serve as a core component.

NEJM report by Kitahata and associates shows early initiation of antiretroviral therapy in 9,155 asymptomatic HIV-infected individuals with >500 CD4 improves survival compared to 94 percent increased risk of death in 6,935 people in the delayed treatment group.

UNAIDS and WHO estimate that 5.25 million people receive ARVs.

Worldwide annual statistics: 33.3 million living with HIV; 2.6 million new infections; 1.8 million died of AIDS.

2010

Malawi proposes beginning HAART treatment for life for all HIV-infected pregnant women regardless of CD4 count (Option B plus). International AIDS Society recommends treating all asymptomatic HIV-infected people with a 500 CD4 count.

NIH reports that a daily dose of ARVs reduces the risk of HIV infection among HIV-negative men who have sex with men by 44 percent, supporting the concept of pre-exposure prophylaxis (PrEP). Subsequent study of the data indicates 90 percent protection with daily adherence.

Eighteenth International AIDS Conference held in Vienna, Austria.

UNAIDS reports that the number of new infections has dropped by 17 percent since 2001.

Global Fund board announces that, due to reduced pledges and unmet or delayed contributions, the funding of "Round 11" would be cancelled.

UNAIDS estimates that more than 350,000 new HIV infections in children have been averted due to prevention of mother-to-child transmission (PMTCT) since 1995.

Worldwide annual statistics: 34 million living with HIV; 2.7 million new infections; 1.8 million died of AIDS.

2011

Malawi initiates HAART for life for all HIV-infected pregnant women regardless of CD4 count (Option B plus). In 2013 they report a 763 percent increase in HIV-infected pregnant women receiving ART.

A large perinatal HIV transmission study in Africa demonstrates that triple antiretroviral treatment is superior to zidovudine and single-dose nevirapine prophylaxis during pregnancy and breastfeeding (Kesho Boro Study Group 2011).

A study of HIV-discordant, mostly heterosexual couples (HPTN 052) shows early treatment of an HIV-infected person greatly reduces transmission to a negative partner, as well as reducing AIDS-related events.

WHO announces 6.6 million HIV infected individuals had access to ART. (But there are 33 million in need of treatment.)

On December 23, the journal *Science* announces that it has chosen the HPTN 052 study as its "2011 Breakthrough of the Year."

Worldwide annual statistics: 34 million living with HIV; 2.7 million new infections; 1.8 million died of AIDS.

2012

Uganda initiates treatment for life of all HIV-infected pregnant women regardless of CD4 count (Option B plus).

New HIV infections in the US reported to have remained at fifty thousand per year for the past decade.

USPHS and HHS recommend that all HIV-infected individuals should be treated with ART.

The International AIDS Society (IAS) recommends treating all HIV-infected individuals with ART.

Global Strategies conducts "Treat All" Campaign in conjunction with International AIDS Conference in Washington, DC.

Nineteenth International AIDS Conference held in Washington, DC.

FDA approves the use of Truvada (emtricitabine/tenofovir disoproxil fumarate) for reducing the risk of HIV infection in uninfected individuals at high risk for HIV (PrPEP). UNAIDS reports nine million people living with HIV had access to antiretroviral therapy in low and middle income countries.

Worldwide annual statistics: 35 million living with HIV; 2.3 million new infections; 1.6 million died of AIDS.

2013

WHO issues recommendation to start HAART at CD4 <500.

UNAIDS reports that there are 300,000 infants infected per year compared to 700,000 prior to use of ARVs for PMTCT.

UNAIDS reports a 52 percent reduction in new HIV infections among children and a combined 33 percent reduction among adults and children since 2001, representing a decrease from 3.4 million infections in 2001 to 2.3 million in 2012.

New HIV infections among adults and adolescents decreased by 50 percent or more in twenty-six countries between 2001 and 2012.

PEPFAR announces that one million infants worldwide have been born HIV-free as a result of PMTCT.

Possible first documented instance of an HIV "cure" in a child reported by Dr. Hannah Gay in Jackson, Mississippi.

UNAIDS estimates global HIV funding totaled $19.1 billion in 2013.

Globally, the number of new HIV infections continues to fall. There were 2.3 million new HIV infections in 2012.

Worldwide annual statistics: 37 million living with HIV; 2.3 million new infections; 1.2 million died of AIDS.

2014

The rate of diagnosis for HIV infections in the US fell by a third between 2002 and 2011. There are more than 1.1 million people in the US who are HIV infected; approximately 16 percent, around 181,000 people, do not know they are infected.

New infections have been stable at 50,000 since 2008, but about 50 percent of new infections result from people who do not know they are infected.

Studies from the United Kingdom report a decrease of perinatal HIV transmission from 2 percent to less than 0.5 percent with early initiation of HAART.

Twentieth International AIDS Conference is held in Melbourne, Australia

Worldwide annual statistics: 37 million living with HIV; 2 million new infections; 1.2 million died of AIDS.

2015

Strategic Timing of AntiRetroviral Treatment (START), a 4,685-patient NIH-sponsored study, concludes that all HIV-infected individuals should be treated with HAART regardless of CD4 count or clinical symptoms.

September 30. WHO recommends treating all HV-infected individuals with HAART.

May 22. NIH announces that all HIV-infected individuals should receive treatment (HAART).

July 7. IMPAACT/Promise tells its researchers that all HIV-infected pregnant women in their studies should be started on HAART "at the earliest possible opportunity."

Vancouver IAS meeting presents its 2015 Consensus document calling for worldwide access to immediate treatment with HAART for all HIV-infected individuals.

San Francisco announces that new HIV infections are down to 302 per year from a 1992 peak of 2,332 per year. Deaths are down to 177 per year from a peak of 1,641. The decrease is attributed largely to "test and treat" and PrEP.

WHO declares that Cuba is joining the US and Canada in "elimination" of perinatal HIV. Elimination is defined as stopping the transmission of a disease in a specific geographic area.

San Francisco, once the epicenter of HIV and the city where AIDS was first reported in infants, has reported no infected infants since 2005.

For the first time in the HIV epidemic, CDC's director Thomas Friedman calls for partner notification (contact tracing) as a "core intervention to stop transmission of communicable diseases."

Worldwide annual statistics: 37 million living with HIV; 2 million new infections; 1.2 million died of AIDS.

2016

Cohen and associates report that early ART versus delayed ART in the HPTN 052 clinical trial was superior in preventing HIV transmission from infected to uninfected sexual partners. Early ART resulted in a 93 percent lower risk of linked partner HIV infection.

Twenty-First International AIDS Conference is held in Durban, South Africa.

NIH launches an estimated $200 million international clinical study of 2,700 men who have sex with men in the US and South America, 1,500 women in sub-Saharan African, and 26 infants born to HIV infected mothers in the US and South Africa. It is the largest and most expensive study of an experimental mono-clonal antibody (VRC01) without prior evidence of efficacy.

African Americans have the highest percentage of HIV infections in the US (47 percent); African American and Hispanic/Latino women continue to be disproportionately affected; the majority of the 2,000 children living with HIV/AIDS are African American; an estimated 5,000 children have died since the beginning of the epidemic; fewer than 150 infants became infected with HIV perinatally.

US annual statistics: 1.2 million living with HIV; 44 thousand new infections; about 7,000 died of AIDS.

Worldwide annual statistics, adults: 37 million living with HIV; 2.1 million new infections; 1.1 million died of AIDS; 78 million people have become infected and 35 million have died since the start of the epidemic; of the 37 million living with HIV fewer than 50 percent are on antiretroviral treatment (17 million).

Worldwide annual statistics, infants and children: 49 percent of all children living with HIV were accessing treatment, up from 21 percent in 2010; 220,000 children were newly infected; an estimated 200,000 children died of AIDS-related illnesses; 77 percent of pregnant women living with HIV had access to ARVs to prevent transmission of HIV to their babies.

ACRONYMS

3TC lamivudine, Epivir

ABC "Abstinence, Be faithful, Condoms" program.

ACTG AIDS Clinical Trial Group

ACTU AIDS Clinical Trial Units

ADCC antibody dependent cellular cytotoxicity

AIDS acquired immune deficiency syndrome

amfAR American Foundation for AIDS Research

ART antiretroviral therapy

ARV antiretroviral (drug)

ARVs antiretrovirals

AZT zidovudine (also known as ZDV), Retrovir

cART combination antiretroviral therapy

CD4 T lymphocyte; the subset of T-cells that are most affected in AIDS

CDC US Centers for Disease Control and Prevention

CIPRA Comprehensive International Program of Research on AIDS

CMV cytomegalovirus

CNS central nervous system

CTL cytotoxic T lymphocytes

CTX co-trimoxazole

DNA deoxyribonucleic acid

DRC Democratic Republic of Congo

DSMB Data and Safety Monitoring Board

EBV Epstein-Barr virus

EGPAF Elizabeth Glaser Pediatric AIDS Foundation

ELISA enzyme-linked immunosorbent assay

FDA US Food and Drug Administration

GHI Global Health Initiative

GRID Gay-Related Immunodeficiency

HAART highly active antiretroviral therapy

HBIG hepatitis B immunoglobulin

HHS US Department of Health and Human Services

HIV human immunodeficiency virus (previously HTLV-3; LAV; ARV)

HHV-8   Kaposi's sarcoma-associated herpes virus (or KSHV)

HIVNET   HIV Network for Prevention Trials

HRSA   Health Resource and Services Administration

HSV   herpes simplex virus

HTLV-1, 2   human T-cell leukemia virus

HTLV-3   human T-cell lymphotropic virus type 3 (Renamed HIV-1)

IAS   International AIDS Society

IAVI   International AIDS Vaccines Initiative

ICN   intensive care nursery

IDU   injecting drug users

IMPAACT   International Maternal, Pediatric, Adolescent AIDS Clinical Trials Network

IPV   intimate partner violence

IRB   Institutional Review Board (IRB); a committee established to review and approve research involving human subjects

JAMA   *Journal of the American Medical Association*

KS   Kaposi's sarcoma

KSHV   Kaposi's sarcoma–associated herpes virus

LAV   lymphadenopathy-associated virus (Renamed HIV-1)

MAI   Mycobacterium avium intracellulare

MC   male circumcision

MDR   multiple drug resistant

MMWR   *Morbidity and Mortality Weekly Report*

MSM   men who have sex with men

MTCT   mother-to-child transmission (of HIV); also called "perinatal HIV transmission" and sometimes "vertical transmission"

NCI   National Cancer Institute

NEJM   *New England Journal of Medicine*

NHF   National Hemophilia Foundation

NIAID   National Institute of Allergy and Infectious Diseases

NICHD   National Institute of Child Health and Human Development

NIH   National Institutes of Health

NNRTI   non-nucleoside reverse transcriptase inhibitor

NVP   nevirapine, Viramune

OGAC   Office of the Global AIDS Coordinator

PACTG   Pediatric AIDS Clinical Trials Group

PCP   Pneumocystis jirovecii pneumonia or Pneumocystis pneumonia

PCR   polymerase chain reaction

PEP	post-exposure prophylaxis
PEPFAR	US President's Emergency Plan for AIDS Relief
PhRMA	Pharmaceutical Research and Manufacturers of America
PI	protease inhibitor
PMTCT	prevention of mother-to-child transmission (of HIV)
PPRU	Pediatric Pharmacology Research Units
PrEP	pre-exposure prophylaxis
PROMISE	Promoting Maternal-Infant Survival Everywhere
RFA	request for application
RNA	ribonucleic acid
RT	reverse transcriptase
RTV	ritonavir, Norvir
SIMBA	stopping infection from mother to child via breastfeeding in Africa
STD	sexually transmitted disease
STI	sexually transmitted infection
TB	tuberculosis
TDL	T-cells
UCSF	University of California San Francisco Medical Center
UN	United Nations
UNAIDS	Joint United Nations Programme on HIV/AIDS
UNICEF	United Nations Children's Fund
USAID	United States Agency for International Development
USPHS	United States Public Health Service
WHO	World Health Organization
WITS	Women and Infants Transmission Study
ZDV	zidovudine, azidothymidine (also known as AZT)

NOTES

1. Dr. Michael Gottlieb first discovered the acquired immunodeficiency syndrome (AIDS) in young gay men, reporting them to the CDC as "Pneumocystis pneumonia—Los Angeles" in the *Morbidity Mortality Weekly Report* (*MMWR*) in 1981. The *MMWR* stated:

    > Pneumocystis pneumonia in the United States is almost exclusively limited to severely immunosuppressed patients. The occurrence of pneumocystosis in these five previously healthy individuals without a clinically apparent underlying immunodeficiency is unusual. The fact that these patients were all homosexuals suggests an association between some aspect of a homosexual lifestyle or disease acquired through sexual contact and Pneumocystis pneumonia in this population. All five patients described in this report had laboratory-confirmed CMV disease or virus shedding within five months of the diagnosis of Pneumocystis pneumonia. CMV infection has been shown to induce transient abnormalities of in vitro cellular-immune function in otherwise healthy human hosts. Although all three patients tested had abnormal cellular-immune function, no definitive conclusion regarding the role of CMV infection in these five cases can be reached because of the lack of published data on cellular-immune function in healthy homosexual males with and without CMV antibody. All the above observations suggest the possibility of a cellular immune dysfunction related to a common exposure that predisposes individuals to opportunistic infections such as pneumocystosis and candidiasis. Although the role of CMV infection in the pathogenesis of pneumocystosis remains unknown, the possibility of P. carinii infection must be carefully considered in a differential diagnosis for previously healthy homosexual males with dyspnea and pneumonia. (CDC 1981c)

2. When AIDS was first discovered in 1981 it was described as an acquired immunodeficiency syndrome, indicating that it was a collection of symptoms and clinical findings without a specific cause. AIDS became the official designation in 1982, prior to the discovery of the Human Immunodeficiency Virus (HIV), the cause of AIDS. Initially the terms AIDS and HIV were used interchangeably or together, such as HIV/AIDS. In this book the terms HIV, AIDS, and HIV/AIDS are used primarily when the source documentation does not differentiate between them. When possible, the specific terms are used. HIV refers to the infection alone. AIDS is defined as a specific set of laboratory and clinical features that define a more advanced stage of HIV infection. AIDS is commonly used when referring to the epidemic caused by HIV (e.g., AIDS epidemic). A person who is HIV infected may be without symptoms or clinical features and therefore does not have AIDS. A person with AIDS is always HIV infected and has specific symptoms and clinical features. A person who has HIV infection may not advance to AIDS.

3. *Kaposi's Sarcoma and Related Opportunistic Infections: Hearing before the Subcommittee on Health and the Environment of the Committee on Energy and Commerce, House of Representatives*, 97th Congress, April 13, 1982. Serial no. 97-125. Washington, DC: USGPO

4. More on the history of AIDS at the University of California can be found in "Oral Histories on the AIDS Epidemic in San Francisco: The San Francisco AIDS Oral History Series, 1981–1984," an archive of the Oral History Project at Berkeley Library (*vm136.1ib.berkeley.edu/BANC/ROHO/collections/subjectarea/sci_tech/aids.html*).

5. *Kaposi's Sarcoma and Related Opportunistic Infections*, 1982.

6. Members of the ad hoc UCSF faculty group that formed in 1981 included Paul Volberding, Marcus Conant, William Wara, John Greenspan, and me. When the epidemic was first recognized in 1981, the availability of physicians with experience treating patients with a combination of malignancy, opportunistic infection, and immunodeficiency was limited, so patients started visiting Volberding by default. Subsequently, he found himself almost exclusively engaged in the emerging AIDS epidemic. Volberding went on to head up the adult AIDS program at UCSF, published extensively in AIDS research, was one of the investigators in the first clinical trial in 1987 that demonstrated that the drug zidovudine (ZDV) could successfully treat HIV infection, developed a center for HIV information, and subsequently went on to become the director of the AIDS Research Institute and UCSF Global Health Sciences at UCSF.

   Dermatologist Marcus Conant had observed an increase in patients, nearly all of whom he noted were young gay males suffering from KS. Subsequent research showed that KS was caused by a herpes virus called Kaposi's sarcoma-associated herpes virus (KSHV or HHV-8) that behaves much like an opportunistic infection in patients with AIDS. With the advent of highly active antiretroviral therapy (HAART) to treat HIV and restore the immune system, KS became an infrequent manifestation of HIV infection in the United States. Conant is credited with being the force behind creating the UCSF ad hoc group to address the AIDS epidemic in San Francisco and nationally. His influence helped raise the concern of California Assembly Speaker Willie Brown about the AIDS epidemic, which resulted in the first significant funding for AIDS research from any governmental body within the United States. As Conant continued to see patients with KS and AIDS, he helped create one of the largest private AIDS clinics in the United States and helped to found the San Francisco AIDS Foundation. Conant retired from his dermatologic practice and moved to New York in 2010.

   Radiation oncologist William Wara also started to observe patients with AIDS-related KS and lymphomas. As the HIV/AIDS epidemic continued to expand, and as treatment for HIV infection diminished the complications of HIV infection, he too experienced a decline in the number of patients he was seeing for AIDS and malignancy. Wara went on to become the chairman of the radiation oncology department at UCSF.

   John Greenspan, an oral biologist, treated patients with oral hairy leukoplakia, which was showing up in an increasing number of young gay men. Subsequently, Greenspan and his group discovered the association of Epstein-Barr virus (EBV) with oral hairy leukoplakia. Greenspan was later appointed Associate Dean for Global Oral Health at UCSF and was founding director of the Oral AIDS Center, the California AIDS Research Center, and the UCSF AIDS Specimen Bank, and director of the AIDS Research Institute at UCSF.

7. A. J. Ammann Pediatric HIV/AIDS Archives, 1981–2016.

8. The names used in this book are real when they have been used publicly in the media or in publications. The names of some of the patients are fictional to protect their identity. Infants and children with HIV infection and AIDS were not excluded from stigma and discrimination. Ryan White, a child with hemophilia and who was HIV-infected, was the most prominent child to suffer from widespread stigma and discrimination. Much of the stigma was facilitated by the media, which nationalized the details of the discrimination. Recently the role of the media in violating confidentiality and fostering stigma was apparent in the reporting of the Ebola and Zika virus epidemics.

CHAPTER 2

1. When the AIDS epidemic began there were few regulations concerning the confidentiality of medical records. Physicians and clinical researchers were able to examine medical records with only the permission of the attending physician and/or the patient. There were no formal procedures for obtaining patient or physician consents for this process. Tracking exposure to an infectious agent was not considered research and, in fact, was considered good medical practice as a means to limit the number of people who might be exposed to an infectious agent or, if already infected, to facilitate access to treatment. A research protocol was not required, nor was a human protection committee's approval necessary. When Drs. Dritz, Perkins, Jaffe, and I suspected blood transfusion of AIDS, we went directly to the University of California blood transfusion records and the Irwin Memorial Blood Bank donor records to identify patients who had received a blood transfusion from an individual reported to the San Francisco Health Department. This resulted in the rapid discovery of the association of blood transfusion and AIDS. There were no known instances of discrimination or stigma that resulted from this process at that time. However, as the epidemic progressed, stigma and discrimination against the gay population and against others with AIDS accelerated, resulting in the implementation of strict prohibitions against name reporting and investigation of individuals with AIDS, or later with HIV, without formal submission of a research proposal approved by a human protection committee. While these measures were important to prevent stigma and discrimination, many felt they allowed the HIV/AIDS epidemic to expand rapidly by omitting the fundamental public health pillar of contact tracing to control infectious disease epidemics—warning individuals that they had been exposed to HIV. If this had occurred, those who were exposed to HIV but not infected could have protected themselves from HIV infection, and those who were already infected could prevent others from becoming infected as well as receive treatment for themselves. While the strict rules and confidentiality protected HIV-infected individuals from stigma and discrimination, the rules eventually resulted in discrimination against and denial of the right to health for those who had been exposed to HIV and were unaware of their risk for infection or, if already infected, unaware that they needed treatment (a full discussion on HIV/AIDS testing can be found in Schochetman and George 1994).

CHAPTER 3

1. American Red Cross, "Directed Donations. Sample Letter to Hospital Physicians," Joint News Release, June 22, 1983. From A. J. Ammann, Pediatric HIV/AIDS Archives, 1981–2016.
2. The following letters are from the A. J. Ammann Pediatric HIV/AIDS Archives, 1981–2016: Alfred Katz, 1983, "To Executive Heads" and 1984, "Letter to Executive Heads. To AABB/ARC/CCBC Regarding Transfusion Associated AIDS." Gerald Sandler, 1982, "To Medical/Scientific Directors by Dr. S. Gerald Sandler" and 1984, "Transfusion-Associated AIDS. To Executive Heads." John Petricciani, March 24, 1983, "Recommendations to Decrease the Risk of Transmitting Acquired Immunodeficiency Syndrome (AIDS) from Blood Donors: To All Establishments Collecting Human Blood for Transfusion."
3. Alfred Katz, 1983, "To Executive Heads" and John Petricciani, March 24, 1983, "Recommendations to Decrease the Risk of Transmitting Acquired Immunodeficiency Syndrome (AIDS) from Blood Donors: To All Establishments Collecting Human Blood for Transfusion." From the A. J. Ammann Pediatric HIV/AIDS Archives, 1981–2016.

CHAPTER 4

1. Helen Kushnick, "A Mother Tells How a Blood Donation, the Gift of Life, Led to Her Young Son's Death from AIDS," *People*, June 4, 1984.

2. Emily Yaffe, "Post-Tragedy," *Slate*, July 30, 2013. *www.slate.com/articles/double_x/dou-blex/2013/07/sara_kushnick_lost_her_whole_family_but_persevered.html*.

3. The meeting of an ad hoc committee on pediatric transfusion practices was held at the American Red Cross national headquarters in Washington, DC, on January 4, 1985. Presentations were made by Richard Schubert, Gerald Sandler, Joseph Bellanti, and Arthur Ammann. The committee acknowledged that newborns were particularly susceptible to complications of blood transfusions, including HIV and cytomegalovirus infection and graft versus host reaction.

CHAPTER 6

1. The AIDS Clinical Trial Group (ACTG 076) study was the most important pediatric clinical research study providing evidence that the pediatric HIV epidemic might be brought to a halt. It was the first study to demonstrate that an antiretroviral drug could prevent HIV transmission from one individual to another. It paved the way for future studies on the use of ARVs for post-exposure prophylaxis (PEP) following rape, accidental inoculation with HIV, and, most recently, the prevention of sexual HIV transmission between HIV-discordant couples, called pre-exposure prophylaxis (PrEP). PrEP consists of an HIV-uninfected sexual partner taking a pill every day, currently Truvada (tenofovir and emtricitabine), to prevent HIV infection. The concept of "treatment as prevention" was also derived from the ACTG 076 study. Cohen and his associates reported the results from a large clinical trial in 2011 demonstrating that treatment with HAART resulted in decreasing viral load and decreasing HIV transmission to uninfected sexual partners, slowing the epidemic (M. S. Cohen et.al. 2011).

   The prevention of mother-to-child HIV transmission study, "Reduction of Maternal-Infant Transmission of Human Immunodeficiency Virus Type 1 with Zidovudine Treatment," was published in the *NEJM* in 1994. It was a well-coordinated and carefully planned study conducted at multiple clinical sites in the United States and Europe and required the effort of many investigators. The individuals conducting the study were Edward M. Connor, Rhoda S. Sperling, Richard Gelber, Pavel Kiselev, Gwendolyn Scott, Mary Jo O'Sullivan, Russell VanDyke, Mohammed Bey, William Shearer, Robert L. Jacobson, Eleanor Jimenez, Edward O'Neill, Brigitte Bazin, Jean-Francois Delfraissy, Mary Culnane, Robert Coombs, Mary Elkins, Jack Moye, Pamela Stratton, and James Balsley.

CHAPTER 7

1. Brian Deer, "Death by Denial: The Campaigners Who Continue to Deny HIV Causes Aids," *Guardian*, February 21, 2012. *www.theguardian.com/science/blog/2012/feb/21/death-denial-hiv-aids*.

2. "HIV-Positive Mom Going to Court to Breast-Feed Son: Oregon Took Custody of Him over Issue," *Seattle Times*, April 16, 1999. *community.seattletimes.nwsource.com/archive/?date=19990416&slug=2955476*.

3. The text of the Durban Declaration states:

   > Seventeen years after the discovery of the human immunodeficiency virus (HIV), thousands of people from around the world are gathered in Durban, South Africa to attend the XIII International AIDS Conference. At the turn of the millennium, an estimated 34 million people worldwide are living with HIV or AIDS, 24 million of them in sub-Saharan Africa. Last year alone, 2.6 million people died of AIDS, the highest rate since the start of the epidemic. If current trends continue, Southern and Southeast Asia, South America, and regions of the former Soviet Union will also bear a heavy burden in the next two decades.

Like many other diseases, such as tuberculosis and malaria, that cause illness and death in underprivileged and impoverished communities, AIDS spreads by infection. HIV-1, the retrovirus that is responsible for the AIDS pandemic, is closely related to a simian immunodeficiency virus (SIV) which infects chimpanzees. HIV-2, which is prevalent in West Africa and has spread to Europe and India, is almost indistinguishable from SIV that infects sooty mangabey monkeys. Although HIV-1 and HIV-2 first arose as infections transmitted from animals to humans, or zoonosis, both are now spread among humans through sexual contact, from mother to infant, and via contaminated blood.

An animal source for a new infection is not unique to HIV. The plague came from rodents. Influenza and the new Nipah virus in Southeast Asia reached humans via pigs. Variant Creutzfeldt-Jakob disease in the United Kingdom came from "mad cows." Once HIV became established in humans, it soon followed human habits and movements. Like other viruses, HIV recognizes no social, political, or geographic boundaries.

The evidence that AIDS is caused by HIV-1 or HIV-2 is clear-cut, exhaustive, and unambiguous. This evidence meets the highest standards of science. The data fulfill exactly the same criteria as for other viral diseases, such as poliomyelitis, measles, and smallpox:

- Patients with acquired immune deficiency syndrome, regardless of where they live, are infected with HIV.
- If not treated, most people with HIV infection show signs of AIDS within five to ten years. HIV infection is identified in blood by detecting antibodies, gene sequences, or viral isolation. These tests are as reliable as any used for detecting other virus infections.
- Persons who received HIV-contaminated blood or blood products develop AIDS, whereas those who received untainted or screened blood do not.
- Most children who develop AIDS are born to HIV-infected mothers. The higher the viral load in the mother the greater the risk of the child becoming infected.
- In the laboratory, HIV infects the exact type of white blood cell (CD4 lymphocytes) that becomes depleted in persons with AIDS.
- Drugs that block HIV replication in the test tube also reduce viral load and delay progression to AIDS. Where available, treatment has reduced AIDS mortality by more than eighty percent.
- Monkeys inoculated with cloned SIV DNA become infected and develop AIDS.

Further compelling data are available. HIV causes AIDS. It is unfortunate that a few vocal people continue to deny the evidence. This position will cost countless lives.

In different regions of the world HIV/AIDS shows altered patterns of spread and symptoms. In Africa, for example, HIV-infected persons are eleven times more likely to die within five years, and more than one hundred times more likely than uninfected persons to develop Kaposi's sarcoma, a cancer linked to yet another virus.

As with any other chronic infection, various co-factors play a role in determining the risk of disease. Persons who are malnourished, who already suffer other infections, or who are older tend to be more susceptible to the rapid development of AIDS following HIV infection. However, none of these factors weaken the scientific evidence that HIV is the sole cause of AIDS.

In this global emergency, prevention of HIV infection must be our greatest worldwide public health priority. The knowledge and tools to prevent infection exist. The sexual spread of HIV can be prevented by monogamy, abstinence, or by using condoms. Blood transmission can be stopped by screening blood products and by not re-using needles. Mother-to-child transmission can be reduced by half or more by short courses of antiviral drugs.

Limited resources and the crushing burden of poverty in parts of the world constitute a formidable challenge to control of HIV infection. People already infected can be helped by treatment with life-saving drugs, but high cost places these treatments out of reach for most. It is crucial to develop new antiviral drugs that are easier to take, have fewer side effects and are much less expensive, so that millions more can benefit from them.

There are many ways to communicate the vital information about HIV/AIDS. What works best in one country may not be appropriate in another. But to tackle the disease, everyone must first understand that HIV is the enemy. Research, not myths, will lead to the development of more effective and cheaper treatments, and hopefully a vaccine. But for now, emphasis must be placed on preventing sexual transmission.

There is no end in sight to the AIDS pandemic. By working together, we have the power to reverse the tide of this epidemic. Science will one day triumph over AIDS, just as it did over smallpox. Curbing the spread of HIV will be the first step. Until then, reason, solidarity, political will, and courage must be our partners.

The declaration was signed by 5,228 physicians and scientists from eighty-four countries who are dedicated to the control of HIV/AIDS.

CHAPTER 8

1. Martha Sherrill, "Cher Sharing," *Washington Post*, June 23, 1989. *www.washingtonpost.com/archive/lifestyle/1989/06/23/cher-sharing/21a3abbc-75fb-4137-a6f4-70ac9266c7fa.*
2. Randy Kennedy, "Elizabeth Glaser Dies at 47: Crusader for Pediatric AIDS," *New York Times*, December 5, 1994. *www.nytimes.com/1994/12/04/obituaries/elizabeth-glaser-dies-at-47-crusader-for-pediatric-aids.html.*

CHAPTER 9

1. Pediatric AIDS Think Tanks held from 1990 to 1998 and attended by more than 350 scientific experts:

    1. Priorities for Pediatric AIDS Research: New Directions. February 1990.
    2. The Role of Immunity in Maternal/Infant HIV Transmission. March 1990.
    3. Interaction of HIV, the Fetal Immune System, and the Placenta. September 1991.
    4. Factors Which Determine Maternal-Infant HIV Transmission. February 1992.
    5. Growth and Nutrition Issues in HIV-Infected Children. September 1992.
    6. Detection of Maternal Cells in Infant Circulation. December 1992.
    7. Priorities in Psychosocial Research in Long-Term Survivors. February 1993.
    8. Acceleration of Drug Evaluation in Women and Children. March 1993.
    9. Mucosal Immunity and HIV Infection: Relevance to Maternal/Infant Transmission. April 1993.
    10. Consensus Workshop on Pediatric AIDS. June 1993.
    11. Zidovudine Resistance in Infants and Children. August 1993.
    12. Mycobacteria as a Paradigm for New Ways to Diagnose, Prevent, and Treat Opportunistic Infections. September 1993.

13. Long-Term Surviving HIV-Infected Children. October 1993.
14. Priorities for Research in HIV-Infected Pregnant Women. October 1993.
15. A Vision for the Future. February 1994.
16. Passive Immunity in HIV. February 1994.
17. Gene Therapy in Pediatric AIDS. April 1994.
18. Immunopathogenesis of HIV Infection in Infants and Children. September 1994.
19. Animal Models in Clinical Trials. January 1995.
20. Development of a Public Service Announcement for Prevention of HIV Infection. January 1995.
21. Pediatric Long-Term Survivors. May 1995.
22. Advancing Perinatal and Early Therapy Trials. September 1995.
23. HIV Exposed but Uninfected Infants. October 1995.
24. Progress in Understanding Long-Term Surviving HIV-Infected Children. April 1996.
25. Gene Therapy for HIV-Infected Children. July 1996.
26. Achievements of the Ariel Project. August 1996.
27. Stem Cell Repository Workshop. October 1996.
28. The Priorities for Pediatric AIDS Research. November 1996.
29. Moving Forward with Gene Therapy for HIV Infection. January 1997.
30. Developing an HIV-1 Vaccine. April 1997.
31. Cellular and Systemic Reservoirs for HIV Replication under Highly Active Antiretroviral Therapy. March 1998.

2. The more than 350 individuals who attended the Think Tanks represented numerous professions, including scientists from diverse specialties, experts in research study design, representatives from the FDA, the NIH, and pharmaceutical companies, and individuals from the activist community. They traveled long distances to attend the meetings, participate in the discussions, contribute to advances, and help with study design, and they often carried out the research that was identified as highest priority. Many of the Think Tank participants continue to work in HIV, advancing prevention and treatment and helping to slow the epidemic and hopefully, eventually, eradicate HIV.

Think Tank Attendees: Abul Abbas, Rafi Ahmed, Myra Alder, Grace Aldrovandi, Nancy Alexander, Jean Pierre Allain, Arthur Ammann, Clark Anderson, Virginia Anderson, Warren Andiman, Daniel Armstrong, Larry Arthur, James Balsley, David Baltimore, Mary Beth Bankson, Arlene Bardeguez, Penny Baron, Alice Baruch, Andreas Bauer, Laurie Bauman, Richard Beach, John Belmont, Phil Berman, Debbie Birx, Roberta Black, Michael Blaese, Kay Blanchard, Barry Bloom, Mary Boland, William Borokowski, Pam Boyer, Thomas Braciale, Samantha Brigham, Corey Brown, Yvonne Bryson, Sandra Burchett, David Burns, Carolyn Burr, Michael Busch, Jan Capper, Antonino Catanzaro, Raymond Chambers, John Chan, Nancy Chang, Irwin Chen, Mallika Chopra, Sheila Clapp, Dan Clemens, Mario Clerici, John Coffin, Fellissa Cohen, Bob Colegrove, Oriel Coll, Edward Conner, Robert Coombs, Susannah Cort, Suzanne Crowe, Clyde Crumpacker, Kenneth Culver, Larry Cummins, Susanna Cunningham-Rundles, Gordon Cutler, Therese Cvetkovich, Joe Dancis, Martin Delaney, Susan DeLaurentis, Bernie Dempsey, Tom Denny, Ron Desrosiers, Paul Deutsch, Yair Devash, Trish Devine, Ruth Dickover, Dimtre Dimitrov, Christine Dobaday, Gordon Douglas, Steven Douglas, Barbara Draimin, Anne Marie Duliege, Lisa Dunkle, Lee Eiden, Leon Epstein, Alejo Erice, Henry Erlich, Alan Ezekowitz, Joanna Fanos, Patricia Fast, Anthony Fauci, David Feigal, Mark Feinberg, John Fitzgibbon, Susan Foster, Mary Glenn Fowler, John Fraser, Lisa Frenkel,

Karen Froebel, Donald Gamin, Ana Garcia, Patricia Garcia, Eileen Garratty, Helene Gayle, Richard Gaynor, Rebeca Gefen, Ronald Germain, Eli Gilboa, Elizabeth Glaser, Mitchell Globus, James Goedert, David Gold, Randall Goldblum, Karen Goldenthal, Aniceto Gonzaga, Maureen Goodenow, Siamon Gordon, Margaret Gorensek, Michael Gottlieb, Jaap Goudsmit, Philip Goulder, Maribeth Gray, Phil Greenberg, Phalguni Gupta, Laura Gutman, Ashley Haase, Nancy Haigwood, Neal Halsey, Hunter Hamill, Scott Hammer, Celine Hanson, Kathy Harmon, Liana Harvath, David Harvey, Esther Hayes, Margo Heath-Chiozzi, Douglas Heiner, Karen Hensch, Belinda Herring, Seth Herrington, Len Herzenberg, William Hickey, Katherine High, Steven Hirschfeld, David Ho, Eddie Holmes, Edward Hoover, Bob Horsburgh, Margaret Hostetter, Dan Hoth, Shui-lok Hu, Chris Hudnall, Eric Hunter, Robert Husson, Margaret Hweagarty, Clark Inderlied, Brooks Jackson, Damir Janigro, Jennifer Jansen, Judy Jansen, Tony Japour, Ann Johanson, Victoria Johnson, Peggy Johnston, Martine Kagnoff, Richard Kaslow, Sam Katz, David Katzenstein, John Kehrl, Amy Keller, Gerald Keusch, Norval King, Mary Klotman, Scott Koenig, Steve Kohl, Donald Kohn, Bette Korbe, Richard Kornbluth, Richard Koup, Mathilde Krim, Paul Krogstad, Dan Kuritzkes, Andrew Lackner, Shenghan Lai, John Lambert, Daniel Landers, Alan Landy, Louisa Laue, Jeffrey Laurence, Norma Letvin, Sandra Lewis, Paul Lietman, Michael Lipson, Stuart Lipton, Ambrosia Louzao, Tom Lowe, Paul Luciw, Margaret Lui, Katherine Luzuriaga, Hermonie Lyall, Catherine Macken, Dean Mann, Richard Marlink, Marta Marthas, Natasha Martin, Angela Martin Amedee, Laurene Mascola, Henry Masur, Bonnie Mathiesson, Douglas Mayer, Justin McArthur, Colin McClaren, Myra McClure, J. Michael McCune, Paul McCurdy, Kenneth McIntosh, Angela McLean, Andrew McMichael, George McSherry, Jim Mestecky, William Meyer, Chris Miller, Joan Milne, Howard Minkoff, Mark Mirochnick, Lynne Mofenson, Luis Montaner, John Moore, Sheldon Morris, Donald Mosier, Howard Moss, Mark Muldoon, James Mullins, Michael Murphy-Corb, Wendy Nehring, Jay Nelson, George Nemo, Hans Ochs, Perry Ogra, Michael Oldstone, James Oleske, Jan Orenstein, Chin-Yih Ou, Maria Pallavicini, Guiseppe Pantaleo, Robert Pass, Roberto Patarca, William Paul, Carol Pearlman, Catherine Peckham, Niels Pedersen, Alan Perelson, Anne Petru, Peter Piot, Philip Pizzo, Susan Plaeger, Edwina Pollack, Henry Pollack, Milissa Pope, Mikulas Popovic, Barbara Potts, Alfred Prince, Paul Pulumbo, Scott Putney, Lee Ratner, Patricia Reichelderfer, Art Reingold, Lionel Resnick, Kenneth Rich, Douglas Richman, Yves Riviere, Merlin Robb, Martha Rogers, Larry Ross, Paolo Rossi, Sarah Rowland-Jones, Beth Roy, Arye Rubinstein, Ruth Ruprecht, Joe Rutledge, Polly Sager, Nava Sarver, Don Schneider, Gwen Scott, Walter Scott, Anita Septimus, George Shaw, Melissa Shepherd, Laurie Sherwin, Fredrick Siegal, Karelynn Siegel, Robert Silicano, Peter Small, Phillip Smith, Dixie Snider, Joseph Sodroski, Stephen Spector, Rhoda Sperling, Jonathan Sprent, Marty St. Clair, Michael St. Louis, Frank Staal, Stuart Starr, Kathy Steimer, Ralph Steinman, Cladd Stevens, E. Richard Stiehm, Jim Stott, Paul Stratton, Jeremy Sugarman, John Sullivan, Robert Suskind, Susan Swain, Richard Sweet, Simon Sweet, Diane Swindel, Susan Taylor-Brown, Michael Thorner, Reed Tuckson, Gareth Tudor-Williams, Ruth Tuomala, John Udal, Christel Uittenbogaart, Michael Usery, Phillippe Van de Perre, Russell Van Dyke, Cindy Vavro, Sten Vermund, Richard Viscarello. Ford Von Reyn, Sam Waksal, Bruce Walker, Charles Wallas, Chip Walter, Jean Wang, Diane Wara, Heather Watts, Jonathan Weber, Chris Weedy, David Weiner, Kent Weinhold, Seth Welles, Raymond Welsh, John Westfall, Timothy Westmoreland, David Wheeler, Lori Wiener, Clayton Wiley, Catherine Wilfert, Christopher Wilson, Darrel Wilson, Robert Winchester, Cheryl Winkler, Harland Winter, Andrew Wiznia, Constance Wofsy, Steve Wolinsky, Joseph Wong, Flossie Wong-Staal, Jonathan Worth, Sumner Yaffe, Lowell Young, Jerome Zack, Susan Zeegen, Ulrike Ziegner, Susan Zolla-Pasner, and Gabriel Zwart.

3. Those who helped organize the Think Tanks and who are deserving of special recognition for their tireless efforts are Natasha Martin, Judy Jansen, Sheila Clapp, Andrea Kloh, Bernie Dempsey, Trish Divine, Carol Pearlman, and Chris Hudnall.

CHAPTER 10

1. Interviews with selected Elizabeth Glaser Scientists were conducted between 2004 and 2012. They were asked to submit a brief summary of what they considered to be their most import discoveries as well as their reflections about Elizabeth Glaser and the Pediatric AIDS Foundation. The final narrative was constructed by the author and reviewed by the scientists through email correspondence.

CHAPTER 11

1. The first clear indication of an association between maternal viral load and HIV transmission was reported by Sperling and collaborators in 1996. Additional reports followed, all confirming the increased transmission of HIV from infected mothers to infants when viral loads were high, and decreased transmission when viral loads were low following treatment. In 1997 the FDA approved viral load as a surrogate marker for efficacy of ART, potentially shortening clinical trials of treatment of HIV infection and treatment to prevent perinatal HIV transmission. More importantly it meant that clinical research end points of advanced disease and death were not required to determine efficacy of an ARV. In spite of the clear documentation of viral load and HIV transmission and the FDA's decision on its use as a surrogate marker, the pediatric AIDS research community continued to plan large, expensive, and prolonged studies using unacceptable variations of inferior treatment. The decision to ignore viral load results and the FDA's approval of accepting viral load as a surrogate marker for research study end points rather than death and progression to AIDS resulted in unnecessary new HIV infections, increased deaths, and prolongation of the pediatric HIV/AIDS epidemic (Sperling et al. 1996).

CHAPTER 12

1. Andrew Budgell. 2016. "HIV/AIDS," Elizabeth Taylor Archives, accessed August 16. *www. dameelizabethtaylor.com/AIDS*.
2. Scot Haller, "The Long Goodbye: Rock Hudson 1925–85," *People*, October 21, 1985. *www.people.com/people/archive/article/0,,20091996,00.html*.
3. Kushnick, "A Mother Tells," 1984.

CHAPTER 13

1. Susan Buchbinder, MD, email message to author, October 25, 2015.

CHAPTER 14

1. "Ritonavir Gets FDA Approval in Record Time," *BioWorld Today*, March 4, 1996.

CHAPTER 15

1. Tim Westmoreland was a legislative aide for Congressman Henry Waxman and was masterful at writing documents and statements that conveyed important issues. I asked Westmoreland to assist in writing a Call to Action (CTA) that would precipitate a movement to end the pediatric AIDS epidemic through prevention and treatment, especially prevention of HIV transmission from mothers to infants. The CTA was an outcome of the 1999 HIVNET 012 clinical study in Uganda, demonstrating that single-dose nevirapine could reduce perinatal HIV transmission by 50 percent. It was the first time that an

inexpensive, easy-to-use treatment for prevention of perinatal HIV transmission was shown to be effective. A press release that I issued as chair of the 1999 conference and president of Global Strategies for HIV Prevention stated, "Since we last met in 1997, we have moved from the ethics of clinical study design in developing countries, to today when we face a more challenging ethical issue of not implementing life-saving prevention therapies— available right now—to save hundreds of thousands of infants' lives from HIV infection."

The Call to Action to Prevent Perinatal HIV Infection

We call for immediate action worldwide to prevent babies from becoming infected with HIV. This action must include: the creation of information programs to raise public awareness of the issue of perinatal transmission and the possibility of reducing it; the establishment and enhancement of programs to deliver perinatal care and medications to pregnant women and babies; the purchase or acquisition of drugs to prevent perinatal transmission for countries that cannot afford them; the delivery of drugs to HIV-infected pregnant women and their babies to prevent perinatal HIV transmission; and continuing research for additional interventions that might further reduce transmission and expanded efforts to prevent infection of all people.

We explicitly call for this action to be in addition to, not in lieu of, prevention programs for adolescents and adults. This call is directed at the governments of all industrial nations. We call on them for immediate support and assistance. We also call on them to negotiate for donations and dramatic discounts from pharmaceutical companies who make the needed drugs and diagnostics and for contributions from all pharmaceutical companies. This call is directed at governments of developing nations. We call on them to create public information and education campaigns to make all potential parents aware of this step toward a healthy baby. We also call on them to strengthen their systems of perinatal care and programs for families. This call is directed at pharmaceutical companies. We call on them to assist directly and indirectly with the cost of implementing programs to reduce infection of babies. We also call on them to donate, discount, and negotiate. Noting that several drug companies have received worldwide acclaim for donations of drugs to cure other diseases in poor nations, we call on all companies to respond to the human need in the HIV/AIDS epidemic.

The global HIV/AIDS epidemic has reached staggering proportions and, at current rates, threatens to transcend all other health problems in the world. It is estimated that more than 33 million people are HIV-infected, 95 percent of these people live in developing nations; 6 million people are infected each year (or about 16,000 per day); half of these newly infected people are young (age 15–24) and 40 percent are women; 600,000 of these newly-infected people are newborns; and more than half a million children die annually from HIV.

At the end of the presentation of the Call to Action, I stated: "We are increasingly frustrated by what appears to us to be indifference to the infection and the ultimate death of hundreds of thousands of children each year. It is ironic that while we work hard to develop better and less expensive prevention treatments, the numbers keep getting larger and larger. This is not a result of lack of research or effective treatment, but a lack of political will."

2. By 1999, as an increasing number of pregnant women were treated with combination antiretroviral therapy to prevent HIV transmission, concerns increased that the drugs might pose a greater danger to the unborn children than did HIV itself and that they would be born with some other damaging side effects. This concern was first seriously voiced in a

report by the French National Epidemiological Network, which for over thirteen years had studied several thousand infants whose mothers had been treated with ZDV during pregnancy at more than ninety obstetrics and pediatric centers throughout France. The study found that eight infants had been born with dysfunctional mitochondria—two of those children died, and the remainder suffered from neurologic abnormalities. While affecting only eight children, the severity of the disorder appropriately aroused considerable concern. The NIH and the CDC immediately initiated a systematic examination of the largest clinical trial groups in the United States—the PACTG, the Women and Infants Transmission Study (WITS), and the Perinatal AIDS Collaborative Transmission Study (PACTS)—to determine whether similar adverse effects had been observed in any children in the United States. After studying more than fifteen thousand infants who had been exposed to antiretroviral drugs perinatally, no similar deaths or disorders were observed. Nonetheless, the French findings provided a crucial impetus both for reviewing toxicity studies of antiretroviral drugs in animal models and for developing a registry of mothers and infants who had been exposed to antiretroviral drugs during pregnancy.

CHAPTER 16

1. David Orr, "Kampala Days: Ghosts That Lurk in Shadows of Hotel's Gory Past," *Independent* (UK), May 20, 1996. *www.independent.co.uk/news/world/kampala-days-ghosts-that-lurk-in-shadows-of-hotels-gory-past-1348320.html*.

2. "Save a Life," *Global Strategies for HIV Prevention Newsletter*, September 2002.

CHAPTER 17

1. "HIV/AIDS in Conflict Situations: Editor's Comment," *AIDS Analysis Africa* 8, no. 5 (1998): 13; "Liberia: Strong Donor Commitment Urged Amid Ongoing War," *IRIN News*, July 30, 2003.

2. "Lyn Lusi: Lyn Lusi, healer of Congo, died on March 17th, aged 62," *Economist*, March 21, 2012. *www.economist.com/node/21551439*.

3. Many individuals and historians were introduced to the accounts of the brutality in the Democratic Republic of Congo through Joseph Conrad's book, *Heart of Darkness* (1899). A more recent book is Adam Hochschild's *King Leopold's Ghost: A Story of Greed, Terror, and Heroism in Colonial Africa*, published in 1998. It recounts the obsession that Belgian King Leopold II had with owning a portion of Africa; the brutal history of the slave trade, high-level deceptions, and denial; and the terrible consequences for the people of the Congo. The reader has to decide who the "ghost of Leopold" is today. Eastern Democratic Republic of Congo continues to be plagued by rebel activity because of its rich mineral resources, but throughout most of Africa there remains the ghost of colonialism seeking and exploiting its resources. The history of colonialism in Africa raises the issue of whether a new form of colonialism exists in the academy in more subtle forms, including the use of the "resource" of vulnerable populations to conduct research not allowed in the United States, research that benefits only those in wealthy countries, or research that is more easily conducted in populations with a high incidence of infection such as HIV. Is it possible that a form of "academic colonialism" seeks and exploits the resource of vulnerable human research subjects without returning commensurate benefit to the peoples of Africa? (A historical profile of the Congo covering the time period from in the 1200s to 2014 is available at *www.bbc.com/news/world-africa-13286306*.)

4. "Congolese Politics: Will Kabila Go?" *Economist*, December 12, 2015. *www.economist.com/news/middle-east-and-africa/21679750-war-weary-citizens-are-scared-joseph-kabila-may-not-retire-gracefully-will*; Conor Gaffey, "Democratic Republic Of Congo: How Do You

Solve a Problem Like Joseph Kabila?" *Newsweek*, February 19, 2016. *www.newsweek.com/dr-congo-how-do-you-solve-problem-kabila-428152*.

5. Christine Oliver, "Worst Places in the World for Women," *Guardian*, June 15, 2011. *www.theguardian.com/world/interactive/2011/jun/15/gender-afghanistan*; Jack Kahorha, "The Worst Places in the World for Women: Congo," *Guardian*, June 14, 2011. *www.theguardian.com/world/2011/jun/14/worst-places-in-the-world-for-women-congo*.

CHAPTER 18

1. "Save a Life," *Global Strategies for HIV Prevention Newsletter*, September 2002.
2. Costa Gazi, "South Africa: ANC Blocks Treatment for HIV Patients," *Green Left Weekly*, June 7, 2000. *www.greenleft.org.au/node/22152*.
3. The visiting scientists from the Chinese Academy of Sciences in Beijing who testified at the 1999 congressional hearing included Dr. Chumming Chen, Chairperson, Advisory Committee on Public Health, Ministry of Public Health; Dr. Jie Shen, Director of Ministry of Health; Dr. Ke-an Wang, President, Chinese Academy of Preventative Medicine; and Dr. Yiquin Wu, Vice President, Chinese Academy of Preventative Medicine for International Cooperation. Also present was Dr. Yunzhen Cao, representing both her position as director of clinical virology at the Chinese Academy of Preventative Medicine as well as her position at Aaron Diamond AIDS Research Center in New York.
4. WHO published their first official guidelines for the treatment of HIV infection in 2002, six years after they had indicated at the International AIDS Conference that they were developing international treatment guidelines, hinting that the recommendations would include starting ARVs at a CD4 count of 500/mm3. To the surprise and shock of many, the 2002 guidelines recommended initiating treatment at CD4 counts of <200/mm3 and only in individuals with the most advanced forms of AIDS. By 2002 the evidence was overwhelming that delaying treatment in HIV-infected individuals was detrimental to their health and, in many cases, failed to reverse the course of HIV infection to fatal disease. The rationale behind these defective recommendations was not clear and can only be deduced as possibly being related to a faulty short-term economic perspective, reasoning that with limited funds it would be best to treat only the most severe and advanced form of the disease. The decision to treat only advanced forms of HIV infection was a historical precedent, previously unheard of in the treatment of infectious diseases and implemented without evidence of benefit, which facilitated the spread of HIV, increased the numbers of newly infected individuals, expand the AIDS orphan epidemic, and increased the long-term economic and health-care burden of HIV.

CHAPTER 19

1. "Scores Killed as Mai-Mai Target Kinyarwanda Speakers," *IRIN News*, June 12, 2012. *www.irinnews.org/report/95626/drc-scores-killed-mai-mai-target-kinyarwanda-speakers*.

CHAPTER 20

1. Laurie McGinley, "In the Line for AIDS Drugs, Children Are Last," *Wall Street Journal*, November 15, 1996.
2. From A. J. Ammann, Pediatric HIV/AIDS Archives, 1981–2016.
3. "Ritonavir Gets FDA Approval in Record Time," *BioWorld Today*, March 4, 1996.
4. Ibid.
5. Ibid.
6. From A. J. Ammann, Pediatric HIV/AIDS Archives, 1981–2016.

CHAPTER 21

1. "Clinton Plans New Rules on Child Drug Safety," *Pharma Letter*, August 19, 1997. *www.thepharmaletter.com/article/clinton-plans-new-rules-on-child-drug-safety*.

2. David Morrow, "New Ranking on Drug Sales in U.S. in '97," *New York Times*, February 27, 1998. *www.nytimes.com/1998/02/27/business/new-ranking-on-drug-sales-in-us-in-97.html*.

3. From A. J. Ammann, Pediatric HIV/AIDS Archives, 1981–2016.

CHAPTER 22

1. The initial members of the National Task Force on AIDS Drug Development, headed by Philip R. Lee, MD, assistant secretary for health and director of the Public Health Service, were the following: Moises Agosto, National Minority AIDS Council Research and Treatment; Arthur Ammann, MD, Pediatric AIDS Foundation; Stephen K. Carter, MD, Bristol-Myers Squibb; Ben Cheng, Project Inform; Deborah J. Cotton, MD, MPH, Harvard Medical School; Mindy Fullilove, PhD, New York State Psychiatric Institute research psychiatrist; David Ho, MD, Aaron Diamond AIDS Research Center; Daniel Hoth, MD, Cell Genesys; David A. Kessler, MD, FDA commissioner; Theresa McGovern, HIV Law Project; Charles Nelson, Morehouse School of Medicine; G. Kirk Raab, Genentech; Robert Schooley, MD, University of Colorado; Edward Scolnick, MD, Merck Research Laboratories; Peter Staley, Treatment Action Group; Harold Varmus, MD, NIH director; Flossie Wong-Staal, PhD, University of California.

2. From A. J. Ammann, Pediatric HIV/AIDS Archives, 1981–2016.

3. Summary and discussion of the Levine Panel recommendations were not without controversy, as summarized by the Treatment Action Group (TAG):

> One of the panel's more controversial recommendations involved pediatric AIDS research. . . ."It's just not clear that, given the reductions in vertical transmission of HIV that have occurred since the completion of ACTG 076, that we will have the statistical power to do large-scale pediatric clinical research in the US." The panel recommended that NIH carefully monitor recruitment into pediatric therapeutic trials, and consider moving funds to overseas efforts if the US does not offer an adequate patient base . . . the panel also recommended melding the existing twelve clinical research networks into one giant clinical research structure. The new network, centered in the National Institute of Allergy and Infectious Diseases (NIAID), would fund a core of sites with the capacity to do intensive laboratory work, including immunology, virology, and pharmacology, as well as a "clinical core" capable of following patients for clinical status, such as rates of opportunistic diseases and death. In addition, the network would be capable of adding investigators, including private physicians, for large-scale phase III/IV studies on an as-needed basis. ("Review and Reform" 1996; NIH 1996)

CHAPTER 23

1. Anthony Banbury, "I Love the UN but It's Failing," *New York Times*, March 18, 2016. *www.nytimes.com/2016/03/20/opinion/sunday/i-love-the-un-but-it-is-failing.html*.

2. From A. J. Ammann, Pediatric HIV/AIDS Archives, 1981–2016.

3. "Heal Thyself: The Ailing International Health Authority Needs a Stronger Organisation," *Economist*, December 13, 2014. *www.economist.com/news/leaders/21636039-ailing-international-health-authority-needs-stronger-organisation-heal-thyself*.

4.   Somini Sengupta, "Panel Calls WHO Unfit to Handle a Crisis Like Ebola," *New York Times*, July 7, 2015. *www.nytimes.com/2015/07/08/world/africa/who-is-not-equipped-to-handle-a-crisis-like-ebola-report-says.html.*

5.   The ability to identify subsets of immunologically competent lymphocytes in blood using laboratory assays was a major step forward in defining how the immune system functioned. The term *T-cell* was applied to lymphocytes that exerted control over immune responses. Two major types were identified—T helper cells, also called CD4 cells, and T suppressor cells, also called CD8 cells. Extensive research revealed that HIV primarily infected CD4 cells, resulting in marked depletion of this subtype of T-cells. Measurement of CD4 cells became widely used as a surrogate of immunologic function in the HIV epidemic because enumeration of CD4 cells was easier and less costly to perform. However, measurement of CD4 cells was never intended to be an absolute indicator of immunologic function. The decision to develop guidelines using CD4 measurements as an indicator of when to initiate ART was a distortion of the principles of infectious-disease treatment. The most critical diagnostic tool for treatment of an infection is to identify the infecting organism and, if treatment is available, to immediately initiate it to prevent the spread of the infecting agent throughout the body, causing permanent and irreversible damage leading to death.

6.   There are theoretical mechanisms for investigating violations of ethical guidelines in clinical research. Research conducted in the United States, in general, undergoes greater scrutiny than research conducted elsewhere. This does not necessarily mean that violations of ethics will not occur. The circumstances in low-income countries require greater scrutiny to prevent exploitation, as most research subjects either lack legal protection or are unaware of their rights to protection. There is also a greater dependence on local IRBs for final approval, which raises the issue of adequate knowledge about a particular research subject as well as ethical guidelines. Approval or disapproval of a research protocol could also be influenced by conflicts of interest—a clinical research study can bring large amounts of funding to a research site to support salaries and infrastructure without benefiting the research subjects themselves. In 2011, Kerry Gough, JD, and I wrote to Amy Gutmann, Chair of the Presidential Commission for the Study of Bioethical Issues, referencing President Obama's 2010 memorandum titled "Review of Human Subjects Protection" (*www.whitehouse.gov/the-press-office/2010/11/24/presidential-memorandum-review-human-subjects-protection*) urging a review of NIH-sponsored studies involving vulnerable HIV-infected women and infants:

> President Obama's charge to the Commission is to 1) review the clinical research conducted by the Tuskegee and Guatemala studies and 2) to determine whether ethical violations currently or potentially exist in the conduct of clinical research sponsored by the US government in low-income countries. If unbiased determinations are to be made, the reviewers and invited presenters of the commission must be free of potential conflicts of interest. Our review of certain NIH-sponsored research studies, and our review of the brief, publically available biographies of commission members and reviewers, raise questions as to whether some individuals may have potential conflicts of interest in reaching unbiased conclusions. (Ammann 2011a)

Although our letter was answered, there was a refusal to review the subject.

7.   Christy Feig and Sonia Shah, "Setting the Record Straight on WHO Funding: Debating the Money Behind the Global Public Health Agenda," *Foreign Affairs*, November 18, 2011. *www.foreignaffairs.com/articles/2011-11-18/setting-record-straight-who-funding.*

CHAPTER 24

1.   The first official guidelines published by WHO for the treatment of HIV infection were released in 2002, six years after the majority of clinicians caring for HIV-infected

individuals were recommending early initiation of HAART in individuals who had minimal impairment of the immune system and who were not at advanced stages of AIDS. As evidence documenting the overwhelming benefits of early initiation of HAART accumulated, WHO remained entrenched in recommending inferior treatment regimens. Although some suspect that this might have been based on economic reasons (e.g., cost of drugs), even when the cost of HAART plummeted from thousands of dollars per year to less than $120 per year, their recommendations remained largely unchanged, denying lifesaving treatment to millions of HIV-infected individuals and perpetuating the HIV epidemic. WHO was the last major health organization to recommend treating all HIV-infected individuals, regardless of immunologic or clinical status, in 2015—more than three years after it had been recommended by the IAS and the US Public Health Service.

2. Banbury, "I Love the UN," 2016.
3. Principles of Treatment. Summary of the Principles of Therapy of HIV Infection from a 1998 Panel of HIV Experts:

   1. Ongoing HIV replication leads to immune system damage and progression to AIDS. HIV infection is always harmful, and true long-term survival free of clinically significant immune dysfunction is unusual.

   2. Plasma HIV RNA levels indicate the magnitude of HIV replication and its associated rate of CD4 T-cell destruction, whereas CD4 T-cell counts indicate the extent of HIV-induced immune damage already suffered. Regular, periodic measurement of plasma HIV RNA levels and CD4 T-cell counts is necessary to determine the risk for disease progression in an HIV-infected person and to determine when to initiate or modify antiretroviral treatment regimens.

   3. As rates of disease progression differ among HIV-infected persons, treatment decisions should be individualized by level of risk indicated by plasma HIV RNA levels and CD4 T-cell counts.

   4. The use of potent combination antiretroviral therapy to suppress HIV replication to below the levels of detection of sensitive plasma HIV RNA assays limits the potential for selection of antiretroviral-resistant HIV variants, the major factor limiting the ability of antiretroviral drugs to inhibit virus replication and delay disease progression. Therefore, maximum achievable suppression of HIV replication should be the goal of therapy.

   5. The most effective means to accomplish durable suppression of HIV replication is the simultaneous initiation of combinations of effective anti-HIV drugs with which the patient has not been previously treated and that are not cross-resistant with antiretroviral agents with which the patient has been treated previously.

   6. Each of the antiretroviral drugs used in combination therapy regimens should always be used according to optimum schedules and dosages.

   7. The available effective antiretroviral drugs are limited in number and mechanism of action, and cross-resistance between specific drugs has been documented. Therefore, any change in antiretroviral therapy increases future therapeutic constraints.

   8. Women should receive optimal antiretroviral therapy regardless of pregnancy status.

   9. The same principles of antiretroviral therapy apply to HIV-infected children, adolescents, and adults, although the treatment of HIV-infected children involves unique pharmacologic, virologic, and immunologic considerations.

   10. Persons identified during acute primary HIV infection should be treated with combination antiretroviral therapy to suppress virus replication to levels below the limit of detection of sensitive plasma HIV RNA assays.

11. HIV-infected persons, even those whose viral loads are below detectable limits, should be considered infectious. Therefore, they should be counseled to avoid sexual and drug-use behaviors that are associated with either transmission or acquisition of HIV and other infectious pathogens. (Report of the NIH Panel to Define Principles of Therapy of HIV Infection 1998)

4. WHO Staging Adults and Adolescents (WHO 2002; 2003 Revision).

Stage I

Asymptomatic

Persistent generalized lymphadenopathy

Performance scale 1: asymptomatic, normal activity

Stage II

Weight loss < 10 percent of body weight

Minor mucocutaneous manifestations (seborrheic dermatitis, purigo, fungal nail infections, recurrent oral ulcerations, angular chalets)

Herpes zoster within the last five years

Recurrent upper respiratory tract infections (i.e., bacterial sinusitis)

Performance scale two: symptomatic, normal activity

Stage III

Weight loss > 10% of body weight

Unexplained chronic diarrhea > one month

Oral candidiasis (thrush)

Oral hairy leukoplakia

Pulmonary tuberculosis within the past year

Severe bacterial infection (i.e., pneumonia, pyomyositis)

And/or performance scale three: bed-ridden < 50% of the day during the past month

Stage IV

HIV wasting syndrome*

Pneumocystis carinii pneumonia

CNS toxoplasmosis

Cryptosporidiosis with diarrhea > one month

Extrapulmonary cryptococcosis

Cytomegalovirus (CMV) disease of an organ other than liver, spleen, or lymph nodes

Herpes simplex virus (HSV) infections, mucocutaneous > one month, or visceral any duration

Progressive multifocal leukoencephalopathy (PML)

Any disseminated endemic mycosis (i.e., histoplasmosis, coccidiodomycosis)

Disseminated atypical mycobacterium

Non-typhoid Salmonella septicemia

Extrapulmonary tuberculosis

Lymphoma

Kaposi's sarcoma (KS)

HIV encephalopathy**

And/or performance scale four: bed-ridden > 50% of the day during the last month

*HIV wasting syndrome: weight loss >10% of body weight plus either unexplained chronic diarrhea > one month or chronic weakness and unexplained prolonged fever > one month.

**HIV encephalopathy: clinical findings of disabling cognitive and/or motor dysfunction inter-
fering with activities of daily living progressing over weeks to months, in the absence of
concurrent illnesses or conditions other than HIV infection that could explain the findings.

CHAPTER 25

1. Sample informed consent from IMPAACT 1077HS. HAART standard version of the
    PROMISE study. The section below is excerpted from the entire informed consent, illus-
    trating the complex nature of the drug names and potential adverse drug effects that would
    be difficult to explain or understand by vulnerable women in low-income settings.

    ### IMPAACT 1077HS. WHAT ARE THE RISKS OF THE STUDY?
    Taking part in this study may involve some risks and discomforts. These include pos-
    sible side effects of the anti-HIV medicines that you and your baby may take, possible
    risks and discomforts from the study tests, and possible risks to your privacy. More
    information is given on each of these types of risks below.

    Side Effects of Anti-HIV Medicines for Women
    Women in the Antepartum Part of the PROMISE Study will take at least three dif-
    ferent anti-HIV medicines. Some of the medicines are combined together in one
    tablet, others come in separate tablets. Until you join the study, we will not know what
    specific medicines you will take. Therefore, this form gives information about all the
    anti-HIV medicines women may take. These are:

    - Atazanavir, taken with or without ritonavir
    - Didanosine (DDI)
    - Efavirenz
    - Emtricitabine
    - Lamivudine (3TC)
    - Lopinavir, taken with ritonavir (Kaletra)
    - Nevirapine (NVP), taken as a single dose during delivery
    - Tenofovir
    - Zidovudine (AZT)

    There are no known side effects of taking a single dose of nevirapine. Each of the other
    medicines can cause side effects, when taken alone and when taken in combination.
    Some side effects are minor, while others can be severe. Some are common, while
    others are rare. If you join the study, the study staff will tell you about the side effects
    of the specific medicines you will take. They will check for side effects during study
    visits and tell you what to do if you have any side effects.

    First you should know about the possible severe side effects. These effects are rare,
    but they can cause serious health problems and can result in death:

    - Severe rash. This can be caused by atazanavir, efavirenz, and lopinavir.
    - Abnormal heart beat, which can result in lightheadedness, fainting, and serious
      heart problems. This can be caused by atazanavir, lopinavir, and ritonavir.
    - Inflammation of the pancreas. The pancreas is an organ near the stomach.
      When the pancreas becomes inflamed, it can cause pain in the belly, nausea,
      vomiting, and increased fats in the blood. This can be caused by didanosine,
      efavirenz, lamivudine, lopinavir, ritonavir, and tenofovir.
    - Inflammation of the liver. The liver is an organ near the stomach. When the
      liver becomes inflamed, it can cause pain and swelling in the belly, nausea, and
      vomiting. This can be caused by efavirenz, lamivudine, lopinavir, ritonavir,
      tenofovir, and zidovudine.

- Lactic acidosis, enlargement of the liver, and fatty liver, which can result in liver failure. Lactic acidosis is an imbalance in the blood that can cause weight loss, pain in the belly, nausea, vomiting, tiredness, weakness and difficulty breathing. When the liver is enlarged, it can cause pain especially on the right side of the belly, swelling in the belly, nausea, vomiting, and loss of appetite. It can also cause bleeding problems that can result in vomiting blood or dark colored stools. Fatty liver is when healthy liver cells are replaced with fat. Sometimes it causes the liver to be enlarged, but doctors usually find out about it from tests of the blood. These effects can be caused by didanosine, emtricitabine, lamivudine, tenofovir, and zidovudine. They occur more often in women, pregnant women, people who are overweight, and people who already have liver problems.
- Kidney damage or failure. The kidneys are organs near the middle of your back (one on each side). Doctors usually find out about kidney damage from tests of the blood. These effects can be caused by tenofovir.
- Severe mental problems, including suicide attempts, aggression, depression, and abnormal thinking. This can be caused by efavirenz. Efavirenz might also cause severe harm to unborn babies if taken during the first month of pregnancy.

2. From A. J. Ammann, Pediatric HIV/AIDS Archives, 1981–2016.

3. There are three "trigger" words that evoke images of unethical clinical research—Tuskegee, Nuremberg, and most recently Guatemala. These represent some of the most egregious, but not the only, violations of medical ethics. Tuskegee involved performing historical observations of untreated syphilis in African Americans; Nuremberg consisted of forced sterilizations, extermination of individuals with mental illness, and medical experiments that resulted in an estimated 200,000 deaths; Guatemala, only recently discovered, involved the deliberate exposure of prisoners and prostitutes to gonorrhea to determine the effectiveness of treatment. All three have in common experiments conducted by academic physicians and scientists, utilization of vulnerable minority populations, experiments which were rationalized as benefiting either the state (Nuremberg) or mankind (Tuskegee and Guatemala), and gradual erosion and an eventual violation of fundamental principles of medical ethics.

In August 2012, *Lancet* published an article titled "Apologizing for Nazi Medicine: A Constructive Starting Point" (Kolb et al 2012). The article presented a written apology by the German Medical Assembly and makes for sobering reading. It is a cautionary warning about how medical science can be seduced into abrogating its role from a patient-oriented approach and an ethically driven philosophy to an authoritarian approach with justification of clinical research for the benefit of the "state." An editorial in the *American Medical Association Journal* agreed (Livingston 2012).

The 115th German Medical Assembly apology begins with the following:

This is the city (Nuremberg) where, sixty-five years ago, twenty physicians were tried for their roles as leading representatives of the state medical authorities of the Nazi regime in committing medical crimes against humanity. Research conducted over the past decades has documented that the extent of human rights violations was vastly greater than documented during the trial. Today, we know considerably more about the goals and practices of various involuntary human experiments, which often ended in death, and the killing of more than 200,000 psychologically ill and disabled people, as well as the forced sterilization of more than 360,000 individuals classified with hereditary illness.

It seems clear that the medical profession, and those engaged in research on humans everywhere, should take seriously the apology and conclusions offered. The apology continues:

> In contrast to still widely accepted views, the initiative for the most serious human rights violations did not originate from the political authorities, but rather from physicians themselves. The crimes were simply not the acts of individual doctors, but rather took place with the substantial involvement of leading representatives of the medical association and medical specialties as institutional bodies, as well as with the considerable participation of eminent representatives of university medicine and renowned biomedical research facilities. These human rights violations perpetrated in the name of medicine under the Nazi regime continue to have repercussions to this day and raise questions concerning the way in which physicians perceive themselves, their professional behavior, and medical ethics. We acknowledge the substantial responsibility of doctors for the medical crimes committed under the Nazi regime and regard these events as a warning for the present and the future.

It would be appropriate to ask whether the trend in current medical research in income-poor and even income-rich countries has already tilted toward the interests of the state (economic) rather than the individual. Offering inferior treatment as a comparative study arm, especially to vulnerable subjects, based on economic interests of the "state" is one example. A perceptible shift in the ethical interpretation of what is standard of care in poor countries is another example and has made it possible to perform clinical research studies that could not be performed in an income-rich country. The impact of such studies is significant, as they have been used by international organizations such as WHO to base their standard of care recommendations on false economic rationales, providing justification for countries to neglect the health of their citizens. The US NIH has also used rationalization based on economics to ethically justify certain research studies in poor countries. It has not gone unnoticed that there are increasing numbers of studies that compare established treatment regimens to shortened treatment regimens to determine if equal efficacy can be attained at a reduced cost, with the research subjects placed at risk in the process, conducting research that has little or no direct benefit to individual research subjects and using studies that do not properly inform participants of risks.

The World Medical Association has revised their international ethical guidelines for research in humans, and at a time when there are increasing questions as to how carefully ethical principles are considered in clinical research studies sponsored by the NIH, it would be wise to closely examine the process of approval of clinical research studies performed both in the United States and in low-income countries to determine if they comply with established scientific and ethical principles (Ammann 2014a).

4.   "Corruption in Kenya: At Long Last, a Prosecution," *Economist*, March 21, 2015. *www.economist.com/news/middle-east-and-africa/21646811-after-long-era-impunity-crooked-politicians-may-now-have-watch-out.*

CHAPTER 26

1.   A further complication was introduced in determining what might be both scientifically and ethically sound when the concept of "for the public good" or "for the good of mankind" was introduced as a justification for performing research in vulnerable subjects in low-income countries. Many ethicists felt that this was a subversion of ethical standards, as the research-study participants would receive no immediate and, in most instances, no long-term benefit from their participation in the research. Some ethicists considered this exploitation of vulnerable populations. In 2002 the Council for International

Organizations of Medical Sciences International Ethical Guidelines for Biomedical Research Involving Human Subjects stated, "If the knowledge gained from the research in such a country is used primarily for the benefit of populations that can afford the tested product, the research may rightly be characterized as exploitative and therefore, unethical" (CIOMS 2002).

2. It is generally assumed that immunization to prevent an infection will result in only one of two outcomes—either failure or success in preventing the targeted infection. However, there is an additional outcome which is not often seen but calls for caution in assuming that immunization can do no harm. Certain vaccines have actually resulted in enhanced disease or enhanced rates of infection when exposed to the natural infection. This is referred to as antibody enhancement. A large clinical trial of an HIV vaccine candidate that increased infection was reported in 2012, which required the study to be discontinued (Duerr et al 2012). A study of passive HIV antibody treatment also demonstrated enhanced infection in infants born to HIV-infected mothers. Although the authors of the study denied that there was an increased rate of infection and death, their own statistical analysis confirmed the fear that some research approaches may actually increase rather than decrease HIV infection (Onyango-Makumbi et al. 2011).

3. There is evidence of widespread indifference in academics and the NIH to ethical concerns raised by advocates seeking to protect vulnerable women and children. Kerry Gough, JD, and I wrote to Francis Collins, director of the NIH, in 2011, calling on him to investigate ethical abuses in NIH studies:

> The Presidential Commission for the Study of Bioethical Issues has recommended that we contact the Office of Human Research Protections (OHRP) regarding our concern about a scientifically and ethically severely flawed NIH-funded research study which needlessly endangered vulnerable Ugandan women and infants (See Onyango-Makumbi, et al, "Safety and Efficacy of HIV Hyperimmune Globulin for Prevention of Mother to Child HIV Transmission in HIV-1-Infected Women in Kampala, Uganda." *JAIDS*, Volume 58, N0.4, 12/1/2011). Our letter to the Presidential Commission, dated November 16, 2011, and its response to us are enclosed. Since OHRP is a part of the NIH, of which you are director, we are addressing our letter to you.

> Feb 12, 2012, Collins replied, "The Office for Human Resource Protections (OHRP), which is not part of NIH, is a component of the Office of the Assistant Secretary for Health in the Department of Health and Human Services. If you also wish to bring your concerns to the attention of OHRP, you can reach the Office at OHRP@hhs.gov or at 866–447–4777." A letter was written to OHRP, which predictably referred us back to the IRBs who had already declined to investigate.

4. On September 15, 2010, Gough and I wrote one of our first letters to Amy Gutmann, Chair of the Presidential National Bioethics Advisory Commission, outlining our increasing concern regarding the ethical conduct of NIH-sponsored studies in low-income countries:

> We are contacting you to express our deep concern regarding ethical issues in certain clinical research studies conducted by the National Institutes of Health in low-income countries. Our purpose is to determine whether your organization will assist in investigating current NIH practices in designing research studies in low-income countries among vulnerable populations. We have been unable to receive a satisfactory response [from NIH].

> We believe that there are specific instances that result in harm to vulnerable women, men, and children placing them at risk for HIV infection and disease

progression. This is a matter of urgent concern as outlined in our most recent letter to NAIAD. Our first inquiries were initiated in 2009. The responses have been unacceptably slow and incomplete and do not adequately address the issues we raised. Below is a brief summary of our concerns.

In the past the NIH has distinguished itself by conducting highly ethical clinical research when enrolling individuals that are particularly vulnerable such as women and children in low-income countries, maintaining high ethical standards and informed consents. These studies provided benefit to research subjects and significantly advanced public health throughout the developing world. Our concerns relate to what appears to be a deviation from previous high ethical standards. (Complete letter available in Ammann, "The Clock Keeps Ticking," in Ethics in Health (blog), September 19, 2016. *ethicsinhealth.org/?p=690*).

5.   John Solomon, 2004, "Research Flawed on Key AIDS Medicine: Bush Had Planned Its Use in Africa," *Washington Post*, December 14, A14. *www.washingtonpost.com/wp-dyn/articles/A62360-2004Dec13.html*.
6.   Susan Buchbinder, MD, email message to author, October 25, 2015.
7.   Serious consideration should be given to whether some IRBs lack the competence to review the ethical and scientific issues related to research in low-income countries. Scientific discovery has advanced to a level where it is difficult even for experts to maintain full knowledge of the impact of research interventions and risks versus benefits. In addition, IRBs are overwhelmed with the sheer number of new research studies that are proposed as well as the requirement to review the studies annually. It has become far too easy to simply rubberstamp proposed research studies. A study that was conducted to evaluate oxygen therapy in premature babies highlights these issues. The informed consent used in the study stated: "Because all of the treatments proposed in the proposed study are standard of care, there is no predictable increase in risk for your baby." However, rather than receiving standard of care, infants were assigned to either the low oxygen value or the high oxygen value, a randomization that would increase the likelihood for the study having significant statistical outcomes—either an increase in retinopathy of prematurity or neurologic complications. The end points of the study were skewed toward complications rather than benefits. The IRBs of multiple academic institutions approved the study, but in all likelihood they lacked the expertise to identify the risks and complications that premature infants would be exposed to (Sabrina Tavernise, "Study of Babies Did Not Disclose Risks, U.S. Finds," *New York Times*, April 10, 2013).
8.   Sam Stein, "Ebola Vaccine Would Likely Have Been Found by Now If Not for Budget Cuts," *Huffington Post*, Oct 16, 2014. *www.huffingtonpost.com/2014/10/12/ebola-vaccine_n_5974148.html*.

CHAPTER 27

1.   Laurie Garrett, "Study: AIDS Funds Often Go Elsewhere," *Newsday*, March 13, 1996.
2.   Laurie Garrett, "Report: AIDS Effort Lacks Vision," *Newsday*, March 14, 1996
3.   From A. J. Ammann, Pediatric HIV/AIDS Archives, 1981–2016.
4.   "AIDS Research Chief Bows Out," *Science Magazine*, October 7, 1997.
5.   Stein, "Ebola Vaccine," 2014.

CHAPTER 28

1.   IMPAACT maintains a list of studies, including the PROMISE studies, on its website at *www.impaactnetwork.org/studies/#promise*.

CHAPTER 31

1. PEPFAR's 2014 goals and five-year strategy were outlined in the publication *The US President's Emergency Plan for AIDS Relief. Five-Year Strategy* ("PEPFAR's Targets" 2014). They are as follows:

    1. Transition from an emergency response to promotion of sustainable country programs.
    2. Strengthen partner government capacity to lead the response to this epidemic and other health demands.
    3. Expand prevention, care, and treatment in both concentrated and generalized epidemics.
    4. Integrate and coordinate HIV/AIDS programs with broader global health and development programs to maximize impact on health systems.
    5. Invest in innovation and operations research to evaluate impact, improve service delivery, and maximize outcomes.

2. In 2014, Deborah Birx was sworn in, replacing Goosby as the new ambassador at large and US global AIDS coordinator to lead all US government international HIV/AIDS efforts to oversee and implement PEPFAR. Details of her view on goals and implementation are available on the PEPFAR website (*www.pepfar.gov*).

CHAPTER 32

1. From A. J. Ammann, Pediatric HIV/AIDS Archives, 1981–2016.
2. Global Strategies for HIV Prevention developed a campaign and a blog urging all organizations to recommend early initiation of HAART for all HIV-infected individuals. The campaign was launched in 2012 at the Nineteenth International AIDS Conference in Washington, DC, stating, "At last! The United States Public Health Service released treatment recommendations for HIV-infected individuals. ART is recommended for all HIV-infected individuals. It's simple, straightforward, and lifesaving. Now is the time to make certain that all HIV-infected individuals throughout the world get treated. It will save lives, it will decrease tens of thousands of new HIV infections, it will decrease the complications and long-term cost of treating HIV infection, and it will decrease hundreds of thousands of new HIV-related children entering orphanhood" (Ammann 2012).
3. Conclusions from *Sixteen Ideas for Addressing Violence against Women in the Context of the HIV Epidemic*:

    • Laws that are based on international human rights standards for addressing violence against women, promoting gender equality, and protecting the rights of communities affected by and living with HIV from discrimination can create an enabling environment for reducing women's vulnerability to violence and HIV.
    • In many countries, law reforms have not necessarily yielded changes on the ground for women, in part because laws are not adequately operationalized or enforced and national policies and implementation plans are not adequately resourced.
    • Improving women's access to justice may require strengthening the broader justice system. This may require strengthening capacities of the police, judiciary, paralegals, and forensic experts to: recognize the problem of violence against women; reflect on their own biases including against key populations affected by HIV; and interpret laws and respond appropriately. Strengthening coordination, referrals, and linkages among different sectors providing services to women who experience violence (e.g., legal, police protection, health care, safe space, psychosocial support) is also necessary.

- Efforts to train police, judiciary forensic experts, and others need buy-in from senior management. Such efforts may need to be integrated into pre- and in-service curricula, and into law enforcement and legal practices in routine procedures and protocols. It is not necessarily true that female police or judges are, by virtue of their sex, automatically more sensitive to women survivors of violence.
- National policies, protocols, and plans are useful mechanisms for guiding, resourcing, coordinating, and ensuring accountability of national responses to violence against women. While a number of good practices are emerging in developing such plans, policies, and protocols, their implementation lags behind due to lack of political will and lack of resources.
- Policies to reduce the harmful consequences of alcohol represent an emerging area of intervention to reduce violence against women and HIV risk. More evaluations are needed to assess the impact of policies and of individual and community interventions to reduce problem drinking on violence and HIV risk, especially in low- and middle-income countries. (WHO and UNAIDS 2013, 45).

4. WHO Definitions of Violence Against Women:

> Violence against women (VAW). Any public or private act of gender-based violence that results in, or is likely to result in, physical, sexual, or psychological harm or suffering to women, including threats of such acts, coercion, or arbitrary deprivation of liberty with the family or general community.
> Gender-based violence (GBV). Violence that establishes, maintains, or attempts to reassert unequal power relationships based on gender.
> Intimate partner violence (IPV). Behavior within an intimate relationship that causes physical, sexual, or psychological harm, including acts of physical aggression, sexual coercion, psychological abuse, and controlling behaviors.
> Sexual violence including rape. Any sexual act, attempt to obtain a sexual act, unwanted sexual comment or advance, or attempts to traffic, or act otherwise directed against a person's sexuality using force or by any person regardless of their relationship to the victim, in any setting including, but not limited to, home and work. (WHO and UNAIDS 2013, 3)

5. Sexual violence against women has long been a recognized consequence of war. There is an emerging consensus that sexual violence and rape during warfare have been integrated into a deliberate and nefarious means of destabilizing opposing populations. The higher rate of HIV infection in individuals who rape and the use of both pregnancy and deliberate HIV infection during genocides support the concept that gender-based violence and HIV infection are synergistic epidemics. The association of protracted conflict with migration lends itself to dissemination of HIV infection during conflict and post-conflict periods. There is sufficient evidence, based on observations in conflict settings and studies of intimate partner violence, of a nexus between violence against women and increased risk for HIV infection. This circumstance should be viewed as an international public-health issue and a crime against humanity that targets women and contributes to the spread of HIV by establishing reservoirs of HIV infection that can ignite or reignite the spread of HIV. The issues of gender-based violence and the increasing use of rape and HIV as weapons of choice for destabilizing populations must be addressed at the international level to develop and fully enforce international laws to restrain sexual violence against women, protect them from fatal HIV infection, and prevent the spread of HIV (Jewkes et al. 2010; Dunkle et al. 2004; Townsend et al. 2011).

6. From A. J. Ammann, Pediatric HIV/AIDS Archives, 1981–2016.

7. Abigail Zuger, "AIDS in Africa: Rising Above the Partisan Babble," *New York Times*, July 3, 2007. *www.nytimes.com/2007/07/03/health/03book.html.*

8. An estimate of how many new HIV infections and HIV-related deaths could have been prevented can be approximated using data derived from research studies and HIV-surveillance information. The rates of death and new infections prior to implementation of HAART can be compared to those in the years following implementation. Additional data comes from surveillance studies conducted by the CDC and local public health departments.

    Dramatic decreases in new HIV infections and in HIV-related mortality in adults were documented by the CDC following increased use of HAART beginning in 1996 (CDC 2015). Within four years, without any additional US research studies beyond the 1994 zidovudine study on perinatal HIV transmission, the number of new perinatal HIV infections decreased from over two thousand per year to fewer than one hundred per year as physicians and other health-care providers implemented early diagnosis and combination antiretroviral treatment for pregnant women (CDC 2006). More recently, the San Francisco public health department reported that new HIV infections in adults decreased from a peak of 2,332 new infections to 302 in 2104. The number of AIDS-related deaths decreased from 1,641 in 1992 to 177 in 2014. The results were attributed primarily to "test and treat," initiated in 2002, in which individuals were tested for HIV and immediately started on treatment with HAART, and the subsequent implementation of pre-exposure prophylaxis. San Francisco, once the epicenter of HIV in California and the city where AIDS was first reported in children, had no HIV-infected infant in ten years.

REFERENCES

"Abbott Protease Inhibitor in Combination: Sustained Viral Load Drop." 1995. *AIDS Treatment News*, no. 231 (Sept. 29). *www.thebody.com/content/art31465.html#Abbott*.

Abrams, Elaine J., R. J. Simonds, Surbhi Modi, et al. 2012. "PEPFAR Scale-up of Pediatric HIV Services: Innovations, Achievements, and Challenges." *Journal of Acquired Immune Deficiency Syndromes* 60 (suppl. 3): S105–12. doi: 10.1097/QAI.0b013e31825cf4f5.

Adler, M. W., and A. M. Johnson. 1988. "Contact Tracing for HIV Infection." *British Medical Journal (Clinical Research Edition)* 296 (6634): 1420–21.

Akiki, Faith Spicer. 2002. "The Focus On Women Kampala Declaration: Ugandan Women Call For Action On HIV / AIDS." *British Medical Journal* 324 (7331): 247. Stable url: *www.jstor.org/stable/25227311*.

Alfano, S. L. 2013. "Conducting Research with Human Subjects in International Settings: Ethical Considerations." *Yale Journal of Biology and Medicine* 86 (3): 315–21.

Allen, C., M. Mbonye, J. Seeley, J. Birungi, B. Wolff, A. Coutinho, and S. Jaffar. 2011. "ABC for People with HIV: Responses to Sexual Behaviour Recommendations among People Receiving Antiretroviral Therapy in Jinja, Uganda." *Culture, Health, and Sexuality* 13 (5): 529–43. doi: 10.1080/13691058.2011.558593.

Allers, K., G. Hutter, J. Hofmann, C. Loddenkemper, K. Rieger, E. Thiel, and T. Schneider. 2010. "Evidence for the Cure of HIV Infection by CCR5delta32/Delta32 Stem Cell Transplantation." *Blood* 117 (10): 2791–99. doi: 10.1182/blood-2010–09–309591.

Altema, R., and L. Bright. 1983. "Only Homosexual Haitians, Not All Haitians." *Annals of Internal Medicine* 99 (6): 877–88.

Altman, Lawrence. 1981. "Rare Cancer Seen in 41 Homosexuals," *New York Times*, July 3. *www.nytimes.com/1981/07/03/us/rare-cancer-seen-in-41-homosexuals.html*.

———. 1996. "Panel Offers Sharp Criticism of AIDS Research Projects." *New York Times*, March 14. *www.nytimes.com/1996/03/14/us/panel-offers-sharp-criticism-of-aids-research-projects.html*.

amfAR. 2012a. "30 Years of HIV/AIDS: Snapshots of an Epidemic." amfAR.org. Accessed March 22, 2016. *www.amfar.org/about_hiv_and_aids/more_about_hiv_and_aids/thirty_years_of_hivaids__snapshots_of_an_epidemic*.

———. 2012b. "Dame Elizabeth Taylor: Founding International Chairman." amfAR. org. Accessed March 22, 2016. *www.amfar.org/about_amfar/trustee_biographies/dame_elizabeth_taylor*.

Ammann, A. J. 1983. "Is There an Acquired Immune Deficiency Syndrome in Infants and Children?" *Pediatrics* 72 (3): 430–32.

———. 1985. "The Acquired Immunodeficiency Syndrome in Infants and Children." *Annals of Internal Medicine* 103 (5): 734–37.

———. 1994. "Human Immunodeficiency Virus Infection / AIDS in Children: The Next Decade." *Pediatrics* 93 (6 Pt 1): 930–35.

———. 1995. "AIDS Leadership Award Acceptance Speech. Harvard AIDS Institute." *Pediatric AIDS and HIV Infection* 6:129–30.

———. 2000a. "HIV in China: An Opportunity to Halt an Emerging Epidemic." *AIDS Patient Care and STDs* 14 (3): 109–12. doi: 10.1089/108729100317885.

———. 2003. "Preventing HIV." *British Medical Journal* 326 (7403): 1342–43. doi: 10.1136/
bmj.326.7403.1342.

———. 2005. "Completing the Public Health HIV/AIDS Alphabet." *PLOS Medicine* 2 (1):
e28. doi: 10.1371/journal.pmed.0020028.

———. 2006. "Saving Lives Globally: Dr. Krim and amfAR." *AIDS Patient Care and STDs* 20
(7): 461–62. doi: 10.1089/apc.2006.20.461.

———. 2009. "Optimal Versus Suboptimal Treatment for HIV-Infected Pregnant Women and
HIV-Exposed Infants in Clinical Research Studies." *Journal of Acquired Immune Deficiency
Syndromes* 51 (5): 509–12. doi: 10.1097/QAI.0b013e3181aa8a3d.

———. 2011a. "An Open Letter to the Presidential Commission for the Study of Bioethical
Issues." *Ethics in Health* (blog), October 17. *ethicsinhealth.org/?p=57.*

———. 2011b. "Who Will Protect Vulnerable Populations from Research Exploitation?" *Ethics
in Health* (blog), December 8. *ethicsinhealth.org/?p=221.*

———. 2012. "Treat All as the Standard of Care: What Now?" *Ethics in Health* (blog),
September 12. *ethicsinhealth.org/?p=395.*

———. 2013. "US Clinical-Research System in Need of Review." *Nature* 498 (7452): 7. doi:
10.1038/498007a.

———. 2014a. "Doing Away with Ethical Guidelines. What's Going On?" *Ethics in Health*
(blog), February 26. *ethicsinhealth.org/?p=527.*

———. 2014b. "From Scarcity to Abundance: Who Decides the Priority for Clinical Trials
in Resource Poor Countries?" Global HIV Vaccine Enterprise. Accessed March 22, 2016.
*www.vaccineenterprise.org/content/scarcity-abundance-who-decides-priority-clinical-trials-
resource-poor-countries.*

———. 2015a. "Are IRBs Uninformed about Informed Consents?" *Ethics in Health* (blog),
March 3. *ethicsinhealth.org/?p=558.*

———. 2015b. "A Hollow Victory." *Ethics in Health* (blog), June 24. *ethicsinhealth.org/?p=572.*

———. 2015c. "The Right to Know vs The Failure to Inform." *Ethics in Health* (blog),
November 10. *ethicsinhealth.org/?p=591.*

———. 2016. "The Calculus of Human Value." *Ethics in Health* (blog), March 23. *ethicsin-
health.org/?p=607.*

Ammann, A. J., D. Abrams, M. Conant, D. Chudwin, M. Cowan, P. Volberding, B. Lewis, and
C. Casavant. 1983. "Acquired Immune Dysfunction in Homosexual Men: Immunologic
Profiles." *Clinical Immunology and Immunopathology* 27 (3): 315–25.

Ammann, A. J., M. J. Cowan, D. W. Wara, P. Weintrub, S. Dritz, H. Goldman, and H. A.
Perkins. 1983. "Acquired Immunodeficiency in an Infant: Possible Transmission by Means
of Blood Products." *Lancet* 1 (8331): 956–58.

Ammann, A. J., K. Gough, and A. Caplan. 2012. "Were the Interests of the Vulnerable
Truly Served? The Predictable Failure of HIVIG." *Journal of Acquired Immune Deficiency
Syndromes* 61 (1): e8-e10. doi: 10.1097/QAI.0b013e318253a5dc.

Ammann, A. J., L. Kaminsky, M. Cowan, and J. A. Levy. 1985. "Antibodies to AIDS-Associated
Retrovirus Distinguish between Pediatric Primary and Acquired Immunodeficiency
Diseases." *Journal of the American Medical Association* 253 (21): 3116–118.

Ammann, A. J., D. W. Wara, and M. J. Cowan. 1984. "Pediatric Acquired Immunodeficiency
Syndrome." *Annals of the New York Academy of Sciences* 437:340–49.

Angell, M. 1997. "The Ethics of Clinical Research in the Third World." *New England Journal of
Medicine* 337 (12): 847–49. doi: 10.1056/NEJM199709183371209.

Arshagouni, Paul. 2002. "Federal Court Invalidates the FDA Pediatric Rule: AAPS v. FDA."
University of Houston Law Center, December 23. Accessed March 22, 2016, *www.law.
uh.edu/healthlaw/perspectives/Children/021223Federal.html.*

Auerbach, D. M., W. W. Darrow, H. W. Jaffe, and J. W. Curran. 1984. "Cluster of Cases of the Acquired Immune Deficiency Syndrome: Patients Linked by Sexual Contact." *American Journal of Medicine* 76 (3): 487–92.

Auvert, B., A. Buvé, B. Ferry, et al. 2001. "Ecological and Individual Level Analysis of Risk Factors for HIV Infection in Four Urban Populations in Sub-Saharan Africa with Different Levels of HIV Infection." *AIDS* 15 (suppl. 4): S15–30.

Bachman, D. M., M. M. Rodrigues, F. C. Chu, S. E. Straus, D. G. Cogan, and A. M. Macher. 1982. "Culture-Proven Cytomegalovirus Retinitis in a Homosexual Man with the Acquired Immunodeficiency Syndrome." *Ophthalmology* 89 (7): 797–804.

Baeten, J., and C. Celum. 2012. "Oral Antiretroviral Chemoprophylaxis: Current Status." *Current Opinion in HIV and AIDS* 7 (6): 514–19. doi: 10.1097/COH.0b013e3283582d30.

Barouch, D. H. 2013. "The Quest for an HIV-1 Vaccine—Moving Forward." *New England Journal of Medicine* 369 (22): 2073–76. doi: 10.1056/NEJMp1312711.

Barre-Sinoussi, F., J. C. Chermann, F. Rey, et al. 1983. "Isolation of a T-Lymphotropic Retrovirus from a Patient at Risk for Acquired Immune Deficiency Syndrome (AIDS)." *Science* 220 (4599): 868–71.

Bartels, S. A., J. A. Scott, J. Leaning, J. T. Kelly, D. Mukwege, N. R. Joyce, and M. J. Vanrooyen. 2011. "Sexual Violence Trends between 2004 and 2008 in South Kivu, Democratic Republic of Congo." *Prehospital and Disaster Medicine* 26 (6): 408–13. doi: 10.1017/s1049023x12000179.

Bateman, C. 2007. "Paying the Price for AIDS Denialism." *South African Medical Journal* 97 (10): 912–14.

BBC. 2014. "Democratic Republic of Congo Profile." *BBC News.* Last updated February 10, 2016. Accessed March 22, 2016, *www.bbc.com/news/world-africa-13283212.*

Becquet, R., and L. M. Mofenson. 2008. "Early Antiretroviral Therapy of HIV-Infected Infants in Resource-Limited Countries: Possible, Feasible, Effective and Challenging." *AIDS* 22 (11): 1365–68. doi: 10.1097/QAD.0b013e32830437f5.

Bemelmans, M., S. Baert, E. Goemaere, et al. 2014. "Community-Supported Models of Care for People on HIV Treatment in Sub-Saharan Africa." *Tropical Medicine and International Health* 19 (8): 968–77. doi: 10.1111/tmi.12332.

Bendavid, E., R. Wood, D. A. Katzenstein, A. M. Bayoumi, and D. K. Owens. 2009. "Expanding Antiretroviral Options in Resource-Limited Settings: A Cost-Effectiveness Analysis." *Journal of Acquired Immune Deficiency Syndromes* 52 (1): 106–13. doi: 10.1097/QAI.0b013e3181a4f9c4.

Beyrer, C., D. L. Birx, L. G. Bekker, et al. 2015. "The Vancouver Consensus: Antiretroviral Medicines, Medical Evidence, and Political Will." *Lancet* 386 (9993): 505–7. doi: 10.1016/s0140–6736(15)61458–1.

Bishop, J. M., N. Jackson, W. E. Levinson, E. Medeiros, N. Quintrell, and H. E. Varmus. 1973. "The Presence and Expression of RNA Tumor Virus Genes in Normal and Infected Cells: Detection by Molecular Hybridization." *American Journal of Clinical Pathology* 60 (1): 31–43.

Blanche, S., M. J. Mayaux, C. Rouzioux, et al. 1994. "Relation of the Course of HIV Infection in Children to the Severity of the Disease in Their Mothers at Delivery." *New England Journal of Medicine* 330 (5): 308–12. doi: 10.1056/nejm199402033300502.

Blanche, S., M. L. Newell, M. J. Mayaux, D. T. Dunn, J. P. Teglas, C. Rouzioux, and C. S. Peckham. 1997. "Morbidity and Mortality in European Children Vertically Infected by HIV-1. The French Pediatric HIV Infection Study Group and European Collaborative Study." *Journal of Acquired Immune Deficiency Syndromes and Human Retrovirology* 14 (5): 442–50.

Blanche, S., M. Tardieu, P. Rustin, et al. 1999. "Persistent Mitochondrial Dysfunction and Perinatal Exposure to Antiretroviral Nucleoside Analogues." *Lancet* 354 (9184): 1084–89. doi: 10.1016/s0140–6736(99)07219–0.

Blaser, N., C. Wettstein, J. Estill, L. S. Vizcaya, G. Wandeler, M. Egger, and O. Keiser. 2014. "Impact of Viral Load and the Duration of Primary Infection on HIV Transmission: Systematic Review and Meta-Analysis." *AIDS* 28 (7): 1021–29. doi: 10.1097/qad.0000000000000135.

Bleicher, Josh. 2014. "Interview with Dr. Goosby." *Master's Corner* (blog), February 18. Global Health Sciences. University of California San Francisco. *globalhealthsciences.ucsf.edu/education-training/blogs/masters-corner/interview-with-dr-goosby*.

Bobat, R., D. Moodley, A. Coutsoudis, and H. Coovadia. 1997. "Breastfeeding by HIV-1-Infected Women and Outcome in Their Infants: A Cohort Study from Durban, South Africa." *AIDS* 11 (13): 1627–33.

Bogart, L. M., B. O. Cowgill, D. Kennedy, G. Ryan, D. A. Murphy, J. Elijah, and M. A. Schuster. 2008. "HIV-Related Stigma among People with HIV and Their Families: A Qualitative Analysis." *AIDS and Behavior* 12 (2): 244–54. doi: 10.1007/s10461–007–9231-x.

Bond, Patrick. 2004. "South Africa's Deadly Decade of HIV Denial." *Solidarity*, July-August. Accessed March 22, 2016, *www.solidarity-us.org/node/1117*.

Brandt, A. M. 2013. "How AIDS Invented Global Health." *New England Journal of Medicine* 368 (23): 2149–52. doi: 10.1056/NEJMp1305297.

Branson, B. M., H. H. Handsfield, M. A. Lampe, R. S. Janssen, A. W. Taylor, S. B. Lyss, and J. E. Clark. 2006. "Revised Recommendations for HIV Testing of Adults, Adolescents, and Pregnant Women in Health-Care Settings." *Morbidity and Mortality Weekly Report Recommendations and Reports* 55 (Rr-14): 1–17; quiz CE1–4.

Broder, S., and R. C. Gallo. 1984. "A Pathogenic Retrovirus (HTLV-III) Linked to AIDS." *New England Journal of Medicine* 311 (20): 1292–97. doi: 10.1056/NEJM198411153112006.

Bulterys, M., S. Nesheim, E. J. Abrams, P. Palumbo, J. Farley, M. Lampe, and M. G. Fowler. 2000. "Lack of Evidence of Mitochondrial Dysfunction in the Offspring of HIV-Infected Women: Retrospective Review of Perinatal Exposure to Antiretroviral Drugs in the Perinatal AIDS Collaborative Transmission Study." *Annals of the New York Academy of Sciences* 918:212–21.

"Call to Action: Towards an HIV-free and AIDS-free Generation." 2005. Prevention of Mother-to-Child Transmission (PMTCT) High Level Global Partners Forum. Abuja, Nigeria, December 3. *www.who.int/hiv/mtct/pmtct_calltoaction.pdf*.

Camus, Albert. (1947) 1972. *The Plague*. Translated by Stuart Gilbert. Reprint, New York: Vintage Books.

Carlo, W. A., E. F. Bell, and M. C. Walsh. 2013. "Oxygen-Saturation Targets in Extremely Preterm Infants." *New England Journal of Medicine* 368 (20): 1949–50. doi: 10.1056/NEJMc1304827.

Carpenter, C. C., M. A. Fischl, S. M. Hammer, et al. 1996. "Antiretroviral Therapy for HIV Infection in 1996: Recommendations of an International Panel. International AIDS Society-USA." *Journal of the American Medical Association* 276 (2): 146–54.

———. 1997. "Antiretroviral Therapy for HIV Infection in 1997. Updated Recommendations of the International AIDS Society-USA Panel." *Journal of the American Medical Association* 277 (24): 1962–69.

Carr, A., and D. A. Cooper. 1996. "Current Clinical Experience with Nevirapine for HIV Infection." *Advances in Experimental Medicine and Biology* 394:299–304.

Casarett, D. J., and J. D. Lantos. 1998. "Have We Treated AIDS Too Well? Rationing and the Future of AIDS Exceptionalism." *Annals of Internal Medicine* 128 (9): 756–59.

CDC (Centers for Disease Control and Prevention). 1981a. "Follow-up on Kaposi's Sarcoma and Pneumocystis Pneumonia." *Morbidity and Mortality Weekly Report* 30 (33): 409–10.

———. 1981b. "Kaposi's Sarcoma and Pneumocystis Pneumonia among Homosexual Men—New York City and California." *Morbidity and Mortality Weekly Report* 30 (25): 305–8.

———. 1981c. "Pneumocystis Pneumonia—Los Angeles." *Morbidity and Mortality Weekly Report* 30 (21): 250–52.

———. 1982a. "Possible Transfusion-Associated Acquired Immune Deficiency Syndrome (AIDS)—California." *Morbidity and Mortality Weekly Report* 31 (48): 652–54.

———. 1982b. "Unexplained Immunodeficiency and Opportunistic Infections in Infants—New York, New Jersey, California." *Morbidity and Mortality Weekly Report* 31 (49): 665–67.

———. 1982c. "Update on Acquired Immune Deficiency Syndrome (AIDS)—United States." *Morbidity and Mortality Weekly Report* 31 (37): 507–8, 513–14.

———. 1982d. "Update on Acquired Immune Deficiency Syndrome (AIDS) among Patients with Hemophilia A." *Morbidity and Mortality Weekly Report* 31 (48): 644–46, 652.

———. 2006. "Achievements in Public Health. Reduction in Perinatal Transmission of HIV Infection—United States, 1985–2005." *Morbidity and Mortality Weekly Report* 55 (21): 592–97.

———. 2015. "HIV Diagnoses Decline Almost 20 Percent, but Progress Is Uneven." NCHHSTP Newsroom, December 6. *www.cdc.gov/nchhstp/newsroom/2015/nhpc-press-release-hiv-diagnoses.html*.

Chamow, S. M., A. M. Duliege, A. Ammann, et al. 1992. "CD4 Immunoadhesins in Anti-HIV Therapy: New Developments." *International Journal of Cancer*, suppl. 7, 69–72.

Check, E. 2005. "Activists Angry at Fallout from AIDS Drug Trial Allegations." *Nature Medicine* 11 (3): 238. doi: 10.1038/nm0305–238a.

Chen, Y., R. Winchester, B. Korber, et al. 1997. "Influence of HLA Alleles on the Rate of Progression of Vertically Transmitted HIV Infection in Children: Association of Several HLA-DR13 Alleles with Long-Term Survivorship and the Potential Association of HLA-A*2301 with Rapid Progression to AIDS. Long-Term Survivor Study." *Human Immunology* 55 (2): 154–62.

Chermann, J. C., F. Barre-Sinoussi, C. Dauguet, F. Brun-Vezinet, C. Rouzioux, W. Rozenbaum, and L. Montagnier. 1983. "Isolation of a New Retrovirus in a Patient at Risk for Acquired Immunodeficiency Syndrome." *Antibiotics and Chemotherapy* 32:48–53.

"Child Cured of HIV." 2013. Forum with Michael Krasny. KQED radio, March 5. *www.kqed.org/a/forum/R201303050900*.

Chigwedere, P., and M. Essex. 2010. "AIDS Denialism and Public Health Practice." *AIDS and Behavior* 14 (2): 237–47. doi: 10.1007/s10461-009-9654-7.

CIOMS (Council for International Organizations of Medical Sciences). 2002. "International Ethical Guidelines for Biomedical Research Involving Human Subjects." Geneva: WHO. *www.cioms.ch/publications/layout_guide2002.pdf*.

ClinicalTrials.gov. 2016a. "Clinical Trials. VRC601: A Phase I, Open-Label, Dose-Escalation Study of the Safety and Pharmacokinetics of a Human Monoclonal Antibody, VRCHIV mab060–00-Ab (VRC01), with Broad HIV-1 Neutralizing Activity, Administered Intravenously or Subcutaneously to HIV-Infected Adults." Sponsor: NIAID. (ClinicalTrials.gov identifier: NCT01950325). Last updated, Aug. 6. *clinicaltrials.gov/ct2/show/NCT01950325*.

————. 2016b. "Evaluating the Safety and Efficacy of the VRC01 Antibody in Reducing Acquisition of HIV-1 Infection in Women." Sponsor: NIAID. (ClinicalTrials.gov identifier: NCT02568215). Accessed March 26. *clinicaltrials.gov/ct2/show/NCT02568215*.

Coetzee, D., K. Hilderbrand, E. Goemaere, F. Matthys, and M. Boelaert. 2004. "Integrating Tuberculosis and HIV Care in the Primary Care Setting in South Africa." *Tropical Medicine and International Health* 9 (6): A11–5. doi: 10.1111/j.1365–3156.2004.01259.x.

Coffin, J., A. Haase, J. A. Levy, et al. 1986. "What to Call the AIDS Virus?" *Nature* 321 (6065): 10.

Cohen, A., D. Doyle, D. W. Martin, Jr., and A. J. Ammann. 1976. "Abnormal Purine Metabolism and Purine Overproduction in a Patient Deficient in Purine Nucleoside Phosphorylase." *New England Journal of Medicine* 295 (26): 1449–54. doi: 10.1056/NEJM197612232952603.

Cohen, I. Glenn. 2003. "Therapeutic Orphans, Pediatric Victims? The Best Pharmaceuticals for Children Act and Existing Pediatric Human Subject Protection." *Food and Drug Law Journal* 58:661–709.

Cohen, J. 1996. "AIDS Task Force Fizzles Out." *Science* 271 (5248): 438–39.

————. 1998. "Exploring How to Get at—and Eradicate—Hidden HIV." *Science* 279 (5358): 1854–55.

————. 2011. "Breakthrough of the Year: HIV Treatment as Prevention." *Science* 334 (6063): 1628. doi: 10.1126/science.334.6063.1628.

————. 2015. "Treat All HIV-Infected People, Says New WHO Guideline." *Science*, September 30. *www.sciencemag.org/news/2015/09/treat-all-hiv-infected-people-says-new-who-guideline*.

Cohen, M. S. 2010. "HIV Treatment as Prevention: To Be or Not to Be?" *Journal of Acquired Immune Deficiency Syndromes* 55 (2): 137–38. doi: 10.1097/QAI.0b013e3181f0cbf3.

Cohen, M. S., Y. Q. Chen, M. McCauley, et al. 2011. "Prevention of HIV-1 Infection with Early Antiretroviral Therapy." *New England Journal of Medicine* 365 (6): 493–505. doi: 10.1056/NEJMoa1105243.

Connor, E. M., R. S. Sperling, R. Gelber, et al. 1994. "Reduction of Maternal-Infant Transmission of Human Immunodeficiency Virus Type 1 with Zidovudine Treatment. Pediatric AIDS Clinical Trials Group Protocol 076 Study Group." *New England Journal of Medicine* 331 (18): 1173–80. doi: 10.1056/nejm199411033311801.

Contopoulos-Ioannidis, D. G., and J. P. Ioannidis. 1998. "Maternal Cell-Free Viremia in the Natural History of Perinatal HIV-1 Transmission: A Meta-Analysis." *Journal of Acquired Immune Deficiency Syndromes and Human Retrovirology* 18 (2): 126–35.

Cooper, E. R., M. Charurat, L. Mofenson, et al. 2002. "Combination Antiretroviral Strategies for the Treatment of Pregnant HIV-1-Infected Women and Prevention of Perinatal HIV-1 Transmission." *Journal of Acquired Immune Deficiency Syndromes* 29 (5): 484–94.

"Court Upholds Mother's Right to Decline Medicines for Son." 1998. *AIDS Policy Law* 13 (22): 3.

Coutsoudis, A., A. Goga, C. Desmond, P. Barron, V. Black, and H. Coovadia. 2013. "Is Option B+ the Best Choice?" *The Lancet* 381 (9863): 269–71.

Culliton, B. J. 1972. "Dual Publication: 'Ingelfinger Rule' Debated by Scientists and Press." *Science* 176 (4042): 1403–5. doi: 10.1126/science.176.4042.1403.

————. 1989. "AIDS Drugs Remain Unavailable for Kids." *Science* 246 (4926): 22. doi: 10.1126/science.246.4926.22.

Curran, J. W. 1985. "The Epidemiology and Prevention of the Acquired Immunodeficiency Syndrome." *Annals of Internal Medicine* 103 (5): 657–62.

Curran, J. W., and H. W. Jaffe. 2011. "AIDS: The Early Years and CDC's Response." *Morbidity and Mortality Weekly Report Surveillance Summaries* 60 (suppl. 4): S64–69.

De Cock, K. M., and W. M. El-Sadr. 2013. "When to Start ART in Africa: An Urgent Research Priority." *New England Journal of Medicine* 368 (10): 886–89. doi: 10.1056/ NEJMp1300458.

De Martino, M., P. A. Tovo, M. Balducci, L. Galli, C. Gabiano, G. Rezza, and P. Pezzotti. 2000. "Reduction in Mortality with Availability of Antiretroviral Therapy for Children with Perinatal HIV-1 Infection: Italian Register for HIV Infection in Children and the Italian National AIDS Registry." *Journal of the American Medical Association* 284 (2): 190–97.

De Mendoza, C., F. Blanco, and V. Soriano. 2003. "Mitochondrial Damage by Antiretrovirals: Diagnosis and Monitoring." *Medicina Clínica (Barcelona)* 121 (8): 310–15.

Del Rio, C., and G. H. Hernandez-Tepichin. 1996. "Optimism Rises on Combination Therapy and Protease Inhibitor Data." *AIDS Clinical Care* 8 (3): 19–20, 23.

Deresinski, S. C., D. P. Cooney, D. M. Auerbach, A. J. Ammann, B. Luft, and H. Goldman. 1984. "AIDS Transmission Via Transfusion Therapy." *Lancet* 323 (8368): 102. (originally published as Volume 1, Issue 8368, January 14, 1984)

Devita, V. T., and E. Devita-Raeburn. 2015. *The Death of Cancer: After Fifty Years on the Front Lines of Medicine, a Pioneering Oncologist Reveals Why the War on Cancer is Winnable—and How We can Get There*. New York: Sarah Crichton Books.

Deyton, L. 1996. "Importance of Surrogate Markers in Evaluation of Antiviral Therapy for HIV Infection." *Journal of the American Medical Association* 276 (2): 159–60.

Dickover, R. E., E. M. Garratty, S. A. Herman, et al. 1996. "Identification of Levels of Maternal HIV-1 RNA Associated with Risk of Perinatal Transmission: Effect of Maternal Zidovudine Treatment on Viral Load." *Journal of the American Medical Association* 275 (8): 599–605.

"Did HIV-Positive Mom's Beliefs Put Her Children at Risk?" 2005. ABC News, December 8. *abcnews.go.com/Primetime/Health/story?id=1386737.*

DHHS Panel on Antiretroviral Guidelines for Adults and Adolescents. 2016. *AIDSinfo: Guidelines for the Use of Antiretroviral Agents in HIV-1-Infected Adults and Adolescents*. Rockville, MD: Office of AIDS Research Advisory Council (OARAC), NIH. Last updated January 16. *aidsinfo.nih.gov/contentfiles/lvguidelines/adultandadolescentgl.pdf.*

Drew, W. L., M. A. Conant, R. C. Miner, et al. 1982. "Cytomegalovirus and Kaposi's Sarcoma in Young Homosexual Men." *Lancet* 320 (8290): 125–27. (Originally published as Volume 2, Issue 8290, July 17, 1982)

Drew, W. L., J. Mills, J. Levy, J. Dylewski, C. Casavant, A. J. Ammann, H. Brodie, and T. Merigan. 1985. "Cytomegalovirus Infection and Abnormal T-Lymphocyte Subset Ratios in Homosexual Men." *Annals of Internal Medicine* 103 (1): 61–63.

Duerr, A., Y. Huang, S. Buchbinder, et al. 2012. "Extended Follow-Up Confirms Early Vaccine-Enhanced Risk of HIV Acquisition and Demonstrates Waning Effect over Time among Participants in a Randomized Trial of Recombinant Adenovirus HIV Vaccine (Step Study)." *Journal of Infectious Diseases* 206 (2): 258–66. doi: 10.1093/infdis/jis342.

Duesberg, P. H. 1990. "AIDS: Non-Infectious Deficiencies Acquired by Drug Consumption and Other Risk Factors." *Research in Immunology* 141 (1): 5–11.

———. 1991. "AIDS Epidemiology: Inconsistencies with Human Immunodeficiency Virus and with Infectious Disease." *Proceedings of the National Academy of Sciences* 88 (4): 1575–79.

———. 1996. *Inventing the AIDS Virus*. Washington: Regnery Publishing

Duesberg, P. H., and D. Rasnick. 1998. "The AIDS Dilemma: Drug Diseases Blamed on a Passenger Virus." *Genetica* 104 (2): 85–132.

Duesberg, P. H., J. M. Nicholson, D. Rasnick, C. Fiala, and H. H. Bauer. 2009. "WITHDRAWN: HIV-AIDS Hypothesis Out of Touch with South African AIDS: A New Perspective." *Medical Hypotheses*, July 19. doi: 10.1016/j.mehy.2009.06.024.

Dunkle, K. L., and M. R. Decker. 2013. "Gender-Based Violence and HIV: Reviewing the Evidence for Links and Causal Pathways in the General Population and High-Risk Groups." *American Journal of Reproductive Immunology* 69 (suppl. 1): S20–26. doi: 10.1111/aji.12039.

Dunkle, K. L., R. K. Jewkes, H. C. Brown, G. E. Gray, J. A. McIntryre, and S. D. Harlow. 2004. "Gender-Based Violence, Relationship Power, and Risk of HIV Infection in Women Attending Antenatal Clinics in South Africa." *Lancet* 363 (9419): 1415–21. doi: 10.1016/s0140–6736(04)16098–4.

"The Durban Declaration." 2000. *Nature* 406 (6791): 15–16. doi: 10.1038/35017662.

"Durban Declaration on HIV and AIDS." 2000. *AIDS Treatment News*, no. 346 (July 7). *www.thebody.com/content/art32103.html.*

EGPAF (Elizabeth Glaser Pediatric AIDS Foundation). 2016a. "Dr. Arthur Ammann." EGPAF. Accessed March 16. *www.pedaids.org/series/entry/ammann.*

———. 2016b "Elizabeth's Story." EGPAF. Accessed March 16. *www.pedaids.org/pages/elizabeths-story.*

"The Elizabeth Glaser Scientist Award Announcement." 1995. *Nature* 375 (6528): n.p.

Ellis, David. 1994. "The Defiant One." *People*, December 19: 46–53. *www.people.com/people/archive/article/0,,20104707,00.html.*

El-Sadr, W. M., J. Lundgren, J. D. Neaton, et al. 2006. "CD4+ Count-Guided Interruption of Antiretroviral Treatment." *New England Journal of Medicine* 355 (22): 2283–96. doi: 10.1056/NEJMoa062360.

Epstein, Helen. 2007. *The Invisible Cure: Why We Are Losing the Fight against AIDS in Africa.* New York: Farrar, Strauss and Giroux.

Erb, P., M. Battegay, W. Zimmerli, M. Rickenbach, and M. Egger. 2000. "Effect of Antiretroviral Therapy on Viral Load, CD4 Cell Count, and Progression to Acquired Immunodeficiency Syndrome in a Community Human Immunodeficiency Virus-Infected Cohort: Swiss HIV Cohort Study." *Archives of Internal Medicine* 160 (8): 1134–40.

Evatt, B. L. 2006. "The Tragic History of AIDS in the Hemophilia Population, 1982–1984." *Journal of Thrombosis and Haemostasis* 4 (11): 2295–301. doi: 10.1111/j.1538–7836.2006.02213.x.

"Experts Rethinking Billions Spent on AIDS: With Lowered Infection Rates, Some Want to Shift Funds to Other Global Ills." 2008. NBC News.com, January 18. Accessed March 22, 2016. *www.nbcnews.com/id/22726852/ns/health-aids/t/experts-rethinking-billions-spent-aids.*

Faden, R. R., T. L. Beauchamp, and N. E. Kass. 2014. "Informed Consent for Comparative Effectiveness Trials." *New England Journal of Medicine* 370 (20): 1959–60. doi: 10.1056/NEJMc1403310.

Fauci, A. S., and G. K. Folkers. 2012. "Toward an AIDS-Free Generation." *Journal of the American Medical Association* 308 (4): 343–44. doi: 10.1001/jama.2012.8142.

Fauci, A. S., and H. D. Marston. 2015. "Ending the HIV-AIDS Pandemic: Follow the Science." *New England Journal of Medicine* 373 (23): 2197–199. doi: 10.1056/NEJMp1502020.

Fawzi, W. W., G. Msamanga, D. Hunter, et al. 2000. "Randomized Trial of Vitamin Supplements in Relation to Vertical Transmission of HIV-1 in Tanzania." *Journal of Acquired Immune Deficiency Syndromes* 23 (3): 246–54.

Fawzi, W. W., G. I. Msamanga, D. Spiegelman, et al. 1998. "Randomised Trial of Effects of Vitamin Supplements on Pregnancy Outcomes and T-Cell Counts in HIV-1-Infected Women in Tanzania." *Lancet* 351 (9114): 1477–82.

FDA. 2011. "Drug Research and Children." FDA.gov, August 24. *www.fda.gov/Drugs/ResourcesForYou/Consumers/ucm143565.htm.*

————. 2014. "HIV/AIDS Historical Time Line 1981–1990." FDA.gov, August 8. *www.fda.gov/ForPatients/Illness/HIVAIDS/History/ucm151074.htm*.

————. 2016. "Prescription Drug User Fee Act (PDUFA)." FDA.gov. Last updated August 17. *www.fda.gov/ForIndustry/UserFees/PrescriptionDrugUserFee*.

FDA. Final Rule. 1994. "Specific Requirements on Content and Format of Labeling for Human Prescription Drugs; Revision of 'Pediatric Use' Subsection in the Labeling; Final Rule (the Pediatric Rule)." *Federal Register* 59, no. 238 (December 13). FR doc. no.: 94-30238. *www.gpo.gov/fdsys/pkg/FR-1994-12-13/html/94-30238.htm*.

"FDA Community Meeting May 16: Clinical Trials and Viral Load." 1997. *AIDS Treatment News*, no. 270 (May 1). *www.thebody.com/content/art31504.html#fda*.

Feldman, Eric. 1999. *Blood Feuds: AIDS, Blood, and the Politics of Medical Disaster*. New York: Oxford University Press.

Feorino, P. M., H. W. Jaffe, E. Palmer, et al. 1985. "Transfusion-Associated Acquired Immunodeficiency Syndrome: Evidence for Persistent Infection in Blood Donors." *New England Journal of Medicine* 312 (20): 1293–96. doi: 10.1056/nejm198505163122005.

Fink, A. J. 1989. "Newborn Circumcision: A Long-Term Strategy for AIDS Prevention." *Journal of the Royal Society of Medicine* 82 (11): 695.

Fischl, M. A., D. D. Richman, D. M. Causey, et al. 1989. "Prolonged Zidovudine Therapy in Patients with AIDS and Advanced AIDS-Related Complex: AZT Collaborative Working Group." *Journal of the American Medical Association* 262 (17): 2405–10.

Fischl, M. A., D. D. Richman, M. H. Grieco, et al. 1987. "The Efficacy of Azidothymidine (AZT) in the Treatment of Patients with AIDS and AIDS-Related Complex: A Double-Blind, Placebo-Controlled Trial." *New England Journal of Medicine* 317 (4): 185–91. doi: 10.1056/NEJM198707233170401.

Flexner, C. 1998. "Post-Exposure Prophylaxis Revisited: New CDC Guidelines." *Hopkins HIV Report* 10 (1): 2–3.

Folkers, G. K., and A. S. Fauci. 2001. "The AIDS Research Model: Implications for Other Infectious Diseases of Global Health Importance." *Journal of the American Medical Association* 286 (4): 458–61.

Forbes, J. M., M. D. Anderson, G. F. Anderson, G. C. Bleecker, E. C. Rossi, and G. S. Moss. 1991. "Blood Transfusion Costs: A Multicenter Study." *Transfusion* 31 (4): 318–23.

Ford, N., D. Wilson, G. Costa Chaves, M. Lotrowska, and K. Kijtiwatchakul. 2007. "Sustaining Access to Antiretroviral Therapy in the Less-Developed World: Lessons from Brazil and Thailand." *AIDS* 21 (suppl. 4): S21–29. doi: 10.1097/01.aids.0000279703.78685.a6.

Fowler, M. G., and M. L. Newell. 2002. "Breast-Feeding and HIV-1 Transmission in Resource-Limited Settings." *Journal of Acquired Immune Deficiency Syndromes* 30 (2): 230–39.

França Junior, Ivan, Gabriela Calazans, and Eliana Miura Zucchi. 2008. "Changes in HIV Testing in Brazil between 1998 and 2005." *Revista de Saúde Pública* 42 (suppl. 1): 84–97. doi: 10.1590/S0034-89102008000800011.

Frederick, T., J. Homans, L. Spencer, F. Kramer, A. Stek, E. Operskalski, and A. Kovacs. 2012. "The Effect of Prenatal Highly Active Antiretroviral Therapy on the Transmission of Congenital and Perinatal / Early Postnatal Cytomegalovirus among HIV-Infected and HIV-Exposed Infants." *Clinical Infectious Diseases* 55 (6): 877–84. doi: 10.1093/cid/cis535.

Frieden, T. R., I. Damon, B. P. Bell, T. Kenyon, and S. Nichol. 2014. "Ebola 2014—New Challenges, New Global Response and Responsibility." *New England Journal of Medicine* 371 (13): 1177–80. doi: 10.1056/NEJMp1409903.

Frieden, T. R., K. E. Foti, and J. Mermin. 2015. "Applying Public Health Principles to the HIV Epidemic—How Are We Doing?" *New England Journal of Medicine* 373 (23): 2281–87. doi: 10.1056/NEJMms1513641.

Friedland, G. H., B. R. Saltzman, M. F. Rogers, P. A. Kahl, M. L. Lesser, M. M. Mayers, and R. S. Klein. 1986. "Lack of Transmission of HTLV-III/LAV Infection to Household Contacts of Patients with AIDS or AIDS-Related Complex with Oral Candidiasis." *New England Journal of Medicine* 314 (6): 344–49. doi: 10.1056/nejm198602063140604.

Gallman, Stephanie. 2015. "FDA Lifts Lifetime Ban on Gay Men Donating Blood." CNN, December 21. *www.cnn.com/2015/12/21/health/fda-gay-men-blood-donation-changes*.

Gallo, R. C., P. S. Sarin, E. P. Gelmann, et al. 1983. "Isolation of Human T-Cell Leukemia Virus in Acquired Immune Deficiency Syndrome (AIDS)." *Science* 220 (4599): 865–67.

Garcia, P. M., L. A. Kalish, J. Pitt, et al. 1999. "Maternal Levels of Plasma Human Immunodeficiency Virus Type 1 RNA and the Risk of Perinatal Transmission. Women and Infants Transmission Study Group." *New England Journal of Medicine* 341 (6): 394–402. doi: 10.1056/nejm199908053410602.

Gatti, R. A., H. J. Meuwissen, H. D. Allen, R. Hong, and R. A. Good. 1968. "Immunological Reconstitution of Sex-Linked Lymphopenic Immunological Deficiency." *Lancet* 292 (7583): 1366–69. (originally published as Volume 2, Issue 7583, Dec. 28, 1968)

Gbowee, L. 2011. *Mighty Be Our Powers: How Sisterhood, Prayer, and Sex Changed a Nation at War*. Philadelphia, PA: Perscus Book Group.

Gendell, S. 1997. "A Dose of Your Own Medicine? Drug Testing on Children and Labeling Drugs for Pediatric Use: Essential Needs." DASH (Digital Access to Scholarship at Harvard). *nrs.harvard.edu/urn-3:HUL.InstRepos:8965627*.

Gerberding, J. L., and M. H. Katz. 1999. "Post-Exposure Prophylaxis for HIV." *Advances in Experimental Medicine and Biology* 458:213–22.

Gisselquist, D. 2008. "Denialism Undermines AIDS Prevention in Sub-Saharan Africa." *International Journal of STD and AIDS* 19 (10): 649–55. doi: 10.1258/ijsa.2008.008180.

Glaser, Elizabeth. 1993. *In the Absence of Angels: A Hollywood Family's Courageous Story*. New York: Putnam.

Gogu, S. R., B. S. Beckman, and K. C. Agrawal. 1989. "Anti-HIV Drugs: Comparative Toxicities in Murine Fetal Liver and Bone Marrow Erythroid Progenitor Cells." *Life Science* 45 (4): iii–vii.

Goosby, E., D. Von Zinkernagel, C. Holmes, D. Haroz, and T. Walsh. 2012. "Raising the Bar: PEPFAR and New Paradigms for Global Health." *Journal of Acquired Immune Deficiency Syndromes* 60 (suppl. 3): S158–62. doi: 10.1097/QAI.0b013e31825d057c.

Goosby, Eric. 2013. "Statement from Ambassador Eric Goosby, MD, US Global AIDS Coordinator, on WHO Guidelines on HIV." PEPFAR, July 2. *www.pepfar.gov/press/releases/2013*.

Gorski, David. 2009. "Christine Maggiore and Eliza Jane Scovill: Living and Dying with HIV/AIDS Denialism." *Science-Based Medicine*, January 5. *www.sciencebasedmedicine.org/christine-maggiore-and-eliza-jane-scovill-living-and-dying-with-hivaids-denialism*.

Gottlieb, M. S., J. E. Groopman, W. M. Weinstein, J. L. Fahey, and R. Detels. 1983. "The Acquired Immunodeficiency Syndrome." *Annals of Internal Medicine* 99 (2): 208–20.

Gottlieb, M. S., R. Schroff, H. M. Schanker, J. D. Weisman, P. T. Fan, R. A. Wolf, and A. Saxon. 1981. "Pneumocystis Carinii Pneumonia and Mucosal Candidiasis in Previously Healthy Homosexual Men: Evidence of a New Acquired Cellular Immunodeficiency." *New England Journal of Medicine* 305 (24): 1425–31. doi: 10.1056/NEJM198112103052401.

Govender, S., K. Otwombe, T. Essien, R. Panchia, G. De Bruyn, L. Mohapi, G. Gray, and N. Martinson. 2014. "CD4 Counts and Viral Loads of Newly Diagnosed HIV-Infected Individuals: Implications for Treatment as Prevention." *PLOS One* 9 (3): e90754. doi: 10.1371/journal.pone.0090754.

Graham, B. "VRC01 in Children and Adults." 2015. Presentation for the HPTN and IMPAACT Annual Meeting, Arlington, VA, June 17. *www.hptn.org/web%20documents/annualmtg15/Presentations/Joint_Plenary/HPTN_IMPAACT_VRC01.pdf.*

Grant, R. M., J. R. Lama, P. L. Anderson, et al. 2010. "Preexposure Chemoprophylaxis for HIV Prevention in Men Who Have Sex with Men." *New England Journal of Medicine* 363 (27): 2587–99. doi: 10.1056/NEJMoa1011205.

Gray, J. M., and D. L. Cohn. 2013. "Tuberculosis and HIV Coinfection." *Seminars in Respiratory and Critical Care Medicine* 34 (1): 32–43. doi: 10.1055/s-0032–1333469.

Greenspan, D. 1985. "Oral Viral Leukoplakia ('Hairy' Leukoplakia): A New Oral Lesion in Association with AIDS." *Compendium of Continuing Education in Dentistry* 6 (3): 204–6, 208.

Greenspan, J. S., D. Greenspan, E. T. Lennette, D. I. Abrams, M. A. Conant, V. Petersen, and U. K. Freese. 1985. "Replication of Epstein-Barr Virus within the Epithelial Cells of Oral 'Hairy' Leukoplakia, an AIDS-Associated Lesion." *New England Journal of Medicine* 313 (25): 1564–71. doi: 10.1056/NEJM198512193132502.

Groopman, J. E., and P. A. Volberding. 1984. "The AIDS Epidemic: Continental Drift." *Nature* 307 (5948): 211–12.

Guay, L. A., P. Musoke, T. Fleming, et al. 1999. "Intrapartum and Neonatal Single-Dose Nevirapine Compared with Zidovudine for Prevention of Mother-to-Child Transmission of HIV-1 in Kampala, Uganda: HIVnet 012 Randomised Trial." *Lancet* 354 (9181): 795–802. doi: 10.1016/s0140–6736(99)80008–7.

Gulick, R. 1998. "Combination Therapy for Patients with HIV-1 Infection: The Use of Dual Nucleoside Analogues with Protease Inhibitors and Other Agents." *AIDS* 12 (suppl. 3): S17–22.

Gulick, R. M., J. W. Mellors, D. Havlir, et al. 1997. "Treatment with Indinavir, Zidovudine, and Lamivudine in Adults with Human Immunodeficiency Virus Infection and Prior Antiretroviral Therapy." *New England Journal of Medicine* 337 (11): 734–39.

Hammer, S. M., K. E. Squires, M. D. Hughes, et al. 1997. "A Controlled Trial of Two Nucleoside Analogues Plus Indinavir in Persons with Human Immunodeficiency Virus Infection and CD4 Cell Counts of 200 Per Cubic Millimeter or Less." *New England Journal of Medicine* 337 (11): 725–33.

Harden, Victoria A. 2012. *AIDS at 30: A History.* Dulles, VA: Potomac Books.

Havlir, D. V., and J. M. Lange. 1998. "New Antiretrovirals and New Combinations." *AIDS* 12 (suppl. A): S165–74.

Hearst, N., P. Kajubi, E. S. Hudes, A. K. Maganda, and E. C. Green. 2012. "Prevention Messages and AIDS Risk Behavior in Kampala, Uganda." *AIDS Care* 24 (1): 87–90. doi: 10.1080/09540121.2011.582478.

Herlihy, J. M., L. Hamomba, R. Bonawitz, et al. 2015. "Implementation and Operational Research: Integration of PMTCT and Antenatal Services Improves Combination Antiretroviral Therapy Uptake for HIV-Positive Pregnant Women in Southern Zambia: A Prototype for Option B+?" *Journal of Acquired Immune Deficiency Syndromes* 70 (4): e123–29. doi: 10.1097/qai.0000000000000760.

HHS (US Department of Health and Human Services). 1995. "FDA Approves First Protease Inhibitor Drug for Treatment of HIV." HHS.gov, December 7. *archive.hhs.gov/news/press/1995pres/951207.html.*

"HIV/AIDS Clinical Trials." 2015. AIDSinfo. Last updated May 13, 2016. *aidsinfo.nih.gov/clinical-trials.*

"HIV/AIDS Mortality Continues to Fall." 1998. *Communicable Disease Report Weekly* 8 (30): 269.

"HIV and AIDS in sub-Saharan Africa Regional Overview." 2013. Avert.org. Last reviewed May 1, 2015. *www.avert.org/professionals/hiv-around-world/sub-saharan-africa/overview*.

HIVInSite. 2016. University of California San Francisco Center for HIV Information. Accessed March 16, 2016. *hivinsite.ucsf.edu*.

"HIV: Science and Stigma." 2014. *Lancet* 384 (9939): 207.

Ho, D. D. 1995. "Time to Hit HIV, Early and Hard." *New England Journal of Medicine* 333 (7): 450–51. doi: 10.1056/nejm199508173330710.

———. 1996a. "Therapy of HIV Infections: Problems and Prospects." *Bulletin of the New York Academy of Medicine* 73 (1): 37–45.

———. 1996b. "Viral Counts Count in HIV Infection." *Science* 272 (5265): 1124–25.

Ho, D. D., A. U. Neumann, A. S. Perelson, W. Chen, J. M. Leonard, and M. Markowitz. 1995. "Rapid Turnover of Plasma Virions and CD4 Lymphocytes in HIV-1 Infection." *Nature* 373 (6510): 123–26. doi: 10.1038/373123a0.

Hochschild, Adam. 1998. *King Leopold's Ghost*. Boston: Mariner Books.

Hodgkinson, N. 2001. "Poisoning Our Babies—The Lethal Dangers of AZT." Alive & Well AIDS Alternatives. *www.aliveandwell.org/html/mothers_babies/poisoning_our_babies.html*. Originally published as "Special Report: HIV, Families, and Medical Justice." 2001. *Mothering Magazine*, September-October.

Holmes, C. B., W. Coggin, D. Jamieson, et al. 2010. "Use of Generic Antiretroviral Agents and Cost Savings in PEPFAR Treatment Programs." *Journal of the American Medical Association* 304 (3): 313–20. doi: 10.1001/jama.2010.993.

HRSA (Health Resources and Services Administration) 2016. "Who Was Ryan White?" HRSA. gov. Accessed March 22. *hab.hrsa.gov/abouthab/ryanwhite.html*.

Hussain, A., D. Moodley, S. Naidoo, and T. M. Esterhuizen. 2011. "Pregnant Women's Access to PMTCT and ART Services in South Africa and Implications for Universal Antiretroviral Treatment." *PLOS One* 6 (12): e27907. doi: 10.1371/journal.pone.0027907.

IMPAACT. 2015. "1077hs (10779): HAART Standard Version of the PROMISE Study (Promoting Maternal and Infant Survival Everywhere)." IMPAACTNetwork.org, October 14. *www.impaactnetwork.org/studies/1077HS.asp*.

Institute for Global Health and Infectious Diseases. 2015. "Malawians for Malawi: Creating a Sustainable Model of Care." UNC Global, Feb. 27. *global.unc.edu/news/malawians-for-malawi-creating-a-sustainable-model-of-care*.

Ioannidis, J. P., and D. G. Contopoulos-Ioannidis. 1999. "Maternal Viral Load and the Risk of Perinatal Transmission of HIV-1." *New England Journal of Medicine* 341 (22): 1698–700. doi: 10.1056/nejm199911253412215.

Ioannidis, J. P., S. Greenland, M. A. Hlatky, M. J. Khoury, M. R. Macleod, D. Moher, K. F. Schulz, and R. Tibshirani. 2014. "Increasing Value and Reducing Waste in Research Design, Conduct, and Analysis." *Lancet* 383 (9912): 166–75. doi: 10.1016/s0140–6736(13)62227–8.

"IOM to Publish Review of Trial Testing Nevirapine Use in HIV-Positive Pregnant Ugandan Women." 2005. KHN (Kaiser Health News) Morning Briefing. March 8. *khn.org/morning-breakout/dr00028513*.

Jacobson, J. M., R. Pat Bucy, J. Spritzler, et al. 2006. "Evidence That Intermittent Structured Treatment Interruption, but Not Immunization with ALVAC-HIV vCP1452, Promotes Host Control of HIV Replication: The Results of AIDS Clinical Trials Group 5068." *Journal of Infectious Diseases* 194 (5): 623–32. doi: 10.1086/506364.

James, J. S. 1995. "Combination Antiretroviral Treatment: New Views, Evolving Practices." *AIDS Treatment News*, no. 226 (July 7), 1–2.

Jansen, J. K., and A. J. Ammann. 1994. "Priorities in Psychosocial Research in Pediatric Human Immunodeficiency Virus Infection." *Journal of Developmental and Behavioral Pediatrics* 15 (suppl. 3): S3–4.

Jervis, Coco. 2012. "Does Obama's 2013 Budget Herald the End of PEPFAR?" Treatment Action Group. Spring. *www.treatmentactiongroup.org/tagline/2012/spring/does-obama's-2013-budget-herald-end-pepfar.*

Jewkes, R. K., K. Dunkle, M. Nduna, and N. Shai. 2010. "Intimate Partner Violence, Relationship Power Inequity, and Incidence of HIV Infection in Young Women in South Africa: A Cohort Study." *Lancet* 376 (9734): 41–48. doi: 10.1016/s0140–6736(10)60548-x.

Johnson, R. E., D. N. Lawrence, B. L. Evatt, D. J. Bregman, L. D. Zyla, J. W. Curran, L. M. Aledort, M. E. Eyster, A. P. Brownstein, and C. J. Carman. 1985. "Acquired Immunodeficiency Syndrome among Patients Attending Hemophilia Treatment Centers and Mortality Experience of Hemophiliacs in the United States." *American Journal of Epidemiology* 121 (6): 797–810.

"Judge Refuses to Let HIV-Positive Mother Breast Feed Son." 1999. *AIDS Policy Law* 14 (9): 13.

Katz, R. V., S. S. Kegeles, N. R. Kressin, B. L. Green, S. A. James, M. Q. Wang, S. L. Russell, and C. Claudio. 2008. "Awareness of the Tuskegee Syphilis Study and the US Presidential Apology and Their Influence on Minority Participation in Biomedical Research." *American Journal of Public Health* 98 (6): 1137–42. doi: 10.2105/ajph.2006.100131.

Katzenstein, D. A., S. M. Hammer, M. D. Hughes, et al. 1996. "The Relation of Virologic and Immunologic Markers to Clinical Outcomes after Nucleoside Therapy in HIV-Infected Adults with 200 to 500 CD4 Cells per Cubic Millimeter: AIDS Clinical Trials Group Study 175 Virology Study Team." *New England Journal of Medicine* 335 (15): 1091–98. doi: 10.1056/nejm199610103351502.

Kelley, B. 2009. "Industrialization of mAb Production Technology: The Bioprocessing Industry at a Crossroads." *mAbs* 1 (5): 443–52.

Kerschberger, B., K. Hilderbrand, A. M. Boulle, D. Coetzee, E. Goemaere, V. De Azevedo, and G. Van Cutsem. 2012. "The Effect of Complete Integration of HIV and TB Services on Time to Initiation of Antiretroviral Therapy: A Before-After Study." *PLOS One* 7 (10): e46988. doi: 10.1371/journal.pone.0046988.

Kesho Boro Study Group. 2011. "Triple Antiretroviral Compared with Zidovudine and Single-Dose Nevirapine Prophylaxis During Pregnancy and Breastfeeding for Prevention of Mother-to-Child Transmission of HIV-1 (Kesho Bora Study): A Randomised Controlled Trial." *Lancet Infectious Diseases* 11 (3): 171–80. doi: 10.1016/S1473-3099(10)70288-7.

Kibrick, S., and R. M. Loria. 1974. "Rubella and Cytomegalovirus: Current Concepts of Congenital and Acquired Infection." *Pediatric Clinics of North America* 21 (2): 513–26.

Kim, J. C., L. J. Martin, and L. Denny. 2003. "Rape and HIV Post-Exposure Prophylaxis: Addressing the Dual Epidemics in South Africa." *Reproductive Health Matters* 11 (22): 101–12.

Kim, S. Y., and F. G. Miller. 2014. "Informed Consent for Pragmatic Trials: The Integrated Consent Model." *New England Journal of Medicine* 370 (8): 769–72. doi: 10.1056/NEJMhle1312508.

King, Martin Luther, Jr. 2004. *Quotations of Martin Luther King*. Bedford, Mass: Applewood Books.

Kintu, K., P. Andrew, P. Musoke, et al. 2013. "Feasibility and Safety of AlVAC-HIV vCP1521 Vaccine in HIV-exposed Infants in Uganda: Results from the First HIV Vaccine Trial in Infants in Africa." *Journal of Acquired Immune Deficiency Syndromes* 63 (1): 1–8. doi: 10.1097/QAI.0b013e31827f1c2d.

Kitahata, M. M., S. J. Gange, A. G. Abraham, et al. 2009. "Effect of Early Versus Deferred Antiretroviral Therapy for HIV on Survival." *New England Journal of Medicine* 360 (18): 1815–26. doi: 1056/NEJM0a0807252.

Kline, M. W., and W. T. Shearer. 1992. "Impact of Human Immunodeficiency Virus Infection on Women and Infants." *Infectious Disease Clinics of North America* 6 (1): 1–17.

Kolata, Gina. 1989. "Hundreds of Children With AIDS Are Unable to Obtain AZT." *New York Times*, September 23. *www.nytimes.com/1989/09/23/us/hundreds-of-children-with-aids-are-unable-to-obtain-azt.html*.

Korschun, H. 1999. "Researchers Outline Pediatric AIDS Ethical Guidelines." *Emory Report* 51 (26). *www.emory.edu/EMORY_REPORT/erarchive/1999/April/erapri1.5/4_5_99pediatrics.html*.

Lallemant, M., G. Jourdain, S. Le Coeur, et al. 2000. "A Trial of Shortened Zidovudine Regimens to Prevent Mother-to-Child Transmission of Human Immunodeficiency Virus Type 1: Perinatal HIV Prevention Trial (Thailand) Investigators." *New England Journal of Medicine* 343 (14): 982–91. doi: 10.1056/NEJM200010053431401.

Lambert, G., D. M. Thea, V. Pliner, et al. 1997. "Effect of Maternal CD4+ Cell Count, Acquired Immunodeficiency Syndrome, and Viral Load on Disease Progression in Infants with Perinatally Acquired Human Immunodeficiency Virus Type 1 Infection: New York City Perinatal HIV Transmission Collaborative Study Group." *Journal of Pediatrics* 130 (6): 890–97.

Landau, E. 2013. "HIV May Be 'Functionally Cured' in Some." CNN, March 18. *www.cnn.com/2013/03/18/health/hiv-functional-cure*.

Lawoyin, T., and O. A. Kehinde. 2006. "Male Circumcision and HIV in Africa." *PLOS Medicine* 3 (1): e74; author reply, e67. doi: 10.1371/journal.pmed.0030074.

Ledford, H. 2014. "Indirect Costs: Keeping the Lights On." *Nature* 515 (7527): 326–29. doi: 10.1038/515326a.

Lallemant, M., G. Jourdain, S. Le Coeur, S. Kim, S. Koetsawang, A. M. Comeau, W. Phoolcharoen, M. Essex, K. McIntosh, and V. Vithayasai. 2000. "A Trial of Shortened Zidovudine Regimens to Prevent Mother-to-Child Transmission of Human Immunodeficiency Virus Type 1: Perinatal HIV Prevention Trial (Thailand) Investigators." *New England Journal of Medicine* 343 (14): 982–91. doi: 10.1056/nejm200010053431401.

Lee, J. S., S. Mullaney, R. Bronson, A. H. Sharpe, R. Jaenisch, J. Balzarini, E. De Clercq, and R. M. Ruprecht. 1991. "Transplacental Antiretroviral Therapy with 9-(2-Phosphonylmethoxyethyl)Adenine Is Embryotoxic in Transgenic Mice." *Journal of Acquired Immune Deficiency Syndromes* 4 (9): 833–38.

Leroy, V., C. Sakarovitch, M. Cortina-Borja, et al. 2005. "Is There a Difference in the Efficacy of Peripartum Antiretroviral Regimens in Reducing Mother-to-Child Transmission of HIV in Africa?" *AIDS* 19 (16): 1865–75. doi: 00002030–200511040–00016.

Leveton, L. B., H. C. Sox, Jr., and M. A. Stoto, eds. 1995. *HIV and the Blood Supply: An Analysis of Crisis Decision Making*. Washington, DC: National Academy Press.

Levy, J. A., A. D. Hoffman, S. M. Kramer, J. A. Landis, J. M. Shimabukuro, and L. S. Oshiro. 1984. "Isolation of Lymphocytopathic Retroviruses from San Francisco Patients with AIDS." *Science* 225 (4664): 840–42.

Lifson, J. D., S. L. Finch, D. T. Sasaki, and E. G. Engleman. 1985. "Variables Affecting T-lymphocyte Subsets in a Volunteer Blood Donor Population." *Clinical Immunology and Immunopathology* 36 (2): 151–60.

Lindegren, M. L., P. Rhodes, L. Gordon, and P. Fleming. 2000. "Drug Safety During Pregnancy and in Infants: Lack of Mortality Related to Mitochondrial Dysfunction among Perinatally HIV-Exposed Children in Pediatric HIV Surveillance." *Annals of the New York Academy of Sciences* 918 (November): 222–35.

Livingston, E. H. 2012. "German Medical Group: Apology for Nazi Physicians' Actions, Warning for Future." *Journal of the American Medical Association* 308 (7): 657–58. doi: 10.1001/jama.2012.9649.

"Look at Me! World AIDS Day 2011." 2011. *Journey with Jesus* (blog). Accessed March 20, 2016. *www.journeywithjesus.net/Essays/20111128JJ.shtml*.

Lorenzo, O., C. M. Beck-Sague, C. Bautista-Soriano, et al. 2012. "Progress Towards Elimination of HIV Mother-to-Child Transmission in the Dominican Republic from 1999 to 2011." *Infectious Diseases in Obstetrics and Gynecology* 2012: article ID 543916. doi: 10.1155/2012/543916.

Loubiere, S., C. Meiners, C. Sloan, K. A. Freedberg, and Y. Yazdanpanah. 2010. "Economic Evaluation of ART in Resource-Limited Countries." *Current Opinion in HIV and AIDS* 5 (3): 225–31. doi: 10.1097/COH.0b013e3283384a9d.

Louwagie, G., B. Girdler-Brown, R. Odendaal, T. Rossouw, S. Johnson, and M. Van der Walt. 2012. "Missed Opportunities for Accessing HIV Care among Tshwane Tuberculosis Patients under Different Models of Care." *International Journal of Tuberculosis and Lung Disease* 16 (8): 1052–58. doi: 10.5588/ijtld.11.0753.

Lundgren, J. D., A. G. Babiker, F. Gordin, et al. 2015. "Initiation of Antiretroviral Therapy in Early Asymptomatic HIV Infection." *New England Journal of Medicine* 373 (9): 795–807. doi: 10.1056/NEJMoa1506816.

Lurie, P., and S. M. Wolfe. 1997. "Unethical Trials of Interventions to Reduce Perinatal Transmission of the Human Immunodeficiency Virus in Developing Countries." *New England Journal of Medicine* 337 (12): 853–56. doi: 10.1056/NEJM199709183371212.

Luzuriaga, K., M. McManus, M. Catalina, S. Mayack, M. Sharkey, M. Stevenson, and J. L. Sullivan. 2000. "Early Therapy of Vertical Human Immunodeficiency Virus Type 1 (HIV-1) Infection: Control of Viral Replication and Absence of Persistent HIV-1-Specific Immune Responses." *Journal of Virology* 74 (15): 6984–91.

"Maintaining Anti-AIDS Commitment Post '3 by 5.'" 2005. *Lancet* 366 (9500): 1828. doi: 10.1016/s0140-6736(05)67735-5.

"Major Report on AIDS Research at NIH." 1996. HHS.gov Archive, March 14. *archive.hhs.gov/news/press/1996pres/960314f.html*.

Mandelbaum-Schmid, J. 2004. "Rwandan Genocide Survivors in Need of HIV Treatment." *Bulletin of the World Health Organization* 82 (6): 472.

Marshall, E. 1993. "Varmus Tapped to Head NIH." *Science* 261 (5123): 820–22.

Martin, N., R. Koup, R. Kaslow, J. Coffin, and A. Ammann. 1996. "Workshop on Perinatally Acquired Human Immunodeficiency Virus Infection in Long-Term Surviving Children: A Collaborative Study of Factors Contributing to Slow Disease Progression. The Long-Term Survivor Project." *AIDS Research and Human Retroviruses* 12 (16): 1565–70.

Mays, V. M. 2012. "Research Challenges and Bioethics Responsibilities in the Aftermath of the Presidential Apology to the Survivors of the US Public Health Services Syphilis Study at Tuskegee." *Ethics and Behavior* 22 (6): 419–30. doi: 10.1080/10508422.2012.730787.

McCarthy, M. 1999. "Judge in USA Bars Breastfeeding by HIV-Infected Mother." *Lancet* 353 (9163): 1506. doi: 10.1016/s0140–6736(05)75123–0.

McFarlane, M. J., A. R. Feinstein, and R. I. Horwitz. 1986. "Diethylstilbestrol and Clear Cell Vaginal Carcinoma: Reappraisal of the Epidemiologic Evidence." *American Journal of Medicine* 81 (5): 855–63.

McNeil, Donald. 2015. "H.I.V. Treatment Should Start at Diagnosis, US Health Officials Say." *New York Times*, May 27. *www.nytimes.com/2015/05/28/health/hiv-treatment-should-start-with-diagnosis-us-health-officials-say.html*.

Medley, A., P. Bachanas, M. Grillo, N. Hasen, and U. Amanyeiwe. 2015. "Integrating Prevention Interventions for People Living with HIV into Care and Treatment Programs: A Systematic Review of the Evidence." *Journal of Acquired Immune Deficiency Syndromes* 68 (suppl. 3): S286–96. doi: 10.1097/qai.0000000000000520.

Mock, P. A., N. Shaffer, C. Bhadrakom, et al. 1999. "Maternal Viral Load and Timing of Mother-to-Child HIV Transmission, Bangkok, Thailand: Bangkok Collaborative Perinatal HIV Transmission Study Group." *AIDS* 13 (3): 407–14.

Mofenson, Lynne. 2009. "Overview of Perinatal Intervention Trials Table." Women, Children, and HIV: Resources for Prevention and Treatment, UCSF. September. *www.womenchildrenhiv.org/wchiv?page=pi-10-02*.

———. 2010. "Protecting the Next Generation: Eliminating Perinatal HIV-1 Infection." *New England Journal of Medicine* 362 (24): 2316–18. doi: 10.1056/NEJMe1004406.

Mok, J. 1993. "Breast Milk and HIV-1 Transmission." *Lancet* 341 (8850): 930–31.

Montaner, J. S., V. D. Lima, P. R. Harrigan, et al. 2014. "Expansion of HAART Coverage is Associated with Sustained Decreases in HIV/AIDS Morbidity, Mortality and HIV Transmission: The 'HIV Treatment as Prevention' Experience in a Canadian Setting." *PLOS One* 9 (2): e87872. doi: 10.1371/journal.pone.0087872.

Montaner, J. S., V. Montessori, R. Harrigan, M. O'Shaughnessy, and R. Hogg. 1999. "Antiretroviral Therapy: 'The State of the Art.'" *Biomedicine and Pharmacotherapy* 53 (2): 63–72.

Moodley, D., J. Moodley, H. Coovadia, et al. 2003. "A Multicenter Randomized Controlled Trial of Nevirapine Versus a Combination of Zidovudine and Lamivudine to Reduce Intrapartum and Early Postpartum Mother-to-Child Transmission of Human Immunodeficiency Virus Type 1." *Journal of Infectious Diseases* 187 (5): 725–35. doi: 10.1086/367898.

Moyle, G., and B. Gazzard. 1996. "Current Knowledge and Future Prospects for the Use of HIV Protease Inhibitors." *Drugs* 51 (5): 701–12.

MSAC (Medical and Scientific Advisory Council of the National Hemophilia Foundation). 1983. *Recommendations to Prevent AIDS in Patients with Hemophilia*. New York: National Hemophilia Foundation.

Mulhall, A., J. de Louvois, and R. Hurley. 1983. "Chloramphenicol Toxicity in Neonates: Its Incidence and Prevention." *British Medical Journal (Clinical Research Edition)* 287 (6403): 1424–27.

Murphy, E. M., M. E. Greene, A. Mihailovic, and P. Olupot-Olupot. 2006. "Was the 'ABC' Approach (Abstinence, Being Faithful, Using Condoms) Responsible for Uganda's Decline in HIV?" *PLOS Medicine* 3 (9): e379. doi: 10.1371/journal.pmed.0030379.

Myer, L., M. Rabkin, E. J. Abrams, A. Rosenfield, and W. M. El-Sadr. 2005. "Focus on Women: Linking HIV Care and Treatment with Reproductive Health Services in the MTCT-Plus Initiative." *Reproductive Health Matters* 13 (25): 136–46.

National Commission for the Protection of Human Subjects and of Biomedical and Behavioral Research. 1979. *The Belmont Report: Ethical Principles and Guidelines for the Protection of Human Subjects of Research*. Washington, DC: Department of Health, Education, and Welfare.

"New Drugs Emerge, but Who Will Pay the Bill?" 1996. *AIDS Policy Law* 11 (3): 4.

"New Trials Reach Same Conclusion: Two Drugs Are Better Than AZT Alone." 1995. *AIDS Alert* 10 (11): 133–36.

NIAID (National Institute of Allergy and Infectious Diseases). 1999. "HIVNET 012 Questions and Answers." AIDSinfo, NIH. July 8. *aidsinfo.nih.gov/news/502/hivnet-012-questions-and-answers*.

———. 2006. "Adult Male Circumcision Significantly Reduces Risk of Acquiring HIV." News release, December 13. *www.nih.gov/news-events/news-releases/adult-male-circumcision-significantly-reduces-risk-acquiring-hiv.*

———. 2016. "NIH Launches Large Clinical Trials of Antibody-Based HIV Prevention." News release, April 7. *www.niaid.nih.gov/news/newsreleases/2016/Pages/AMP-studies-launch.aspx.*

Nielsen, K., G. McSherry, A. Petru, et al. 1997. "A Descriptive Survey of Pediatric Human Immunodeficiency Virus-Infected Long-Term Survivors." *Pediatrics* 99 (4): E4.

NIH (National Institute of Health). 1996. "Proceedings: Office of AIDS Research Advisory Council Meeting, (3rd: 1996, Bethesda, Maryland)." Jon Cohen AIDS Research Collection, University of Michigan. *quod.lib.umich.edu/c/cohenaids/5571095.0109.004.*

———. 2015. "Starting Antiretroviral Treatment Early Improves Outcomes for HIV-Infected Individuals." News release, May 27. *www.niaid.nih.gov/news/newsreleases/2015/Pages/START.aspx.*

Novitsky, V., and M. Essex. 2012. "Using HIV Viral Load to Guide Treatment-for-Prevention Interventions." *Current Opinion in HIV and AIDS* 7 (2): 117–24. doi: 10.1097/COH.0b013e32834fe8ff.

Nuffield Council on Bioethics Working Group. *The Ethics of Research Related to Healthcare in Developing Countries.* 2016. London: Nuffield Council on Bioethics. *nuffieldbioethics.org/wp-content/uploads/2014/07/Ethics-of-research-related-to-healthcare-in-developing-countries-I.pdf.*

O'Farrell, N., L. Morison, P. Moodley, K. Pillay, T. Vanmali, M. Quigley, R. Hayes, and A. W. Sturm. 2006. "Association between HIV and Subpreputial Penile Wetness in Uncircumcised Men in South Africa." *Journal of Acquired Immune Deficiency Syndromes* 43 (1): 69–77. doi: 10.1097/01.qai.0000225014.61192.98.

Office for Human Research Protections. 2016. "Federal Policy for the Protection of Human Subjects." HHS.gov, March 18. *www.hhs.gov/ohrp/regulations-and-policy/regulations/common-rule/index.html.*

Okware, S., J. Kinsman, S. Onyango, A. Opio, and P. Kaggwa. 2005. "Revisiting the ABC Strategy: HIV Prevention in Uganda in the Era of Antiretroviral Therapy." *Postgraduate Medical Journal* 81 (960): 625–28. doi: 10.1136/pgmj.2005.032425.

Oleske, J., A. Minnefor, R. Cooper, Jr., K. Thomas, A. Dela Cruz, H. Ahdieh, I. Guerrero, V. V. Joshi, and F. Desposito. 1983. "Immune Deficiency Syndrome in Children." *Journal of the American Medical Association* 249 (17): 2345–49.

Onyango-Makumbi, C., S. B. Omer, M. Mubiru, et al. 2011. "Safety and Efficacy of HIV Hyperimmune Globulin for Prevention of Mother-to-Child HIV Transmission in HIV-1-Infected Pregnant Women and Their Infants in Kampala, Uganda (HIVIGLOB/NVP Study)." *Journal of Acquired Immune Deficiency Syndromes* 58 (4): 399–407. doi: 10.1097/QAI.0b013e31822f8914.

Orbinski, J., C. Beyrer, and S. Singh. 2007. "Violations of Human Rights: Health Practitioners as Witnesses." *Lancet* 370 (9588): 698–704. doi: 10.1016/s0140–6736(07)61346–4.

Ornstein, Charles, and Daniel Costello. 2005. "A Mother's Denial, a Daughter's Death." *LA Times*, September 24. *articles.latimes.com/2005/sep/24/local/me-eliza24.*

Pace, C., and M. Markowitz. 2015. "Monoclonal Antibodies to Host Cellular Receptors for the Treatment and Prevention of HIV-1 Infection." *Current Opinion in HIV and AIDS* 10 (3): 144–50. doi: 10.1097/coh.0000000000000146.

Pape, J. W., B. Liautaud, F. Thomas, et al. 1983. "Characteristics of the Acquired Immunodeficiency Syndrome (AIDS) in Haiti." *New England Journal of Medicine* 309 (16): 945–50. doi: 10.1056/NEJM198310203091603.

Parikh, S. A. 2007. "The Political Economy of Marriage and HIV: The ABC Approach, 'Safe' Infidelity, and Managing Moral Risk in Uganda." *American Journal of Public Health* 97 (7): 1198–208. doi: 10.2105/ajph.2006.088682.

Pawar, S., and A. Kumar. 2002. "Issues in the Formulation of Drugs for Oral Use in Children: Role of Excipients." *Paediatric Drugs* 4 (6): 371–79.

Paxton, W. A., S. Kang, and R. A. Koup. 1998. "The HIV Type 1 Coreceptor CCR5 and Its Role in Viral Transmission and Disease Progression." *AIDS Research and Human Retroviruses* 14 (suppl. 1): S89–92.

PCB (President's Council On Bioethics). 2008. *Human Dignity and Bioethics: Essays Commissioned by the President's Council on Bioethics.* Washington, DC: The President's Council on Bioethics.

Pear, Robert. 1997a. "President to Order Drug Makers to Conduct Pediatric Studies," *New York Times*, August 13. *www.nytimes.com/1997/08/13/us/president-to-order-drug-makers-to-conduct-pediatric-studies.html.*

———. 1997b. "Proposal to Test Drugs in Children Meets with Resistance." *New York Times*, November 30. *www.nytimes.com/1997/11/30/us/proposal-to-test-drugs-in-children-meets-resistance.html.*

PEPFAR. 2016. "United States President's Emergency Plan for AIDS Relief: Home Page." USA. gov. Accessed March 22. *www.pepfar.gov/index.htm.*

"PEPFAR's Targets from Fiscal Year (FY) 2010—FY 2014." 2016. PEPFAR. Accessed March 22. *www.pepfar.gov/about/138278.htm.*

Pepin, J. 2013. "The Origins of AIDS: From Patient Zero to Ground Zero." *Journal of Epidemiology and Community Health* 67 (6): 473–75. doi: 10.1136/jech-2012–201423.

Perez-Then, E., R. Pena, M. Tavarez-Rojas, et al. 2003. "Preventing Mother-to-Child HIV Transmission in a Developing Country: The Dominican Republic Experience." *Journal of Acquired Immune Deficiency Syndromes* 34 (5): 506–11.

"Perinatal HIV Down as Treatment Increases." 1997. *AIDS Alert* 12 (11): 126–27.

Persaud, D., H. Gay, C. Ziemniak, Y. H. Chen, M. Piatak, Jr., T. W. Chun, M. Strain, D. Richman, and K. Luzuriaga. 2013. "Absence of Detectable HIV-1 Viremia after Treatment Cessation in an Infant." *New England Journal of Medicine* 369 (19): 1828–35. doi: 10.1056/NEJMoa1302976.

Petra Study Team. 2002. "Efficacy of Three Short-Course Regimens of Zidovudine and Lamivudine in Preventing Early and Late Transmission of HIV-1 from Mother to Child in Tanzania, South Africa, and Uganda (Petra Study): A Randomised, Double-Blind, Placebo-Controlled Trial." *Lancet* 359 (9313): 1178–86. doi: 10.1016/S0140–6736(02)08214–4.

Pfeiffer, J., P. Montoya, A. J. Baptista, et al. 2010. "Integration of HIV/AIDS Services into African Primary Health Care: Lessons Learned for Health System Strengthening in Mozambique—a Case Study." *Journal of the International AIDS Society* 13 (Jan. 20): 3. doi: 10.1186/1758–2652–13–3.

Phelps, B. R., and N. Rakhmanina. 2011. "Antiretroviral Drugs in Pediatric HIV-Infected Patients: Pharmacokinetic and Practical Challenges." *Paediatric Drugs* 13 (3): 175–92. doi: 10.2165/11587300-000000000-00000.

Piot, P., and T. C. Quinn. 2013. "Response to the AIDS Pandemic—A Global Health Model." *New England Journal of Medicine* 368 (23): 2210–18. doi: 10.1056/NEJMra1201533.

Pitchenik, A. E., M. A. Fischl, G. M. Dickinson, D. M. Becker, A. M. Fournier, M. T. O'Connell, R. M. Colton, and T. J. Spira. 1983. "Opportunistic Infections and Kaposi's Sarcoma among Haitians: Evidence of a New Acquired Immunodeficiency State." *Annals of Internal Medicine* 98 (3): 277–84.

Ploch, L. 2011. *South Africa: Current Issues and US Relations* (CRS report no. RL31697). Washington, DC: Congressional Research Service. *www.fas.org/sgp/crs/row/RL31697.pdf.*

Presidential Commission on the Human Immunodeficiency Virus Epidemic. 1988. *Report of the Presidential Commission on the Human Immunodeficiency Virus Epidemic: Submitted to the President of the United States, June 24, 1988* (GPO: 1988 0-214-701: QL3). Washington, DC: US Government Printing Office. *archive.org/details/reportofpresiden00pres*

"Protease Inhibitor Trials Moving to Next Phase: Roche Announces 'Compassionate Use' Program." 1995. *AIDS Alert* 10 (8): 100–101.

Raju, T. N. 2000. "The Nobel Chronicles. 1989: John Michael Bishop (B 1936) and Harold Eliot Varmus (B 1939)." *Lancet* 355 (9209): 1106.

Rathe, M., and A. Moline. 2011. "[The Health System of the Dominican Republic]." *Salud Pública de México* 53 (suppl. 2): S255–64.

Ratner, L., R. C. Gallo, and F. Wong-Staal. 1985. "HTLV-III, LAV, ARV Are Variants of Same AIDS Virus." *Nature* 313 (6004): 636–37.

"Report of a Consensus Workshop, Siena, Italy, January 17–18, 1992. Maternal Factors Involved in Mother-to-Child Transmission of HIV-1." 1992. *Journal of Acquired Immune Deficiency Syndromes* 5 (10): 1019–29.

"Report of the NIH Panel to Define Principles of Therapy of HIV Infection." 1998. *Annals of Internal Medicine* 128 (12, Pt. 2): 1057–78.

Reverby, S. M. 2011. "Listening to Narratives from the Tuskegee Syphilis Study." *Lancet* 377 (9778): 1646–47.

"Review and Reform: OAR Advisory Panel Would Meld Twelve Trials Networks into One and Requests Improved Institute Collaboration." 1996. Treatment Action Group, June. *www.treatmentactiongroup.org/tagline/1996/june/review-and-reform.*

Richman, D. D., and D. Havlir. 1995. "Early Versus Delayed Treatment of HIV Infection. Zidovudine Should be Given before Symptoms Develop." *Drugs* 49 (suppl. 1): 9–16; discussion, 38–40.

Richter, Ruthann. 2013. "Blood Quest: The Battle to Protect Transfusions from HIV." *Stanford Medicine* 13 (Spring). *sm.stanford.edu/archive/stanmed/2013spring/article4.html.*

Rogers, M. F., A. W. Taylor, and S. R. Nesheim. 2010. "Preventing Perinatal Transmission of HIV: The National Perspective." *Journal of Public Health Management and Practice* 16 (6): 505–8. doi: 10.1097/PHH.0b013e3181ef1964.

Rosenfield, A., and E. Figdor. 2001. "Where Is the M in MTCT? The Broader Issues in Mother-to-Child Transmission of HIV." *American Journal of Public Health* 91 (5): 703–4.

Rubinstein, A., M. Sicklick, A. Gupta, et al. 1983. "Acquired Immunodeficiency with Reversed T4/T8 Ratios in Infants Born to Promiscuous and Drug-Addicted Mothers." *Journal of the American Medical Association* 249 (17): 2350–56.

Ruprecht, R. M., L. D. Bernard, M. A. Gama Sosa, M. A. Sosa, F. Fazely, J. Koch, P. L. Sharma, and S. Mullaney. 1990. "Murine Models for Evaluating Antiretroviral Therapy." *Cancer Research* 50 (suppl. 17): S5618–27.

Russell, S. L., R. V. Katz, M. Q. Wang, R. Lee, B. L. Green, N. R. Kressin, and C. Claudio. 2011. "Belief in AIDS Origin Conspiracy Theory and Willingness to Participate in Biomedical Research Studies: Findings in Whites, Blacks, and Hispanics in Seven Cities across Two Surveys." *HIV Clinical Trials* 12 (1): 37–47. doi: 10.1310/hct1201-37.

Salmon, D. A., M. Z. Dudley, J. M. Glanz, and S. B. Omer. 2015. "Vaccine Hesitancy: Causes, Consequences, and a Call to Action." *American Journal of Preventative Medicine* 49 (6 suppl. 4): S391–98. doi: 10.1016/j.amepre.2015.06.009.

Sacks, C. A., and C. E. Warren. 2015. "Foreseeable Risks? Informed Consent for Studies within the Standard of Care." *New England Journal of Medicine* 372 (4): 306–7. doi: 10.1056/NEJMp1415113.

Sande, M. A., C. C. Carpenter, C. G. Cobbs, K. K. Holmes, and J. P. Sanford. 1993. "Antiretroviral Therapy for Adult HIV-Infected Patients. Recommendations from a State-of-the-Art Conference. National Institute of Allergy and Infectious Diseases State-of-the-Art Panel on Anti-Retroviral Therapy for Adult HIV-Infected Patients." *Journal of the American Medical Association* 270 (21): 2583–89.

Schachter, A. D., and M. F. Ramoni. 2007. "Paediatric Drug Development." *Nature Reviews Drug Discovery* 6 (6): 429–30. doi: 10.1038/nrd2333.

Schneider, H., and D. Fassin. 2002. "Denial and Defiance: A Socio-Political Analysis of AIDS in South Africa." *AIDS* 16 (suppl. 4): S45–51.

Schochetman, G., and J. R. George. 1994. *AIDS Testing*. New York: Springer Verlag.

Scudellari, M. 2010. "State of Denial." *Nature Medicine* 16 (3): 248. doi: 10.1038/nm0310–248a.

Semeniuk, I., and S. Reverby. 2010. "A Shocking Discovery." *Nature* 467 (7316): 645. doi: 10.1038/467645a.

Sendi, P. P., H. C. Bucher, T. Harr, B. A. Craig, M. Schwietert, D. Pfluger, A. Gafni, and M. Battegay. 1999. "Cost Effectiveness of Highly Active Antiretroviral Therapy in HIV-Infected Patients: Swiss HIV Cohort Study." *AIDS* 13 (9): 1115–22.

Sepulveda, J., C. Carpenter, J. Curran, W. Holzemer, H. Smits, K. Scott, and M. Orza, eds. 2007. *PEPFAR Implementation: Progress and Promise*. Washington, DE: National Academy Press. *www.nap.edu/catalog/11905/pepfar-implementation-progress-and-promise*.

Settle, Edmund. 2003. *AIDS in China: An Annotated Chronology 1985–2003*. Monterey, CA: China AIDS Survey.

Shah, S., and C. Grady. 2013. "When to Start ART in Africa." *New England Journal of Medicine* 368 (23): 2238. doi: 10.1056/NEJMc1304494#SA1.

Sharp, P. M., and B. H. Hahn. 2010. "The Evolution of HIV-1 and the Origin of AIDS." *Philosophical Transactions of the Royal Society of London Series B: Biological Sciences* 365 (1552): 2487–94. doi: 10.1098/rstb.2010.0031.

Sharpe, A. H., R. Jaenisch, and R. M. Ruprecht. 1987. "Retroviruses and Mouse Embryos: A Rapid Model for Neurovirulence and Transplacental Antiviral Therapy." *Science* 236 (4809): 1671–74.

Sharpe, A. H., J. J. Hunter, R. M. Ruprecht, and R. Jaenisch. 1988. "Maternal Transmission of Retroviral Disease: Transgenic Mice as a Rapid Test System for Evaluating Perinatal and Transplacental Antiretroviral Therapy." *Proceedings of the National Academy of Sciences USA* 85 (24): 9792–96.

Shilts, Randy. 1987. *And the Band Played On*, twentieth anniversary edition. New York: St. Martins.

Slater, M., E. M. Stringer, and J. S. Stringer. 2010. "Breastfeeding in HIV-Positive Women: What Can Be Recommended?" *Paediatric Drugs* 12 (1): 1–9. doi: 10.2165/11316130–000000000–00000.

Smith, Michael. 2015. "Fauci: HIV Science 'Has Spoken': 'No Excuse' Left for Not Using Anti-HIV Drugs to Treat and Prevent Infection." *MedPage Today*, December 1. *www.medpagetoday.com/HIVAIDS/HIVAIDS/54951*.

Soderlund, N., J. Lavis, J. Broomberg, and A. Mills. 1993. "The Costs of HIV Prevention Strategies in Developing Countries." *Bulletin of the World Health Organization* 71 (5): 595–604.

Solinger, Dorothy. 1999. "China's Floating Population." In *The Paradox of China's Post-Mao Reforms*, edited by Merle Goldman and Roderick MacFarquhar, 220–40. Cambridge, MA: Harvard University Press. *www.socsci.uci.edu/~dorjsoli/China's%20Floating%20Population.pdf*.

"South African Treatment Action Campaign Defamation Lawsuit against Vitamin Advocate Rath Opens Amid Protests." 2009. KHN (Kaiser Health News) Morning Briefing, June 11. *khn.org/morning-breakout/dr00030100*.

Sperling, R. S., D. E. Shapiro, R. W. Coombs, et al. 1996. "Maternal Viral Load, Zidovudine Treatment, and the Risk of Transmission of Human Immunodeficiency Virus Type 1 from Mother to Infant: Pediatric AIDS Clinical Trials Group Protocol 076 Study Group." *New England Journal of Medicine* 335 (22): 1621–29. doi: 10.1056/NEJM199611283352201.

Starr, Douglas. 1998. *Blood: An Epic History of Medicine and Commerce*. NY: Alfred Knopf.

"State-of-the-Art Conference on Azidothymidine Therapy for Early HIV Infection." 1990. *American Journal of Medicine* 89 (3): 335–44. doi: 10.1016/0002-9343(90)90347-G.

Stephenson, K. E., and D. H. Barouch. 2016. "Broadly Neutralizing Antibodies for HIV Eradication." *Current HIV/AIDS Reports* 13 (1): 31–37. doi: 10.1007/s11904-016-0299-7.

Stiehm, E. R. 1991. "New Uses for Intravenous Immune Globulin." *New England Journal of Medicine* 325 (2): 123–25. doi: 10.1056/nejm199107113250209.

Stiehm, E. R., A. J. Ammann, and J. D. Cherry. 1966. "Elevated Cord Macroglobulins in the Diagnosis of Intrauterine Infections." *New England Journal of Medicine* 275 (18): 971–77. doi: 10.1056/nejm196611032751801.

Stiehm, E. R., C. V. Fletcher, L. M. Mofenson, et al. 2000. "Use of Human Immunodeficiency Virus (HIV) Human Hyperimmune Immunoglobulin in HIV Type 1-Infected Children (Pediatric AIDS Clinical Trials Group Protocol 273)." *Journal of Infectious Diseases* 181 (2): 548–54. doi: 10.1086/315224.

Stiehm, E. R., and P. Vink. 1991. "Transmission of Human Immunodeficiency Virus Infection by Breast-feeding." *Journal of Pediatrics* 118 (3): 410–12.

Stolberg, Sheryl. 1997. "A Revolution in AIDS Drugs Excludes the Tiniest Patients." *New York Times*, September 8. *www.nytimes.com/1997/09/08/us/a-revolution-in-aids-drugs-excludes-the-tiniest-patients.html*.

Stoto, M. A., D. A. Almario, and M. C. McCormick, eds. 1999. *Reducing the Odds: Preventing Perinatal Transmission of HIV in the United States*. Washington, DC: National Academy Press.

Taylor, G. P., and N. Low-Beer. 2001. "Antiretroviral Therapy in Pregnancy: A Focus on Safety." *Drug Safety* 24 (9): 683–702.

Thaul, Susan. 2012. *FDA's Authority to Ensure That Drugs Prescribed to Children Are Safe and Effective* (CRS report no. RL33986). Washington, DC: Congressional Research Service. *www.fas.org/sgp/crs/misc/RL33986.pdf*.

Thea, D. M., R. W. Steketee, V. Pliner, et al. 1997. "The Effect of Maternal Viral Load on the Risk of Perinatal Transmission of HIV-1: New York City Perinatal HIV Transmission Collaborative Study Group." *AIDS* 11 (4): 437–44.

Thistle, P., R. F. Spitzer, R. H. Glazier, et al. 2007. "A Randomized, Double-Blind, Placebo-Controlled Trial of Combined Nevirapine and Zidovudine Compared with Nevirapine Alone in the Prevention of Perinatal Transmission of HIV in Zimbabwe." *Clinical Infectious Diseases* 44 (1): 111–19. doi: 10.1086/508869.

Thompson, M. A., J. A. Aberg, J. F. Hoy, et al. 2012. "Antiretroviral Treatment of Adult HIV Infection: 2012 Recommendations of the International Antiviral Society–USA Panel." *Journal of the American Medical Association* 308 (4): 387–402. doi: 10.1001/jama.2012.7961.

Timberg, Craig, and Daniel Halperin. 2012. *Tinderbox*. New York: Penguin Press.

"A Timeline of HIV/AIDS." 2016. AIDS.gov. Accessed March 26. *www.aids.gov/hiv-aids-basics/hiv-aids-101/aids-timeline*.

Toltzis, P., C. M. Marx, N. Kleinman, E. M. Levine, and E. V. Schmidt. 1991. "Zidovudine-Associated Embryonic Toxicity in Mice." *Journal of Infectious Diseases* 163 (6): 1212–18.

Townsend, C. L., L. Byrne, M. Cortina-Borja, C. Thorne, A. De Ruiter, H. Lyall, G. P. Taylor, C. S. Peckham, and P. A. Tookey. 2014. "Earlier Initiation of ART and Further Decline in Mother-to-Child HIV Transmission Rates, 2000–2011." *AIDS* 28 (7): 1049–57. doi: 10.1097/qad.0000000000000212.

Townsend, L., R. Jewkes, C. Mathews, L. G. Johnston, A. J. Flisher, Y. Zembe, and M. Chopra. 2011. "HIV Risk Behaviours and Their Relationship to Intimate Partner Violence (IPV) among Men Who Have Multiple Female Sexual Partners in Cape Town, South Africa." *AIDS and Behavior* 15 (1): 132–41. doi: 10.1007/s10461–010–9680–5.

Tudor Car, L., M. H. Van-Velthoven, S. Brusamento, H. Elmoniry, J. Car, A. Majeed, and R. Atun. 2011. "Integrating Prevention of Mother-to-Child HIV Transmission (PMTCT) Programmes with Other Health Services for Preventing HIV Infection and Improving HIV Outcomes in Developing Countries." *Cochrane Database of Systematic Reviews* 15 (6): Cd008741. doi: 10.1002/14651858.CD008741.pub2.

Tumushabe, Joseph. 2006. *The Politics of HIV/AIDS in Uganda*. Social Policy and Development Programme Paper 28 (August). Geneva: UN Research Institute for Social Development.

UNAIDS. 2016. *How AIDS Changed Everything—MDG6: Fifteen Years, Fifteen Lessons of Hope from the AIDS Response*. Geneva: UNAIDS. *www.unaids.org/sites/default/files/media_asset/MDG6Report_en.pdf*.

———. 2014a. *90–90–90: An Ambitious Treatment Target to Help End the AIDS Epidemic*. Geneva: UNAIDS. *www.unaids.org/en/resources/documents/2014/90-90-90*.

———. 2014b. "UNAIDS Report Shows That 19 Million of the 35 Million People Living with HIV Globally Do Not Know Their HIV-Positive Status." News release, July 16. *www.unaids.org/en/resources/presscentre/pressreleaseandstatementarchive/2014/july/20140716prgapreport*.

UNAIDS and WHO. 1998. *Report on the Global HIV/AIDS Epidemic: June 1998*. Geneva: Joint United Nations Programme on HIV/AIDS. *data.unaids.org/pub/Report/1998/19981125_global_epidemic_report_en.pdf*.

UNAIDS, WHO, and UNICEF. 2004. "Joint WHO/UNAIDS/UNICEF Statement on Use of Cotrimoxazole as Prophylaxis in HIV Exposed and HIV Infected Children." Statement, November 22. *www.unaids.org/sites/default/files/web_story/ps_cotrimoxazole_22nov04_en_2.pdf*.

UNICEF. 2012. *Options B and B+: Key Considerations for Countries to Implement an Equity-Focused Approach* (Draft for Discussion). New York: UNICEF. *www.unicef.org/aids/files/hiv_Key_considerations_options_B.pdf*.

USAID. 2016. "Orphans and Vulnerable Children Affected by HIV and AIDS." USAID.gov. Last updated, February 23. *www.usaid.gov/what-we-do/global-health/hiv-and-aids/technical-areas/orphans-and-vulnerable-children-affected-hiv*.

US Public Health Service Task Force. 1994. "Recommendations of the US Public Health Service Task Force on the Use of Zidovudine to Reduce Perinatal Transmission of Human Immunodeficiency Virus." *Morbidity and Mortality Weekly Report Recommendations and Reports* 43 (RR-11): 1–20.

———. 1998. "Public Health Service Task Force Recommendations for the Use of Antiretroviral Drugs in Pregnant Women Infected with HIV-1 for Maternal Health and for Reducing Perinatal HIV-1 Transmission in the United States." *Morbidity and Mortality Weekly Report Recommendations and Reports* 47 (RR-2): 1–30.

Van Der Westhuizen, Janis. 2005. "Arms over AIDS in South Africa: Why the Boys Had to Have Their Toys." *Alternatives: Global, Local, Political* 30 (3): 275–95.

Van Dyke, R. B., B. T. Korber, E. Popek, et al. 1999. "The Ariel Project: A Prospective Cohort Study of Maternal-Child Transmission of Human Immunodeficiency Virus Type 1 in the Era of Maternal Antiretroviral Therapy." *Journal of Infectious Diseases* 179 (2): 319–28. doi: 10.1086/314580.

Varmus, H. E., J. Stavnezer, E. Medeiros, and J. M. Bishop. 1975. "Detection and Characterization of RNA Tumor Virus-Specific DNA in Cells." *Bibliotheca Haematologica* (40): 451–61.

Varmus, H., and D. Satcher. 1997. "Ethical Complexities of Conducting Research in Developing Countries." *New England Journal of Medicine* 337 (14): 1003–5. doi: 10.1056/NEJM199710023371411.

Vermund, S. H., and R. J. Hayes. 2013. "Combination Prevention: New Hope for Stopping the Epidemic." *Current HIV/AIDS Reports* 10 (2): 169–86. doi: 10.1007/s11904–013–0155-y.

Vernazza, P., B. Hirschel, E. Bernasconi, and M. Flepp. 2008. "HIV Transmission under Highly Active Antiretroviral Therapy." *Lancet* 372 (9652): 1806–7; author reply, 1807. doi: 10.1016/s0140–6736(08)61753–5.

Violari, A., M. F. Cotton, D. M. Gibb, A. G. Babiker, J. Steyn, S. A. Madhi, P. Jean-Philippe, and J. A. McIntyre. 2008. "Early Antiretroviral Therapy and Mortality among HIV-Infected Infants." *New England Journal of Medicine* 359 (21): 2233–44. doi: 10.1056/NEJMoa0800971.

Wade, N. A., G. S. Birkhead, B. L. Warren, T. T. Charbonneau, P. T. French, L. Wang, J. B. Baum, J. M. Tesoriero, and R. Savicki. 1998. "Abbreviated Regimens of Zidovudine Prophylaxis and Perinatal Transmission of the Human Immunodeficiency Virus." *New England Journal of Medicine* 339 (20): 1409–14. doi: 10.1056/NEJM199811123392001.

Wagner, B. G., and S. Blower. 2012. "Universal Access to HIV Treatment versus Universal 'Test and Treat': Transmission, Drug Resistance, and Treatment Costs." *PLOS One* 7 (9): e41212. doi: 10.1371/journal.pone.0041212.

Wain-Hobson, S., M. Alizon, and L. Montagnier. 1985. "Relationship of AIDS to Other Retroviruses." *Nature* 313 (6005): 743.

Watanabe, Myrna. 1999. "China Confronts AIDS." *The Scientist Magazine* 13, no. 1 (January 4). *www.the-scientist.com/?articles.view/articleNo/19222/title/China-Confronts-AIDS*.

Weintrub, P. S., M. A. Koerper, J. E. Addiego, Jr., W. L. Drew, E. T. Lennette, R. Miner, M. J. Cowan, and A. J. Ammann. 1983. "Immunologic Abnormalities in Patients with Hemophilia A." *Journal of Pediatrics* 103 (5): 692–95.

Weis, R., and Mazade, L., eds. 1990. *Surrogate Endpoints in Evaluating the Effectiveness of Drugs against HIV Infection and AIDS: September 11–12, 1989, Conference Summary*. Washington, DC: National Academy Press.

White-Junod, Suzanne 2008. "FDA and Clinical Drug Trials: A Short History." In *A Quick Guide to Clinical Trials*, edited by Madhu Davies and Faiz Kerimani, 25–55. Washington, DC: Bioplan.

WHO. 2002. *Scaling up Antiretroviral Therapy in Resource Limited Settings: Guidelines for a Public Health Approach*. Geneva: World Health Organization. Revised in 2003.

———. 2009. *Screening Donated Blood for Transfusion-Transmissible Infections: Recommendations*. Geneva: WHO. *apps.who.int/iris/bitstream/10665/44202/1/9789241547888_eng.pdf*.

———. 2016. "About WHO: Funding WHO." World Health Organization. Accessed March 22. *www.who.int/about/finances-accountability/funding/en*.

WHO and UNAIDS. 2013. *Sixteen Ideas for Addressing Violence against Women in the Context of the HIV Epidemic: A Programming Tool*. Geneva: WHO. *apps.who.int/iris/bitstream/10665/95156/1/9789241506533_eng.pdf*.

Wibmer, C. K., P. L. Moore, and L. Morris. 2015. "HIV Broadly Neutralizing Antibody Targets." *Current Opinion in HIV and AIDS* 10 (3): 135–43. doi: 10.1097/coh.0000000000000153.

Wilson, R. 2009. "Is It Wrong to Highlight the Deaths of HIV-Positive AIDS Denialists Who Reject Medications and Urge Others to Do the Same?" *Richard Wilson's Blog* (blog), January 15. *richardwilsonauthor.com/2009/01/15/vue-weeklys-connie-howard-accuses-aids-activists-of-celebrating-maggiores-passing-but-is-it-wrong-to-highlight-the-deaths-of-hiv-positive-aids-denialists-who-reject-life-saving-drugs-and-wh.*

WMA. 2013. "WMA Declaration of Helsinki: Ethical Principles for Medical Research Involving Human Subjects." World Medical Association, October. *www.wma.net/en/30publications/10policies/b3.*

Wong, L. H., H. V. Rooyen, P. Modiba, L. Richter, G. Gray, J. A. McIntyre, C. D. Schetter, and T. Coates. 2009. "Test and Tell: Correlates and Consequences of Testing and Disclosure of HIV Status in South Africa (Hptn 043 Project Accept)." *Journal of Acquired Immune Deficiency Syndromes* 50 (2): 215–22. doi: 10.1097/QAI.0b013e3181900172.

Yin, N., S. Mei, L. Li, F. L. Wei, L. Q. Zhang, and Y. Z. Cao. 2003. "[Study on the Epidemiology and Distribution of Human Immunodeficiency Virus-1 and Hepatitis C Virus Infection among Intravenous Drug Users and Illegal Blood Donors in China]." *Zhonghua Liu Xing Bing Xue Za Zhi* 24 (11): 962–65.

Zakowski, P., S. Fligiel, G. W. Berlin, and L. Johnson, Jr. 1982. "Disseminated Mycobacterium Avium-Intracellulare Infection in Homosexual Men Dying of Acquired Immunodeficiency." *Journal of the American Medical Association* 248 (22): 2980–82.

INDEX